IMMUNOLOGY
Basic Concepts

Edited by
Dr. B K Gupta
MBBS, DTCD, Ph D
Professor and Head
Department of Biochemistry, Subharti Medical College
Swami Vivekanand Subharti University
Meerut - 250005, India

and

Dr. Alpana Sharma
Ph D
Additional Professor
Department of Biochemistry
All India Institute of Medical Sciences
New Delhi - 110029, India

PEEPEE
PUBLISHERS AND DISTRIBUTORS (P) LTD.

This book has been subsidised by the Government of India through the National Book Trust, India for the benefit of students.

Immunology: Basic Concepts

Published by
Pawaninder P. Vij

Peepee Publishers and Distributors (P) Ltd.
Head Office: 160, Shakti Vihar, Pitam Pura
Delhi-110034 (India)

Correspondence Address: 7/31, First Floor, Ansari Road, Daryaganj
New Delhi-110002 (India)

Ph: 65195868, 9811156083, 23246245

e-mail: peepee160@yahoo.co.in

e-mail: peepee160@rediffmail.com

e-mail: peepee160@gmail.com

www.peepeepub.com

First Edition: **2012**

ISBN: 978-81-8445-107-8

Dedicated to

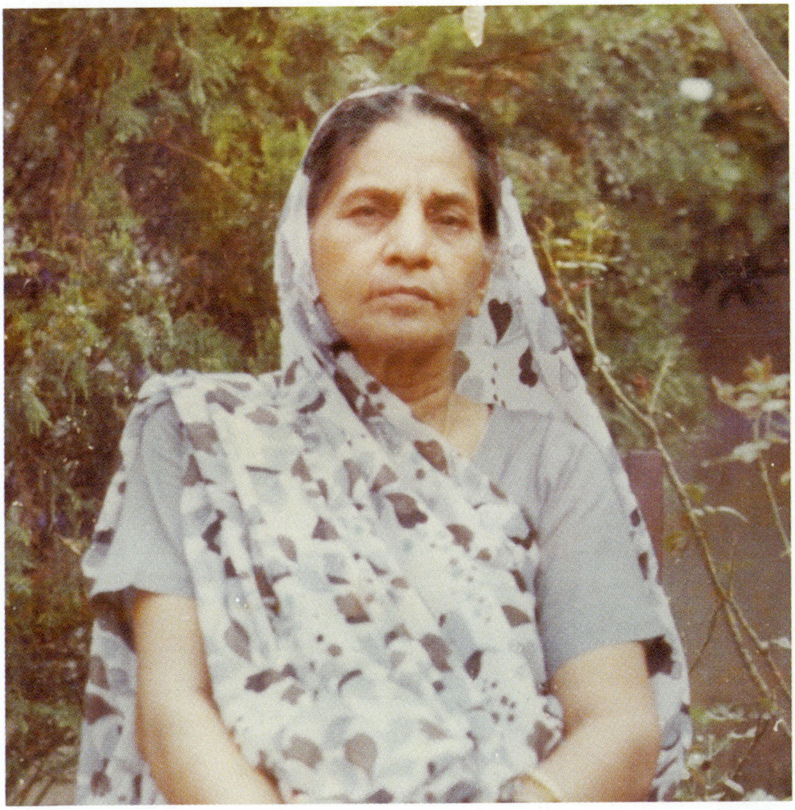

मेरी माँ,

(1916–1988)

and

those who are suffering

for no fault

and are alone

FOREWORD

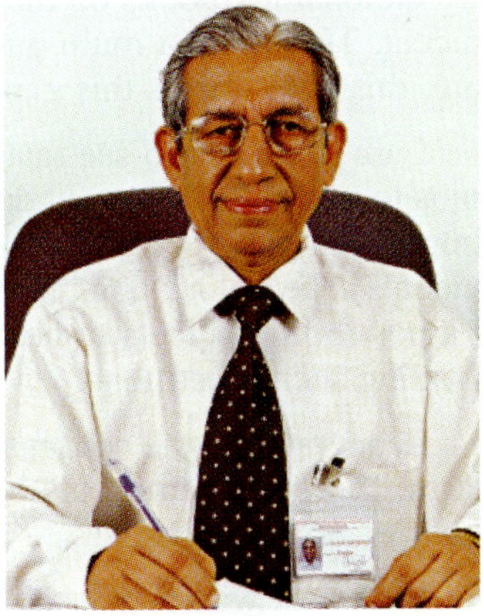

It is my privilege to write the foreword to this masterly work, the **Immunology: Basic Concepts,** edited by Dr. B.K. Gupta and Dr. Alpana Sharma. Immunology is one of the rapidly advancing branches of medical science. I remember, when I was a student of MBBS about 50 years back, the textbooks of physiology and pathology described the morphology of lymphocytes, but told that the function of lymphocyte was obscure. At that time, it was postulated that the lymphocytes are bystander cells or mere visitors at the site of inflammation. Within the short span of another 10 years, by the time when I was an MD student, things have been rapidly changed, and lymphocytes were considered as the pivotal players of immunological system. Within another 5 years, when I was a postdoctoral fellow in Switzerland, my work was on tumour immunology. The rapid progress in the field of immunology was truly phenomenal. Nowadays, the impact of immunology is not only in medicine, but in agriculture, environmental sciences and so many other branches of science.

The concept of immunity was prevalent from ancient times itself. The father of Indian medicine, Charaka (? 400 BC to 100 BC) says that diseases are of three types, endogenous, exogenous (contagious) and cosmic. Out of this endogenous variety he again classifies into those caused by hereditary factors and those caused by reduction of natural strength (immunity). Thus conceptual knowledge of immunology was available to our ancestors. Was it a mere theoretical concept, or was it applied in Ancient India?

Smallpox has been completely eradicated from the world by 1985, which can be considered as the triumph of applied immunology. In this connection, we generally accept the fact that Edward Jenner discovered the vaccination in 1796. Jenner's work is widely regarded as the foundation of immunology, despite the fact that he was neither the first to suggest that infection with cowpox conferred specific immunity to smallpox nor the first to attempt cowpox inoculation for this purpose.

Smallpox is believed to have appeared in prehistorical time. The skin lesions of smallpox are found on faces of Egyptian mummies from the period 1570-1085 BC. The concept of vaccination, although primitive, was very effectively practised in Ancient India, from early historical times. The earliest record of inoculation is to be found in 8th century in India, when Madhav's medicinal treatise which included a special chapter on smallpox (masurik?) and described the method of inoculation to protect against smallpox.

It is interesting, then, to find a detailed account by Holwell, then Governor of Bengal and a practising surgeon written in 1767 (30 years before Jenner), describing the widespread practice of inoculation in Bengal. His letter to the College of Physicians in London is entitled, "an account of the manner of inoculating for the smallpox in India". He wrote: "When the before-recited treatment of the inoculation is strictly followed, it is next to a miracle, that only one in a million fails. This practice of the East has been followed without variation and with uniform success from the remotest known times."

Ancient Indian vaccination was to take pustules of smallpox, keep it for one whole year in damp surroundings, and powder it by next year. In this way, a live attenuated vaccine was prepared. Just before the starting of the smallpox season, practitioners will come to villages and along with rituals, sprinkle the powder in houses. Considerable amount of immunity against smallpox was achieved in this manner.

There are only limited number of books on Immunology written by Indian authors. Some of the international textbooks on the subject are so elaborate that it may not be digested easily by an average student. Therefore, a multi-authored textbook by Indian authors is the necessity of the time. And I am sure, this book fulfils this gap.

I am delighted to see that the book deals with all aspects of Immunology. The authors have taken pains to explain both the fundamentals as well as the recent advances in the knowledge. The language is simple, straightforward and easily understandable. The diagrams are lucid, and clarify the idea to the students. The colour combination looks bright and catchy. In books written by different authors, there is a possibility of facts to be overlapped. The editors of this textbook have done an excellent work in avoiding such repetitions.

I congratulate the editors and the authors in bringing out a world-class textbook. With much enthusiasm, I am submitting this book to the students of Immunology. I am sure, this book will serve the needs of both undergraduate and postgraduate students.

With best wishes !

Dated: 16 June 2009

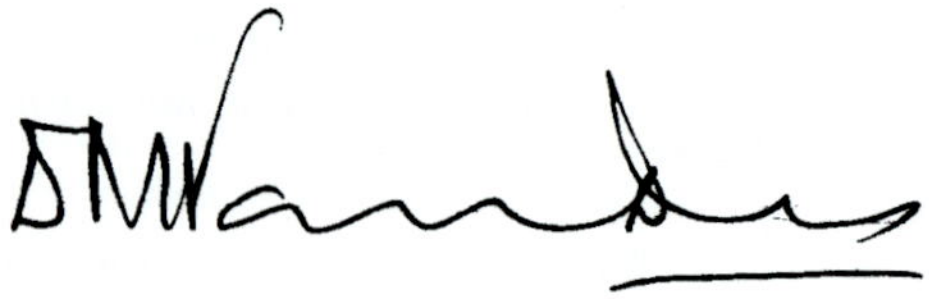

Prof. D.M. Vasudeven
MD, FRCPath
Professor of Biochemistry
Chairman, Amrita Laboratory Medicine
Dean, Faculty of Medicine, Amrita University
Amrita Institute of Medical Sciences
Kochi-682041
Email: dmvasudevan@yahoo.co.in

PREFACE - I

This book is designed as a concept book of Immunology for medical students as well as for graduate students who require a broad introduction to the fundamentals of immunology. It is also suitable for postgraduate courses and competitive entrance examinations including state and all India PGME, USMLE and PLAB. Recent and everyday advances have profoundly influenced the manner in which immunology can and should be learnt. Since immunology first and foremost seeks to explain basics of life and disease, the book has tried to provide the requisite inputs in this direction.

There are limited books on basic immunology. The few textbooks available are written by single author. We felt the need of a book which can make immunology understandable; can clear the basic concepts on the subject in simple language and remove the terror of "Immunology being a difficult subject", from the minds of our students. So, we worked over it and this manuscript is the outcome of the multi-author write-up.

Instead of compartmentalizing this interconnected subject, we decentralized different components and correlated it with every organ / part and to every action / response of human body and thus we tried to discuss immunology in its real sense.

The invited contributors have expertise and professional involvement in their respective areas. This book differs from the other usual textbooks of immunology in that it provides an overall perception of all the aspects of immunity. The book covers a wide range of topics relevant to medical students beginning from an overview, Innate Immunity, Complement System and Its Receptors, Antigen, Immunoglobulin – Structure and Function, Iso-, Allo- and Idiotypes, Genetics, Antigen-Antibody Interactions, Biogenesis of Antibodies, Cells Involved, Major Histocompatibility Complex and T-Cell Receptors, Response to Antigen and Cell Interaction in Specific Immune Response.

Immune Regulation, Immunization, Genetics and Role in Transplantation, Tolerance and Autoimmunity, Hypersensitivity Reactions, Tumor Immunology, Immunodeficiency and Human Immunodeficiency Virus / Acquired Immunodeficiency Syndrome have been sufficiently documented and covered quite comprehensively.

The relevance of immunology to society has never been greater; the impact of immunological concepts on advances in understanding medicine, agricultural, environmental sciences, forensic sciences and in various other fields have profound implications for the future of mankind. On one hand, scientists all over the world are trying to conquer **"GOD"** by trying to understand life completely and advance their capability to alter it while on the other hand, medical and science students want to feel its real and intellectual excitement. Hence, this knowledge of immunology would be of paramount importance for all including well informed citizens.

The chapters on emerging areas, such as Immunocytochemistry, Immunologically Privileged Sites have been adequately covered for the first time. The present day knowledge in Immune response and its relevance to diseases have been dealt with appropriately in this book.

I am grateful to all my colleagues and seniors who accepted my invitation to contribute chapter(s) for the book without which this project would not have been completed successfully. A project of this nature required cooperation and assistance from colleagues within and outside the working place. I was fortunate to get cooperation from one and all, not only within Uttar Pradesh but throughout India and also from Ethiopia and USA.

I will fail in my duties, if I do not thank **Professor Dr. Atul Krishana**, a great visionary and a foresighted living legend, not only in building "सुभारती" (Good India) but he is the one who brought me in teaching profession and made me a teacher. I am also thankful to **Professor Dr. Mukti Narayan**, a burning fire behind Subharti and President of Subharti education and training Universe, who has taken me too, on the path of light, without whose inspiration this work would never have been completed. I am especially thankful to **Dr. V B Sahai**, Vice-Chancellor, Swami Vivekanand Subharti University, Meerut for even taking the trouble of coming to my house and pulling my ears whenever it was required. I am specially thankful to **Professor Dr. A K Asthana**, Principal, Subharti Medical College, Swami Vivekanand Subharti University, Meerut for encouraging, helping and guiding me every time whenever I went to him with one or the other difficulty.

I am particularly thankful to my co-editor **Dr. Alpana Sharma** and **Dr. Ankit Bharat** for their precious suggestions and comments from time to time during the preparation of this book. I am also thankful to **Prof. Mohd. Suhail,** Former Professor and Head, Department of Biochemistry, University of Allahabad, Allahabad and **Dr. Molly Madan**, Professor and Head, Department of Microbiology, Subharti Medical College for extending help in reviewing different chapters. I must also thank **Dr. Debapriya Bandyopadhyay** for helping me in proofreading and **Dr. Madhvi Gupta** and **Dr. Yashu Tyagi** for secretarial assistance. I thank one and all who directly or indirectly helped me in any way in preparation and completion of this literature.

Finally, I express my deepest appreciation to my wife **Vinay** and my younger son **Anchit,** for their continuous encouragement, for performing even in bad times and when I am alone, without which this tremendous work would never have seen the light of the day.

Our readers would ultimately judge our work and we expect, that they will give us a chance to improve; by sending their feedback, comments and suggestions.

B K Gupta

PREFACE - II

Human suffering is the result of failure of human body defense, may it be of any origin, communicable, non-communicable, malignant, degenerative or any other. With the milestones of discoveries in medicine, the scientists are now compelled to think that every event of disease and its cure; is somehow related to immunity of the human body.

With the surge of immunedeficiency and autoimmune disorders and hunt for vaccines for all kinds of diseases, including cancer, it is imperative that the knowledge of immunology and its acceptance as a full-fledged subject even at undergraduate level has become a necessity. Immunology inadvertently or insidiously has entered our lives in form of prevention and early detection of diseases even before the appearance of symptoms or diagnosis; serological or immunocytochemistry in biopsy: required for achieving cure.

This textbook presents this intricate subject with utter simplicity in order to introduce, even the beginner – undergraduate or the postgraduate, medical, dental and life science student to these concepts.

I acknowledge the effort and help of our learned and experienced contributors who gave us their valuable time for transforming this book into a compendium that covers on various aspects. I extend my sincere thanks to all of them. My earnest gratitude to the editor **Dr. B K Gupta**, who spent his days and nights in editing the book, coordinating with the contributors and publisher and completed this flawless work.

I express my sincere gratitude to **Dr. Subrata Sinha**, Head, Department of Biochemistry, All India Institute of Medical Sciences, New Delhi for his kind support. I am thankful to all my friends and colleagues for their constant encouragement.

I extend my heartfelt thanks to my husband **Dr. Manoj Sharma** and my loving daughters **Aparna** and **Vrinda** who were always be the constant source of inspiration in fulfilling my dream to complete this book.

I hope this book will be a ready reference for all our readers. The comments and suggestions on the shortcomings of this book shall be highly appreciated and would give us a chance to improve.

Alpana Sharma

CONTRIBUTORS

Alpana Sharma, Ph. D.,
Additional Professor,
Department of Biochemistry,
All India Institute of Medical Sciences,
New Delhi, India

Ankit Bharat, M.D.,
Fellow, Cardiothoracic Surgery,
Department of Surgery,
Washington University, School of Medicine,
Saint Louis, MO 63108, USA

B. K. Gupta, M.B;B.S; D.T.C.D; Ph. D.,
Professor and Head,
Department of Biochemistry,
Subharti Medical College,
Swami Vivekanand Subharti University,
Subhartipurum, Meerut, India

Debapriya Bandyopadhyay, M.D.,
Assistant Professor,
Department of Biochemistry,
Subharti Medical College,
Swami Vivekanand Subharti University,
Subhartipurum, Meerut, India

Hasan Kammal, Ph. D.,
Formerly Assistant Professor,
Department of Biochemistry,
Hindustan Institute of Dental Sciences,
Greater Noida, India

Jawed Iqbal
Research Scholar,
Department of Biochemistry,
Faculty of Medicine, J. N. Medical College,
Aligarh Muslim University,
Aligarh, India

Jayashree Bhattacharjee, M.D.,
Director, Professor and Head,
Department of Biochemistry,
Lady Hardinge Medical College,
New Delhi, India

Krithika N. Kodumudi, Ph. D.,
Post Doctoral Fellow,
Moffitt Cancer Center, 12902
Maguolia Drive, SRB-4, Room 24314
Tampa, FL 33612 USA

L. M. Srivastava, Ph. D., FAMS, FCBI.,
Professor, Senior Consultant and Head,
Department of Biochemistry,
Sir Ganga Ram Hospital,
New Delhi, India
Formerly Professor & Head,
Department of Biochemistry,
All India Institute of Medical Sciences,
New Delhi, India

M. V. R. Reddy, Ph. D.,
Professor and Head,
Department of Biochemistry and
JB Tropical Disease Research Centre,
Mahatma Gandhi Institute of Medical Sciences,
Sevagram, India

Madhvi Gupta, Ph. D.,
Formerly Assistant Professor,
Department of Biochemistry,
Subharti Medical College,
Swami Vivekanand Subharti University,
Subhartipurum, Meerut, India

Man Updesh Singh Sachdeva, M.D., D.N.B.,
Assistant Professor,
Department of Hematology,
Postgraduate Institute of Medical Education and Research,
Chandigarh, India

Mohammad Suhail, M. Phil., Ph. D.,
Formerly Professor and Head,
Department of Biochemistry,
University of Allahabad,
Allahabad, India

Mythily Srinivasan, M.D.S., Ph. D.,
Associate Professor,
Dentistry Immunology,
Center for Autoimmune Diseases,
Indiana University Purdue University Indianapolis (Indianapolis, IN);
Contact Information: 1121, West Michigan Street,
Room 290, Indianapolis,
Indiana 46202 - 5186, USA

Najmul Islam, Ph. D.,
Professor, Chairman and Head,
Department of Biochemistry
Faculty of Medicine, J. N. Medical College,
Aligarh Muslim University,
Aligarh, India

Nalini Gupta, M.D., D.N.B.,
Associate Professor,
Department of Cytology and Gynaecological Pathology,
Postgraduate Institute of Medical Education and Research,
Chandigarh, India

Parul Goel, M.D.,
Assistant Professor,
Department of Biochemistry,
Subharti Medical College,
Swami Vivekanand Subharti University,
Subhartipurum, Meerut, India

Parul Tripathi, Ph. D.,
Research Scientist,
Department of Biochemistry,
K G Medical University,
Lucknow, India

Poonam Elhence, M.D., PDCC, D.N.B., MNAMS.,
Associate Professor,
Department of Pathology,
Subharti Medical College,
Swami Vivekanand Subharti University,
Subhartipurum, Meerut, India

Rajinder Chawla, Ph. D.,
Professor Biochemistry,
Christian Medical College and Hospital,
Ludhiana, India.
Ex-Professor Biochemistry,
Faculty of Medicine, Addis Ababa University,
Addis Ababa, Ethiopia

R. K. Singh, Ph. D.,
Professor and Head,
Guru Ram Rai Institute of Medical Sciences,
Dehradun, India
Formerly Senior Professor and Head,
Department of Biochemistry,
K G Medical University,
Lucknow, India

Ranjana Singh, Ph. D.,
Assistant Professor,
Department of Biochemistry,
K. G. Medical University,
Lucknow, India

Rashid Ali, Ph. D.,
Formerly Professor, Chairman & Head,
Department of Biochemistry,
J. N. Medical College,
Aligarh Muslim University,
Aligarh, India

Rekha Gupta, Ph. D.,
Assistant Professor,
Department of Biochemistry,
Hindustan Institute of Dental Sciences,
Greater Noida, India

S. C. Parija, M.D., Ph. D., D. Sc., FRCPath.,
Director-Professor and Head,
Department of Microbiology,
JIPMER, Pondicherry

S. K. Patra, M.B;B.S.,
M.D. Resident,
Department of Biochemistry,
Lady Hardinge Medical College,
New Delhi, India

Seema Garg, M.D.,
Assistant Professor,
Department of Biochemistry,
University College of Medical Sciences,
New Delhi, India

Vinay Bharat, M.D., D.C.P.,
Professor,
Department of Pathology,
Subharti Medical College,
Swami Vivekanand Subharti University,
Subhartipurum, Meerut, India

Vinod Singh, Ph. D.,
Reader,
Department of Microbiology,
Barkatullah University,
Bhopal, MP, India

CONTENTS

1

CHAPTER

An Overview of Immune System

(Dr. Ankit Bharat ankitbharat@hotmail.com)

OBJECTIVES

1. To introduce readers to the immune system.
2. To understand the significance of natural and acquired defense.
3. To understand the basic components of the defense system of human body.

INTRODUCTION

The ambience around human body is replete with an enormous variety of micro- and macro-organisms. All human interactions with the natural environment, including respiration and alimentation, are bound to cause entry of these organisms into the body, many of which are pathogenic. The epithelial surfaces of skin, respiratory, gastrointestinal and genitourinary tract, which are continuously exposed to these organisms, provide the first line of defense for the body. The epithelium has several properties which help carry out this function. For instance, the stratified squamous epithelium of the skin contains a dead cornified layer which is unfavorable for microbial growth. The secretions present on the skin surface including sebum have antimicrobial properties. Similarly, lysozyme in the saliva is bactericidal and the gastrointestinal mucous layer prevents bacterial invasion of the epithelial surface. Despite the constant exposure to these pathogenic organisms, it is commendable that the human body stays disease free and infection is an exceptional phenomenon.

Immune System and Its Components

"Immunity" was derived from the Latin word immunitas, which referred to the protection offered to the Roman senators from legal prosecution during their tenures in office. In medical terms, it refers to the phenomenon by which the human body protects itself from foreign substances, particularly infectious agents. It involves a series of extremely complex interactions between the components of immune system and molecules (antigens) present in the internal milieu.

An antigen is any moiety present within the body capable of generating an immune response (i.e. it is immunogenic). Most antigens are proteins, although carbohydrates and lipids may, in some cases, act as antigen(s) too. The immune system perceives antigens as "self" (belonging to the host and thereby safe) or "foreign", and works to eliminate the latter. Hence, foreign antigens are immunogenic while self antigens are not. Occasionally, the immune system finds new antigens being expressed on cells within the body as a result of genetic alterations, for example in tumors, which may or may not be immunogenic. However, it is important to understand here that even self-antigens can occasionally become immunogenic, an unusual occurrence leading to the phenomenon of autoimmunity.

The immune system can broadly be divided into innate or acquired. The innate system is phylogenetically the oldest form of host defense while the acquired system developed later in evolution. Hence invertebrates lack the acquired system and their defense against foreign substances primarily consists of innate immune mechanisms. Innate immunity (also called natural or native immunity) consists of cellular and biochemical components which are present even before any infection takes place. The components of innate immunity respond only to infectious substances; the response being rapid and essentially same for repeated infections which makes this system non-specific **(Figure 1.1)**. Innate system comprises:

i. Physical barriers in the form of epithelial surfaces lining the different organ system of the body along with the antimicrobial substances produced at these surfaces.
ii. Phagocytic cells (including the neutrophils and macrophages) and Natural Killer (NK) cells.
iii. Complement system; and
iv. Cytokines and other inflammatory mediators which regulate the immune response.

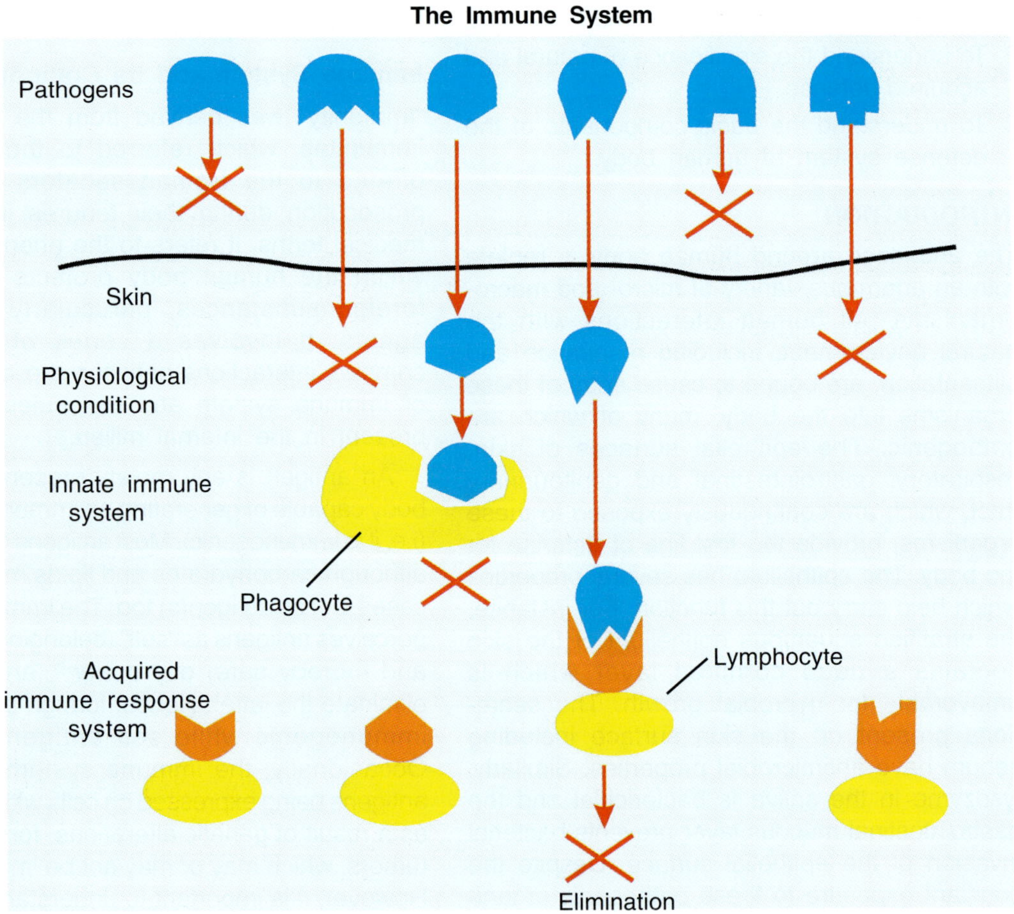

Fig. 1.1: Immune system defenses are multifold

The acquired immune response, on the other hand, is stimulated by exposure to both infectious and non-infectious agents and increases in magnitude with subsequent exposures to the same agent. Since this response develops and adapts in response to an antigen, it is referred to as adaptive immunity. The adaptive response is unique since it can distinguish even between closely related molecules reacting only to the one that originally stimulated it and for this reason it is also called specific immunity.

Innate and adaptive immunity are integrated and work cooperatively to generate an extremely potent and effective immune system. The innate system is essential to stimulate the adaptive immune response against infectious agents. The adaptive immune system, in turn, augments the innate system and activates certain effector mechanisms for more effective and rapid elimination of the microbe.

Acquired Immunity (Adaptive Immunity/ Specific Immunity)

Adaptive immunity involves highly specialised, systemic cells and processes that eliminate or prevent pathogenic challenges. Adaptive immunity consists of two arms–humoral (antibody) and cellular. The humoral or antibody arm consists of B-lymphocytes along with their secretory products called antibodies. The cellular arm consists of a special group of cells called T-lymphocytes which are now believed to be crucial in regulating the adaptive immune response. This type of immunity occurs in response to an agent and is called ADAPTIVE as the immune system must adapt itself to previously "unseen" molecules. Adaptive immunity can be acquired by direct exposure to the antigen (active immunity) or transferred passively (passive immunity) in the form of antibodies in immunized animal sera (vaccination) or from mother to fetus (vertical transmission).

Both T- and B-lymphocytes originate in the bone marrow. However, the B-cells mature in bone marrow while the T-cells migrate to the thymus for further maturation.

The B-lymphocytes are the predominant component of the humoral system. They mainly serve to identify extracellular antigens and produce antibodies, a group of specialized proteins which neutralize antigens by various effector mechanisms. The first evidence of humoral immunity was proved in 1890 by experiments conducted by von Behring and Kitasato. They showed that sera from animals who had recovered from diphtheria transferred to non-immune recipients' conferred immunity to the latter against the diphtheria infection. It was hypothesized that the sera contained certain "anti-toxins" which neutralized the pathogenic effects of the diphtheria toxin. Later, it was found that these "anti-toxins" were produced even to nonmicrobial substances and hence a general term "antibodies" was introduced.

Antibodies are specialized in the sense that they bring about activation of specific effector mechanisms depending on the type of antibody involved. For example, formation antigen-antibody complexes involving the IgE variety of antibodies causes release of inflammatory mediators through mast cells. Other mechanisms which are activated through antibodies include complement activation and opsonization enhanced phagocytosis. The interaction between an antigen and its specific antibody results in the formation of an antigen-antibody complex, which may alter the properties of the antigen. For example, binding of an antibody to a toxin may alter its shape so that it can no longer bind to the target cells. The antibody may also bind to active sites on the toxin, thereby neutralizing it. We shall discuss these mechanisms in more detail in subsequent chapters.

The cellular immunity is mediated by T-lymphocytes alongwith certain specialized "antigen presenting cells" (APCs) and "effector cells". The T-lymphocytes consist of functionally diverse varieties called T-helper (Th) and cytolytic or cytotoxic T-cells (CTLs). T-cells can only recognize antigenic substances when present as an attachment of host cell proteins called Major Histocompatibility Complexes (MHC), also known as Human Leukocytic Antigen (HLA) in humans. These are unique set of proteins expressed on the surface of host cells which provide the self-identity to these cells. T-cells don't recognize soluble antigens. A lymphocyte has over 100,000 receptors on its surface, but because all these receptors have the same structure (a lymphocyte is monoclonal); hence only one lymphocyte can bind to this antigen **(Figure 1.2)** although there is some inherent degeneracy.

APCs are specialized cells which capture infectious agent and process it, thereafter and express it on the cell surface in context of MHC molecule so that T-cell can recognize this. The most characterized of APCs are the dendritic cells. After capturing the foreign antigens, these dendritic cells migrate to the lymphoid tissues and stimulate the naïve T-cells. In response to an antigenic stimulation, the Th cells get activated and release a series of biochemical substances called cytokines which act by activating other cells involved in the immune response including the other T-cells (both helper and CTLs), B-cells, macrophages, and even dendritic cells. Hence it is a phenomenon of "mutual augmentation". Activation of effector mechanisms and certain effector cells which include mononuclear phagocytes and CTLs aid in the elimination of the infectious agent.

Characteristics of the Adaptive Immune Response

1. Immune specificity.
2. Diversity.
3. Self-tolerance.
4. Immune memory and affinity maturation.
5. Self-limitation.

Immune specificity: The antibodies have regions which bind to a specific site on a particular antigen. Since each antibody molecule can only recognize a specific type of antigen it is said to be specific. Similarly, the T-cells have surface molecules called T-cell receptors (TCR) which bind to a specific antigenic site (epitope) which has been processed and expressed in context of the MHC molecules of the APCs. Hence the adaptive system is said to be immunologically specific.

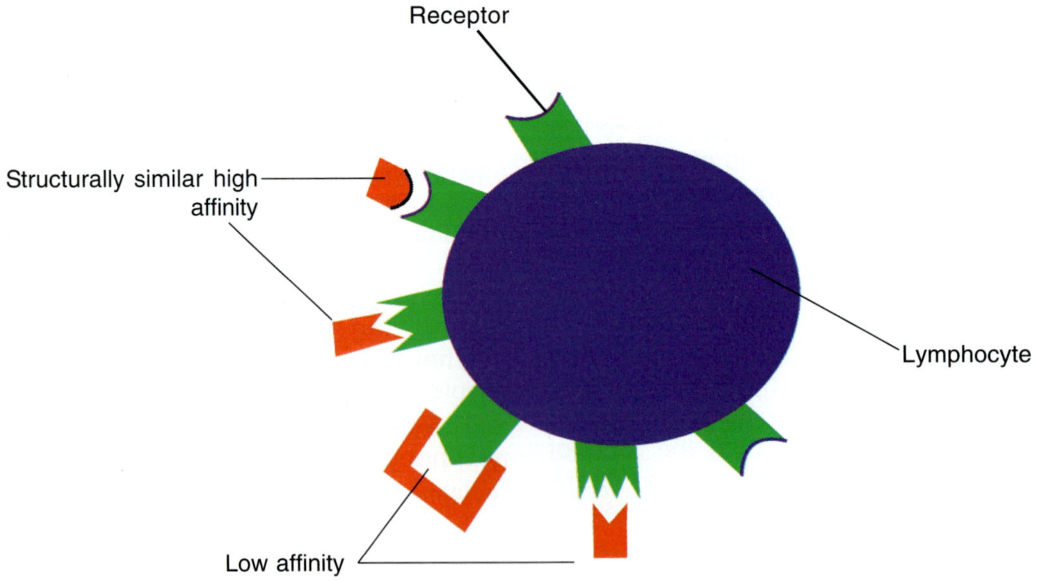

Fig. 1.2: T-cell recognition

Diversity: There are clones of lymphocytes with different specificities already present even in nonimmune individuals. This, as we shall see later, is a result of random combinations of genes involved in the generation of TCRs or antibodies **(Figure 1.3)**. A specific clone will get expanded on encountering its antigen. The entire gamut of antigenic specificities that the lymphocytes of any one individual can recognize is called the lymphocytic repertoire. It is estimated that this is anywhere in the order of 10^7 to 10^9. Hence the adaptive immune system is said to be diverse.

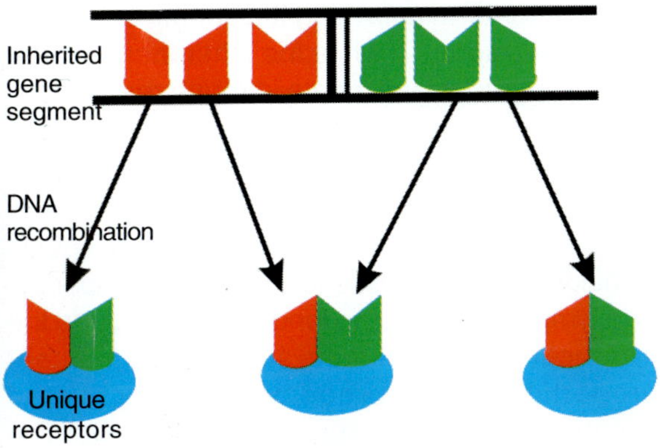

Fig. 1.3: Receptor diversity

Self-tolerance: Self-tolerance is one of the most intriguing and unique characteristics of the immune system which prevents it from reacting to the body's own molecules while still effectively eliminating foreign agents. Multiple mechanisms exist to ensure self-tolerance. These include elimination or inactivation of lymphocytes which can react to self antigens (auto-reactive lymphocytes). Failure of these mechanisms leads to the unusual occurrence of auto-immunity.

Immune memory and affinity maturation: After the first exposure, all subsequent encounters of the adaptive immune system with the antigen lead to a much stronger and a more rapid response. Hence the immune system has mechanisms to remember the nature of each antigen that it encounters. The first immune response is called the primary response and all subsequent encounters are known as secondary immune responses. The primary response leads to the expansion of the antigen-specific lymphocyte clone and generation of special "memory cells" which are much more efficient in eliminating the antigen than naïve cells. For instance, B-cells lead to the formation of memory cells which in secondary response produce antibodies with a much higher binding affinity to the antigen (a phenomenon known as affinity maturation). Affinity maturation occurs due to preferential stimulation of B cells producing higher affinity antibodies with each subsequent exposure. All these factors lead to the secondary response being much rapid and stronger than the primary response **(Figure 1.4)**.

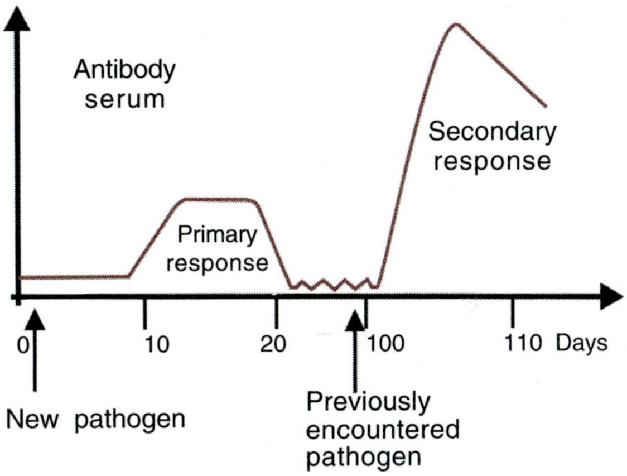

Fig. 1.4: Primary immune response and affinity maturation

Self-limitation: After elimination of the antigen, the immune response subsides thus returning the immune system to its basal state. This happens because elimination of the antigen removes the necessary stimulus for immune activation. Also, the immune system has integral regulatory mechanisms which inhibit the response. This is an important phenomenon to maintain homeostasis within the body.

Phases of the Immune Response

As mentioned earlier, the primary response is the first immune response against an antigen.

The secondary responses are all subsequent encounters of the immune response with that specific antigen. The secondary response is much rapid and stronger than the primary response due to various mechanisms, viz. expansion of the specific lymphocytic clone, immune memory and affinity maturation. This became the concept of inoculation later.

The immune response can be divided into various phases. These include:

1. Antigenic recognition.
2. Lymphocytic activation.
3. Antigen elimination or effector phase.
4. Self-limitation.

Antigenic recognition: A clone of lymphocytes specific to an antigen exists in the body even before the immune system has ever "seen" that antigen. The cells constituting any one clone have identical antigen receptors, which differ from the receptors present on all other clones. Hence the lymphocytes of any individual can recognize a set of different antigenic determinants which is called the lymphocytic repertoire of that individual. As mentioned before, this is estimated to be anywhere in the order of 10^7 to 10^9. During development of lymphocytes, random combinations of genes responsible for lymphocyte antigen receptors leads to the generation of such diversity (**Figure 1.3**). This shall be discussed in more details in subsequent chapters.

Whenever any antigen is encountered it selects and preferentially actives its specific pre-existing clone and this is called the clonal selection hypothesis, which has been validated by various experiments.

Lymphocytic activation: This second phase of immune response requires two distinct signals. Signal 1 is the antigen which ensures that the response is specific and Signal 2 is an additional stimulus, either directly from the microbe or from the innate immune system. The latter ensures that the immune response is activated only when it is required (i.e. only against foreign agents) and not against self-molecules. Lymphocytic activation then leads to cellular proliferation, cytokine production and initiation of effector mechanisms.

Antigen elimination: Lymphocytic activation leads to effector mechanisms for antigen elimination. This includes antibody production and activation of cytolytic lymphocytes which eliminates extracellular and intracellular agents respectively. It is to be noted here, that the effector mechanisms also involve components of innate immunity which we shall discuss in subsequent chapters. Thus the innate and adaptive immune responses perform an integrated function by means of mutual co-operation. The innate system is instrumental in activating the adaptive immune response (Signal 2) while the latter then, in turn, further augments the innate immune response.

Self-limitation: After elimination of the antigen, the immune response subsides restoring homeostasis. Since the immune response is antigen dependent, the elimination of antigenic stimulus leads to quiescence of immune response. The lymphocytes are no longer activated and the production of cytokines stops. A significant proportion of the progeny of the activated lymphocytic clone(s) dies due to apoptosis. The antibody titers also reduce over time. However, memory cells exist in the system for prolonged periods. And the stimulated clone still remains expanded than the basal levels. This is important for more effective elimination of the antigen in subsequent encounters.

Intracellular Pathogens

The immune system is much more complex than described here. An important facet which is worth mentioning is the elimination of intracellular pathogens which mainly include viruses and certain intracellular bacteria like Mycobacterium tuberculosis. Such pathogens are not directly "visible" to B-cells. This function is carried out by the T-lymphocytes. An intracellular pathogen is the one, which invades the cell directly often using the cells mechanisms for its own use—as is the case with viruses which have no replication machinery of their own and therefore cannot survive very long outside a host cell.

All cells in the body have mechanisms to collect fragments of proteins synthesized within the cell, and transport them to the surface, where they can be displayed to the rest of the body. The molecules involved in the transport and surface expression are known as major histocompatibility molecules (MHC) molecules. If, for example, a virus infects a host cell, MHC molecules can carry processed viral proteins from within the cytoplasm to the cell surface where their expression can be detected by the lymphocytes **(Figure 1.5)**. The other mechanism in which foreign antigens are expressed on the host cell surface involves ingestion of foreign particles by APCs. The APCs then process the antigens present on these foreign particles and then express them on their cell surface in the context of MHC molecules. The types of MHC molecules involved in these two unique processes are different. Foreign antigens from infected cells (non-APCs) are presented in the context of MHC class I molecules while the APCs express the processed antigens of the captured foreign particles in context of MHC class II molecules. This shall be discussed in greater details in subsequent chapters. However, these mechanisms have been mentioned here as an overview of T-cells recognition of foreign antigens.

At this time you should know the following:

1. Basics of innate and acquired immunity.
2. Functions of the immune system.
3. Characteristic features of adaptive immune response.
4. Body defenses against pathogens.

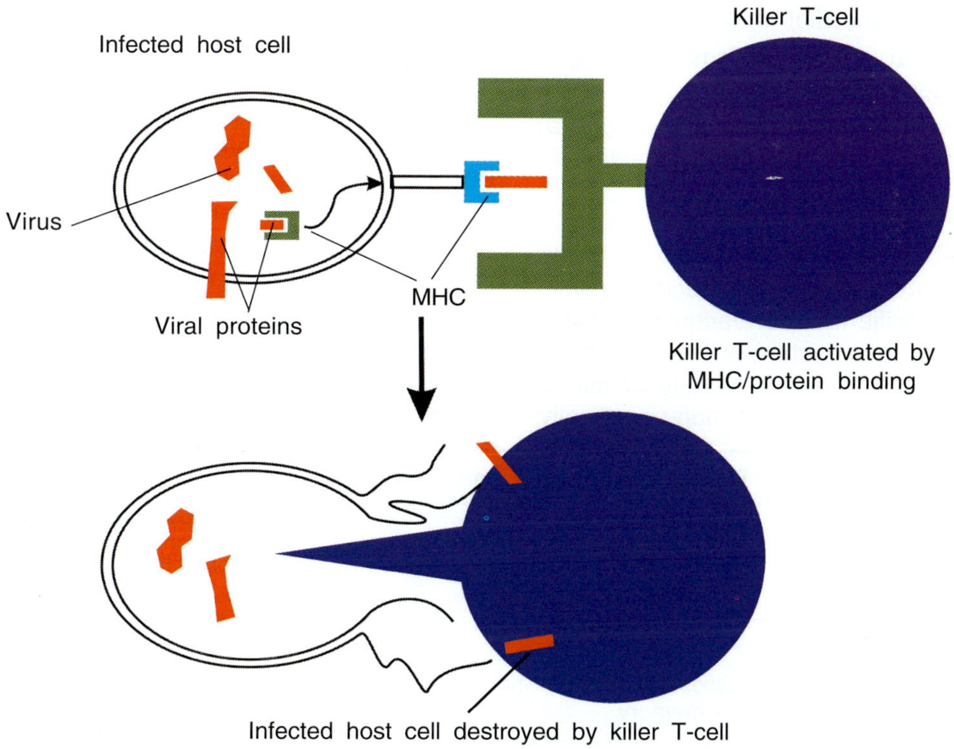

Fig. 1.5: T-cells and intracellular pathogens

2
CHAPTER
Innate (Non-Specific) Immunity

(Dr. Vinay Bharat and Dr. Parul Goel *anchitbharat@hotmail.com*)

OBJECTIVES

1. To know the significance of immune system in defending the human body from infection and disease.
2. To differentiate between innate (non-specific) and adaptive (specific) immune systems.
3. To understand the mechanisms of killing of the pathogens.
4. To know the humoral and cellular components of the non-specific immunity.

INTRODUCTION

The immune system can be divided into two major categories: Non-specific (innate/native) and specific (adaptive/acquired) **(Table 2.1)**. Innate immune system is the first line of defense that acts against a variety of stimuli and is considered to function non-specifically. It is considered to be critical in activating the adaptive immune system that mediates a more specific reaction.

The elements of the innate immune system include anatomical barriers, secretory molecules and cellular components **(Table 2.2)**.

Anatomical Barriers

There are several anatomical mechanisms that can be included in the innate immune system. For example, intact skin provides resistance against invasion of pathogens. The constant gastrointestinal peristalsis and oscillation of bronchopulmonary cilia help to eliminate the pathogens. Elevation of body temperature (fever) that occurs in response to the release of several bacterial products is inhibitory to bacterial growth.

Table 2.1: Differences between innate and adaptive immunity

Differences	*Innate immunity*	*Adaptive immunity*
Antigen-specificity	Non-specific	Specific
Initiation of response	Immediate	A short lag period between exposure and maximal response
Memory	Does not result in induction of memory	Exposure results in induction of memory
Interaction	Critical for the induction of adaptive immunity	Augments innate immunity
Allergic reaction	None	Hypersensitive

Table 2.2: Biological barriers to infections

System organ	*Active component*	*Effector mechanism*
Skin	Squamous cells; Salt of sweat glands; Sebaceous glands; (Long chain fatty acids and Lactic acid)	Desquamation; flushing, organic acids, bactericidal pH (3-5) retard bacterial growth
Mouth	Saliva	Bathing, flushing, a wide spectrum of antimicrobial agents such as lactoferrin, lysozyme, histatins, cystatins, mucins, agglutinins, secretory leukocyte proteinase inhibitor, tissue inhibitors of proteinases, chitinase, peroxidases and calprotectin
GI tract	Wall Gastric secretions Biliary system	Peristalsis, mucus, gastric acid, pancreatic fluids, proteolytic enzymes, bile salts, IgA, low pH
Respiratory system	Tracheal cilia Coughing reflex	Mucociliary elevator, surfactant Forcible removal
Nasopharynx	Nasal hair, Mucus	Mechanical barrier Entrap and swallow
Eye	Tears	Flushing, lysozyme
Circulation and lymphoid organs	Phagocytic cells NK cells and K-cell LAK	Phagocytosis, intracellular killing direct and antibody dependent cytolysis IL-2 activated cytolysis
Serum	Lactoferrin and transferrin Interferons TNF-α Lysozyme Fibronectin Complement CRP α-1 acid glycoproteins Serum amyloidal P component	Iron binding Anti-viral proteins Anti-viral, phagocyte activation Peptidoglycan hydrolysis Opsonization and phagocytosis Opsonization, enhanced phagocytosis and intracellular killing, inflammation
Female genitalia: Vagina	Acidic pH (5) Surfactant protein A (SP-A)	Retards bacterial growth Facilitate phagocytosis by opsonizing bacteria, fungi and viruses, stimulate the oxidative burst by phagocytes and modulate pro-inflammatory cytokine production by phagocytic cells
Male reproduction: Semen	Spermin and zinc	Anti-bacterial activity
Urinary system	Acidic pH and flow	Retards bacterial growth, flushing, epithelia lining the urinary tract prevent adhesion of bacteria by release of Tamm-Horsfall protein, lactoferrin, lipocalin, and constitutive and inducible bactericidal antimicrobial peptides such as alpha and beta defensins and cathelicidin
Mammary glands: Milk	Antibodies, binding proteins, fatty acids, fibronectin, hormones, interferon, lactoferrin, lysozyme, mucin, oligosaccharides	Protection of newborn

Secretory Molecules

These include organic acids in skin secretions, lysozyme in oronasopharyngeal and lacrimal secretions, thiocyanate in saliva, bile acids and low molecular weight fatty acids in the lower bowel, transferrin, lactoferrin, lysozyme, interferons, fibronectin, complement and acute phase proteins in serum, interferons and tumor necrosis factor at the site of inflammation.

Transferrin and lactoferrin deprive organisms of iron. Interferons inhibit viral replication and activate other cells which kill pathogens. Lysozyme, in serum and tears, breaks down the bacterial cell wall (peptidoglycan); fibronectin coats (opsonizes) bacteria and promotes their rapid phagocytosis. Complement components and their products cause destruction of microorganism directly or with the help of phagocytic cells. Acute phase proteins interact with the complement system proteins to combat infections. TNF-α suppresses viral replication and activates phagocytes through nitric oxide pathway.

Cellular Components

Phagocytic cells: Neutrophils (polymorphonuclear, PMN), macrophages and monocytes are important cellular components of the non-specific immune system.

a. Neutrophils are most important cellular components in bacterial destruction. They are relatively large and most abundant white blood cells with multi-lobed nuclei and cytoplasmic granules (lysosomes). They are identified by their characteristic morphology although monoclonal antibodies against cell surface cluster differentiation (CD) markers are becoming available to identify these cells.

   PMN granules are of two kinds: Primary (azurophilic) and secondary (specific) **(Table 2.3)**.

   Primary (large) azurophilic granules are characteristic of immature and very young neutrophils. They contain NADPH oxidase cofactors, cationic proteins, defensins (small molecular weight proteins), proteases (elastase, cathepsin G, etc.), lysozyme and myeloperoxidase (characteristic of primary granules).

   Secondary (specific) granules are the characteristic of mature neutrophils. Lactoferrin and B-12-binding protein are their two important constituents but they also contain lysozyme and NADPH oxidase cofactors.

Table 2.3: Differences between large and specific granules

Primary (large) azurophilic granules	*Secondary (specific) granules*
Lactoferrin	Myeloperoxidase
Lysozyme	Lysozyme-bacterial factors
Alkaline phosphatase	Cationic proteins
Type IV collagenase	Acid hydrolases
Leukocyte adhesion molecules	Elastase
Plasminogen activator	Non-specific collagenase
Phospholipase A2	Defensins, Cathepsin G, Phospholipase A2

b. Mononuclear phagocytes are the other population of phagocytic cells and include monocytes in circulation, histiocytes in tissues, microglial cells in the brain, kupffer cells in the liver and macrophages in serous cavities and lymphoid organs. They also have granules similar to those found in neutrophils, although not as abundant. They are recognized by their morphology, ability to adhere on glass/plastic surface and phagocytic property.

All phagocytic cells have receptors for a variety of molecules. Most pertinent to non-specific immunity are scavenger and TOLL-like receptors and receptors for the Fc part of IgG, complement, interferons, TNF and certain bacterial components. Interaction of organisms with these receptors promotes phagocytosis and phagocyte activation for a more efficient killing of pathogens.

Monocyte (12-15 micron) are derived from precursor stem cell within 6 days and thereafter leave circulation in 1-3 days and become macrophage (15-20 micron) and are the first line of defense associated with innate immunity.

Dendritic/Langerhans Cells

Dendritic/Langerhans cells are bone marrow derived APCs that are distinct from monocytes-macrophages and are derived from both lymphoid and myeloid lineages. They generally lack the standard T, B, NK and monocyte cell markers but do express CD83 and other molecules that aid in their identification. These cells are potent and effective APCs, because of their high levels of expression of MHC class II and costimulatory molecules. Dendritic cells in response to viral infections, produces high levels of interferon INF-α, which in turn activates NK cell to kill virally infected cell and activates monocytes-macrophages and other APCs to recruit antigen-specific T and B-cells. The APC for T-cells is called dendritic cells while APC for B-cells is called follicular dendritic cell. Immature dendritic cells are important component of innate immunity and mature dendritic cells are important component of adaptive immunity. Dendritic cells are referred to as Langerhans cells when they are present in the skin and beneath the mucosal surface.

Phagocyte Response to Infection

Chemotaxis

Bacteria produce N-formyl-methionine containing peptides and some endogenous substances like C5a of complement system, leukotriene B4 and cytokine IL-8, which are powerful attractants (chemotactic) for phagocytic cells. Many bacteria also act on proteins of the complement and clotting systems to produce peptides that cause vasodilation, vascular permeability and expression of adherence molecules on vascular endothelial cells. They also induce, in phagocytic cells, expression of proteins (e.g. integrins) that promote binding to endothelial cells. Phagocytic cells respond to chemotactic peptides of bacterial and host origin and migrate across the capillary wall (diapedesis) to the site of infection/ inflammation.

Attachment

Once at the site of infection, phagocytes can attach to bacteria via a number of receptors for bacterial components (scavenger receptor, LPS receptor, mannose receptor, TOLL-like receptors, etc.) or host proteins (opsonins) that coat (opsonize) bacteria (e.g., fibronectin, complement, IgG antibody, etc.). This attachment triggers the activation of respiratory burst (hexose monophosphate shunt), internalization of the organisms (phagosome formation), and phagosome lysosome fusion (phagolysosome) etc.

Respiratory Burst and Phagocytosis

The process of attachment and phagosome formation is accompanied by the activation of the respiratory burst (hexose monophosphate shunt) which results in the production of superoxide anion, singlet oxygen, hydroxyl ion and hydrogen peroxide. These molecules are microbicidal and cause killing of organisms in the phagosome.

Phagosome-lysosome Fusion

Phagosome soon after its formation fuses with granules (lysosomes) to form a phago-lysosome. As mentioned earlier, lysosomes contain a variety of antimicrobial substances (e.g., lysozyme, defensins, proteases, lactoferrin, transferrin, etc.) and phago-lysosome fusion results in the exposure of microorganisms to these substances and their destruction. Also, fusion of phagosome with primary granules (in newly recruited phagocytes) that contain myeloperoxidase results in the production of OCl^- (or other halides: I and Br) and halogenation of bacterial proteins. This ultimately lead to bacterial killing.

Three Modes of Intracellular Killing

It should be apparent from the preceding discussion that there are three pathways of killing by phagocytes:

1. By lysosomal antibacterial substances (lactoferrin, cationic proteins, lysozyme, defensins, proteases, etc.) without the requirement of respiratory burst (oxygen-independent killing) **(Table 2.4)**;
2. By products of respiratory burst (superoxide, singlet oxygen, hydroxyl radical, hydrogen peroxide, etc.) without the need for myeloperoxidase (oxygen-dependent, myeloperoxidase-independent killing); and
3. By halogenation of bacterial proteins catalyzed by myeloperoxidase (oxygen-dependent, myeloperoxidase-dependent killing).

These processes occur simultaneously and act synergistically. A defect in any of these pathways, for example, a deficiency of NADPH oxidase (cytochrome b558) components (p91, p22 and p61-phox), myeloperoxidase, etc. would impair the killing activity of phagocytes and render the host more susceptible to pyogenic infections. NADPH oxidase deficiency is the most serious of all these defects.

Table 2.4: Oxygen independent mechanisms of intracellular killing

Effector molecule	*Function*
Cationic proteins (including cathepsin)	Damage to microbial membranes
Lysozyme	Splits mucopeptide in bacterial cell wall
Lactoferrin	Deprives proliferating bacteria of iron
Proteolytic and hydrolytic enzymes	Digestion of killed organisms

Neutrophils also contain catalase and glutathione (GS) which detoxify excess of H_2O_2. Glutathione in its reduced form (GSSH) also recycles $NADPH^+$ to $NADP^+$.

Interaction of phagocytic cells with certain humoral factors (e.g. interferons, TNF, C5a, IL-2, etc.) can increase their phagocytic function, respiratory burst and intracellular killing. Certain proteins (cytokines) secreted by various cells can also induce phagocytic cells, particularly macrophages, to produce nitric oxide (NO) that is toxic to microorganism and malignant cells. Thus, certain bacterial products can cause macrophages to produce TNF that can, in turn, activate NO production. Likewise, interferon-α produced by NK (natural killer) cells (and T-cells) can also activate the NO pathway for killing pathogens.

Other Cells

A number of other cells are also involved in non-specific immune response include **(Table 2.5)**:

- NK cells.
- Antibody dependent cytotoxic cells (ADCC) also referred to as K-cells.
- Lymphokines (proteins secreted by lymphocytes) activated killer (LAK) cells.
- Eosinophils.

NK cells: 5-10% circulating lymphocytes do not contain marker of B or T-cell, hence are called NULL cell and are important in defense against viral infections and malignancies. They resemble lymphocytes in morphology but are larger (double the size) and granular, hence also known as large granular lymphocytes (LGL). The granules contain cytolytic proteins such as perforin. NK cells recognize the difference between normal and malignant or virus-infected cells in a nonspecific manner via sugar-lectin interaction and kill them following intimate contact. They also have low affinity Fc (γ III) receptor (CD16) by which they can interact with antibody-coated cells and cause their death. NK cells also have receptors for interleukin-2 (IL-2) and interferon and interaction with these cytokines leads to their activation. The presence of CD56 and CD16 and absence of CD3 is currently used as characteristic markers for NK cells.

Interaction with IL-2 (or interferon-γ) causes activation of NK cells. These activated cells are referred to as LAK (lymphokine-activated killer) cells. LAK cells function the same way as NK cells except that they are more potent killers and are capable of killing not only malignant but also transformed cells.

K-cells are morphologically undefined cells which attach to target cells coated with IgG antibody via the Fc receptor (Fc-γR) and cause their lysis; thus, they require interaction of specific antibody with target. Macrophages can also function as K-cells since they also have Fc receptors. Macrophages, when activated by a variety of cytokines, can kill malignant cells without the aid of antibody. CD16 is an Fc receptor of IgG and enhances the activity to lyse IgG coated target cell and this phenomenon is known as antibody dependant cell mediated cytotoxicity (ADCC).

Eosinophils have Fc receptor for IgE (Fc-εR) and cause cytotoxicity to large multi-cellular parasites coated with specific IgE antibody, analogous to K-cells.

There is no memory or specificity in the components of non-specific immunity. However, cells of the non-specific immune system become functionally more efficient following exposure to a pathogen because of interaction with products of the specific immune system (e.g., antibodies and cytokines).

Table 2.5: Cells of innate immune system and their major roles in triggering adaptive immunity

	Major role in innate immunity	*Major role in adaptive immunity*
Macrophages	Phagocytize and kill bacteria; produce antimicrobial peptides; bind lipopolysaccharide (LPS); produce inflammatory cytokines.	Produce interleukin (IL) 1 and tumor necrosis factor (TNF) α to upregulate lymphocyte adhesion molecules and chemokines to attract antigen-specific lymphocytes; produce IL-12 to recruit T_H1 helper T-cell responses; upregulate costimulatory and MHC molecules to facilitate T & B lymphocyte recognition and activation; macrophages and dendritic cells, after LPS signaling, upregulate co-stimulatory molecules B7-1 (CD80) and B7-2 (CD86) required for activation of antigen specific antipathogen T-cells; there are also Toll-like proteins on B-cells and dendritic cells that after LPS ligation induce CD80 and CD86 on these cells for T-cell antigen presentation.
Precursors of dendritic cells or immature dendritic cells	Produce large amounts of interferon (INF) α, which has antitumor and antiviral activity.	INF-α is a potent activator of macrophage and mature dendritic cells to phagocytose invading pathogens and present pathogen antigen to T and B-cells.

Contd.

Contd.

Natural killer (NK) cells	Kill foreign and host cells that have low levels of MHC+ self peptides. Express NK receptors that inhibit NK function in the presence of high expression of self-MHC.	Produce TNF-α and IFN-γ that recruit T_H1 helper T-cell responses.
NK-T-cells	Lymphocytes with both T-cell and NK surface markers that recognize lipid antigens of intracellular bacteria such as M tuberculosis by CD1 molecules and kill host cells infected with intracellular bacteria.	Produce IL-4 to recruit T_H2 helper T-cell responses. IgG1 and IgE production.
Neutrophils	Phagocytize and kill bacteria, produce antimicrobial peptides.	Produce nitric oxide synthase and nitric oxide that inhibit apoptosis in lymphocytes and can prolong adaptive immune responses.
Eosinophils	Kill invading parasites.	Produce IL-5 that recruits Ig-specific antibody responses.
Mast cells and basophils	Release TNF-α, IL-6, IFN-γ in response to a variety of bacterial PAMPs.	Produce IL-4 that recruits T_H2 helper T-cell responses and recruit IgG1 and IgE specific antibody responses.
Epithelial cells	Produce anti-microbial peptides; tissue specific epithelia produce mediator of local innate immunity, e.g. lung epithelial cells produce surfactant proteins (proteins within the collectin family) that bind and promote clearance of lung invading microbes.	Produce TGF-β that triggers IgA specific antibody responses.

At this time you should know the following:

1. Differences between the non-specific and specific immune functions.
2. Humoral components of the non-specific immune system and their action.
3. Cellular components of the non-specific immune function and their action.
4. Pathways of intracellular killing of bacteria and their features.
5. Effect of humoral components of the non-specific immune system.

Further Reading

1. Roitt's Essential Immunology: Delves, Martin, Burton and Roitt.
2. Cellular and Molecular Immunology: Abbas, Lichtman, Pillai.
3. Janeway's Immunobiology: Murphy, Travers, Walport.

3 CHAPTER

Complement System and Its Receptors

(Dr. L M Srivastava lalitmohan67@hotmail.com)

OBJECTIVES

1. To learn about complement system.
2. To know about different complement pathways and mechanisms involved in their activation and regulation.
3. To learn about the biological functions of different complements and their breakdown products and consequences of their activation.
4. To know about complement receptors and their functional role.
5. To discuss about the diseases associated with complements and their receptors.

INTRODUCTION

Historical Perspective

The complement proteins were initially discovered in late 19th century by Jules Bordet as heat labile substances, which could complement the bactericidal activity of a heat stable substance (antibody). Subsequently, it was shown that erythrocytes could be lysed in a similar manner and the basis of a hemolytic indicatory system for the heat labile factor designated complement C was established. The term complement was originally proposed by Paul Ehrlich in 1899 to describe the activity of serum that combined with specific antibody to evoke bacterial lysis. Since then, the system has hence been characterized into three distinct activation pathways–Classical pathway, Alternative pathway and Lectin pathway.

While the classical pathway was the first to be characterized, the alternative pathway appears to have phylogenetically preceded not only the classical but the immunoglobulin system. The terminal components probably developed later as an effector arm of the alternative pathway. The classical pathway, along with IgM, developed subsequently.

Complement cascade acts through a potent amplification mechanism based on serine protease dependent cleavages of inactive zymogen forms of proteins to active proteins. Each protease molecule can cleave many substrate molecules, hence amplifying the cascade. Another feature of the complement system is presence of multimolecular complexes formed by sequential additions of proteins.

Complement Nomenclature

Components of the classical pathway and the terminal sequence are indicated by the letter 'C' followed by a number (e.g., C1, C2). Due to variances in the chronology of their discoveries, the reactive order is not identical to the numerical order. Thus, the reaction sequence is C1, C4, C2, C3, C5, C6, C7, C8 and C9. Proteins of the alternative pathway as well as certain regulatory components are termed 'factors' and are symbolized by letters (e.g., B.P.D.). Constituents cleaved from the precursor protein are designated with the suffixed 'a', 'b'

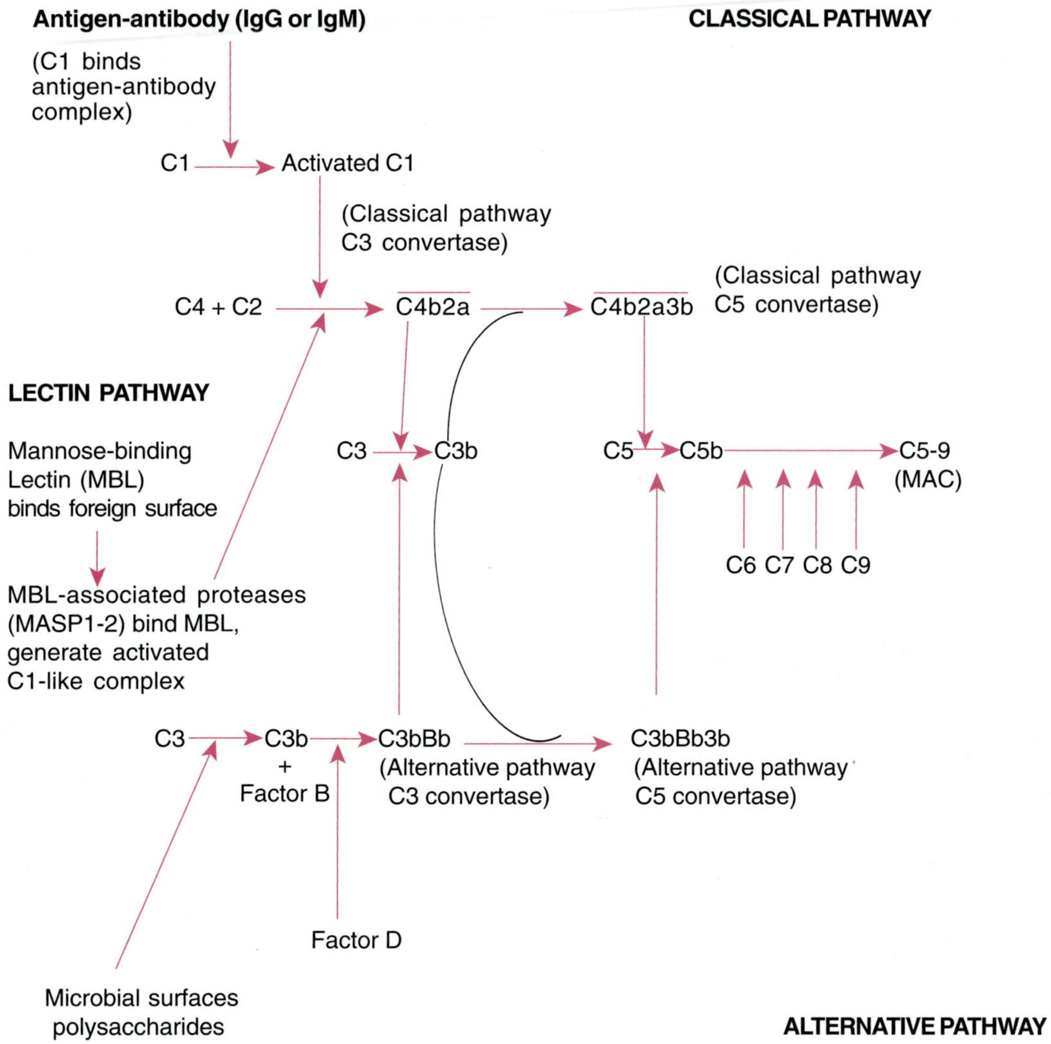

Fig. 3.1: A schematic outline of complement pathway

prevents insertion of the MAC into the inner membrane. Nucleated cells tend to be more resistant to complement-mediated lysis than red blood cells. Lysis of nucleated cells requires formation of multiple MACs, whereas a single MAC can lyse a red blood cell.

Inflammation

Complement is the major mediator at the site of inflammation. The inflammatory response is characterized by localized vasodilation and increased capillary permeability resulting in leakage of fluid into tissue site and migration of phagocytic cells to the area. The complement activation by an infectious agent induces release of three anaphylatoxins C4a, C3a and C5a, which can induce vasodilation and increase vascular permeability. C3a, C4a and C5a are 77 amino acid fragments derived from α chain of C3, C4 and C5 respectively. Both C3a and

C4a are nonglycosylated proteins. C5a bears complex oligosaccharide moiety attached to its Asn 64. C3a induces smooth muscle contraction, enhances vascular permeability and causes degranulation of basophils with consequent release of histamines and other vasoactive substances.

C5a is twofold more potent on a molar basis than C3a. Unlike C3a, C5a is strongly chemotactic for phagocytic cells, increase neutrophil adhesiveness and evoke aggregation. In addition, C5a dramatically stimulates neutrophils oxidative metabolism, the production of toxic oxygen species and release of lysosomal enzymes from a variety of phagocytic cells. Once at the inflammatory site, C5a can stimulate release of leukotriene and reactive oxygen metabolities enhancing the cytotoxicity of neutrophils.

Insertion of the MAC (C5b-9) in sublytic amounts into membranes of nucleated cells and platelets stimulate arachidonate metabolism and can cause release of prostaglandins E2, leukotriene B4 and thromboxane, and secondary mediators that are postulated to contribute to inflammation induced by complement activation in tissues. Lastly, certain complement cascade enzymes may interact, albeit inefficiently, with substrates in the kinin, coagulation and fibrinolytic system and vice versa.

Antigen Processing and Lymphocyte Activation

Complement and its receptors play an important role in controlling initial traffic of Immune Complexes and facilitates their binding to circulating erythrocytes via CR1. CR1/E levels have been shown to be diminished in diseases like SLE, characterized by excessive circulation of ICs. The decrease may be a consequence of excessive processing and proteolysis of Complement Receptor 1 during the passage of erythrocytes through reticuloendothelial system. There is also evidence for increased risk of Systemic Lupus Erythematosus for individuals with low hereditary CR1 levels.

Opsonization and Phagocytosis

C3b is the major opsonin of the complement system. The amplification that occurs with C3 activation results in a coating of C3b on ICs and particulate antigens. Each of the phagocytic cells expresses complement receptors (CR1, CR3 and CR4) that bind C3b, C4b or their degradation products. When antigen has been coated with C3b during complement activation by either pathway, the coated antigen binds to cells bearing CR1. Once C3b-coated antigen has bound to CR1, some of the C3b is degraded into C3bi and C3f. This enables the antigen to bind to CR3, which triggers phagocytosis more effectively than CRI.

Viral Neutralization

The complement system plays an important role in host defence by neutralizing viral infectivity. Some viruses (e.g., retroviruses, Epstein-Barr virus, Newcastle disease virus and rubella virus) can activate the alternative or even the classical pathway in the absence of antibody. For most viruses, the binding of serum antibody to the repeating subunits of the viral structural proteins creates particulate ICs ideally suited for complement activation by classical pathway.

The complement system mediates viral neutralization by a number of mechanisms. Some degree of neutralization is achieved through the formation of larger viral aggregates, simply because these aggregates reduce the net number of infectious viral particles. Although antibody does play a role in the formation of viral aggregates, in vitro studies show that the C3b component facilitates aggregate formation in the presence of as little as two molecules of antibody per virion. The binding of antibody and/or complement to the surface of a viral particle creates a thick protein coating. This coating neutralizes viral infectivity by blocking attachment to susceptible host cells. The deposits of antibody and complement on viral particles also facilitate binding of the viral particle to cells possessing Fc or CR1. In the case of phagocytic cells, such binding can be followed by phagocytosis and intracellular destruction of the ingested viral particle. Finally, complement is effective in lysing most, if not all, enveloped viruses, resulting in fragmentation of the envelop and disintegration of the nucleocapsid.

Significance of Third Component of Complement (C3)

The third component of complement, C3, is arguably the most important protein of the complement system. It is the most abundant of the complement components, being present in the plasma at a concentration of 1-1.2 mg/ml. It is the point at which the reaction sequences of the classical and alternative pathways converge.

The C3b, one of the split products of C3, is a bivalent molecule which can interact simultaneously via covalent binding with various acceptor sites (suitably placed hydroxyl or amino group on various molecules in the fluid phase and on cell surface that forms covalent ester or amide bond with activated internal thioester of C3b) and CR1 present on the membrane of various cells. It is evident that C3 is necessary for normal antibody response to thymus dependent and thymus independent antigens and induction of immunological memory.

The role of C3 in antigen processing and presentation has been demonstrated in the recent studies **(Figure 3.2)**. To maintain memory B-cell clones, the continued stimulation with antigen that persist on follicular dendritic cells is necessary. For this, the antigen has to be trapped in the folliculi, a process shown to be absolutely complement dependent.

In the germinal centre, where the fate of antigen selected B-cells are decided, C3 fragment deposited on the surface of macrophages may influence, directly or via lymphokines induction, the growth and differentiation of pre-activated B-cells to develop into plasma cell. Immobilized C3b and C3d on B-cells (via CR1 and CR2 respectively) have been shown to be capable of controlling the entry of activated B-cells into S-phase. Thus, any cell particles or ICs that display C3 fragments as a consequence of systemic or local complement activation could provide the necessary signal for B-cells activation in certain micro-environments.

Organization of the host cell responses by complement is achieved through the interaction of cell membrane receptors with the activation products of the complement proteins. Although a number of different complement components are involved in this complex process, C3 plays a pivotal role. During complement activation, a number of fluid phase and membrane bound products are generated from C3. The fluid phase fragments function to induce leukocytosis (C3c), increase vascular permeability (C3a) and suppress antibody synthesis (C3a) whereas the bound C3 fragments participate in the assembly of convertase enzymes that amplify C3 activation, enable further progression of the complement cascade and serve as opsonins.

In both natural killer (NK) system and in antibody-dependent cellular cytotoxicity (ADCC), where target cells are sensitized with suboptimal amounts of antibody, C3 fragments serve as accessory or adhesion molecules, strengthening the contact between the effector and target cells **(Figure 3.3)**.

The biological functions of complement and its breakdown products are mentioned in **(Table 3.1)**.

COMPLEMENT BINDING RECEPTORS

A wide variety of biologic effects of complement are mediated by high-affinity specific receptors for fragments of complement proteins **(Table 3.2)**. The fragments are generated by specific cleavage reactions that occur during the activation process. These biologic effects include not only the clearance of antigens that are coated with complement but also the activation of cells of the immune system. This process, in general, promotes the clearance of antigens through the maturation of both the cellular and the humoral immune responses. Also, for some proteins, such as C3, different receptors exist that are relatively specific for different activation fragments of the molecule (C3b, C3bi, C3d) and therefore interact with unique sites on the fragments. By this mechanism the immune response can be modulated with a higher degree of specificity.

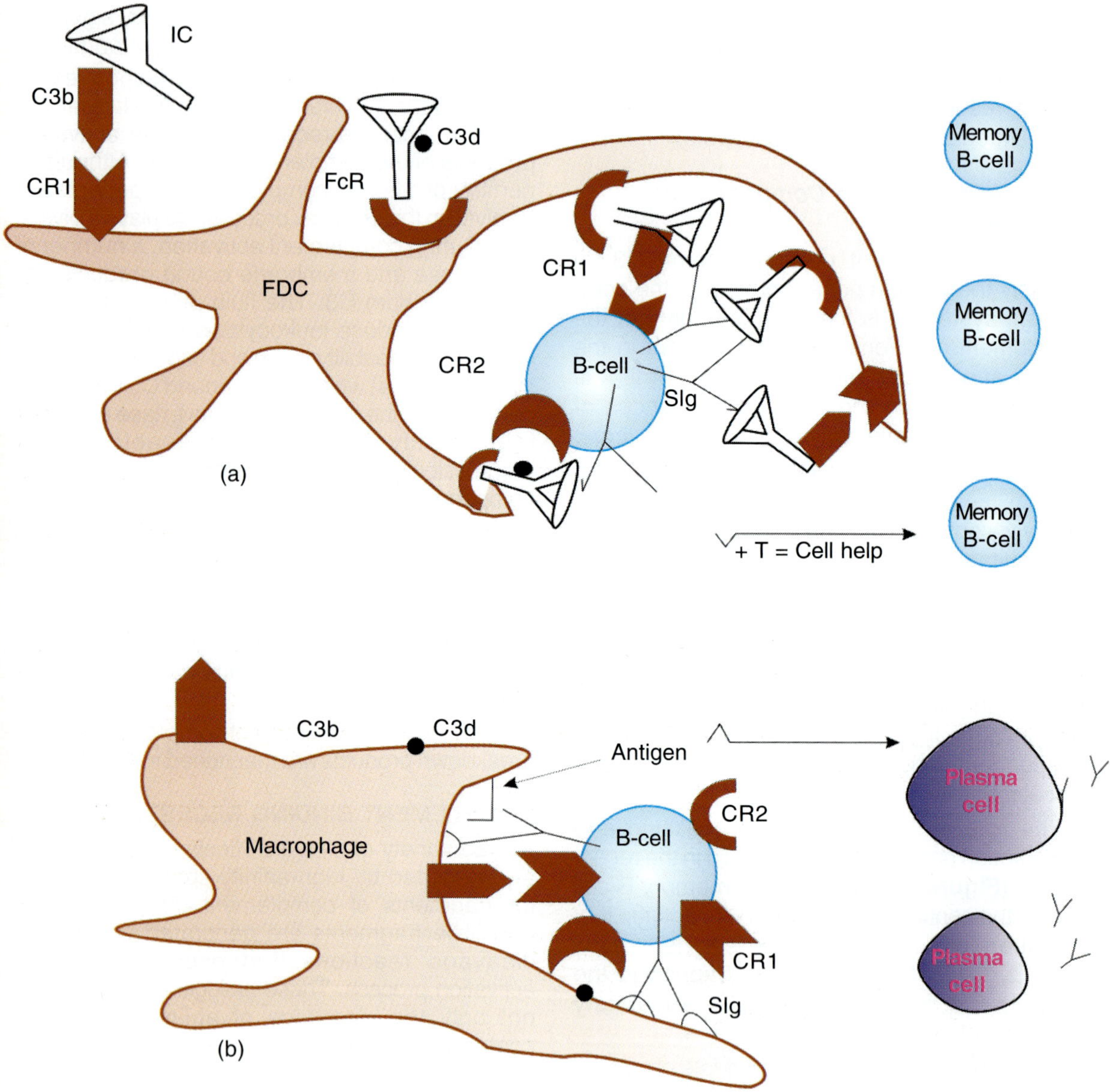

Fig. 3.2: Possible involvement of C3 in antigen processing and presentation

a. The development of memory B-cells; follicular dendritic cells (FDC) possessing FcR and CR1 trap antigen-antibody C3b/C3d complexes. B-cells make contact with FDC via their antigen-binding receptors and CR1/CR2. Cross-linking of these membrane structures and help from T-cells lead to the development of memory cells.

b. The activation of B-cells; activated macrophages display antigenic peptides on their cell membrane together with covalently-bound C3 split product. Cross-linking sIg, CR1/CR2 on B-cells together with the help of T-cells derived factor induce the development of antibody producing plasma cells.

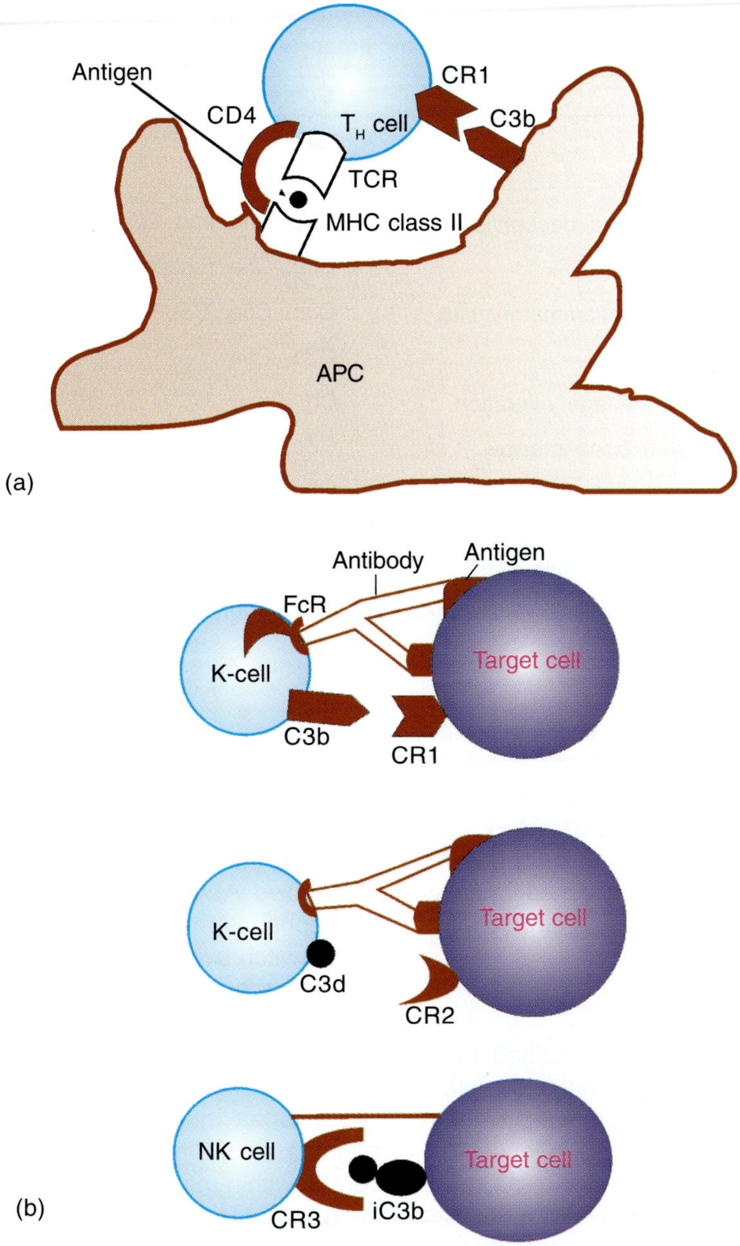

Fig. 3.3: C3 fragment as adhesion molecules

a. During antigen presentation; in addition to the antigen-specific contact between APC and T-helper cells, C3b may promote the interaction by forming a non-antigen specific second bridge between the two cells.
b. In cytotoxic reaction; K and NK – cells mediated lysis of target cells is significantly enhanced by C3 fragments that promote the contact between effector and target cells possessing the relevant C3-binding structures.

Table 3.1: Biological functions of complement and its breakdown products

Effect	*Complement product mediating functions*
Cell lysis.	C5b-9, the membrane-attack complex (MAC)
Inflammatory response.	
Degranulation of mast cells and basophils.	C3a, C4a and C5a (anaphylatoxins)
Degranulation of eosinophils.	C3a, C5a (anaphylatoxins)
Chemotaxis of leukocytes at inflammatory site.	C3a, C5a, C5b67
Aggregation of platelets.	C3a, C5a
Inhibition of monocyte/macrophage migration.	Bb
Release of neutrophils from bone marrow.	C3c
Release of hydrolytic enzymes from neutrophils.	C5a
Enhanced expression of complement receptors type 1 and 3 (CR1 and CR3) on neutrophils.	C5a
Opsonization of particulate antigens and enhancing their phagocytosis.	C3b, C4b, iC3b
Viral neutralization.	C3b, C5b-9 (MAC)
Solubilization and clearance of immune complexes.	C3b

Complement activation fragments for which receptors have been well described include Clq, C3, C4, C5a, C3a, C4a, factor B (both Ba and Bb), and factor H. Some have been cloned, whereas others are still only functionally and/or biochemically described.

Clq Receptor

Receptors for Clq have been described on a wide variety of cells, including most leukocytes, endothelial cells, fibroblasts, platelets, smooth muscle cells, and epithelial cells. Monocytes, neutrophils, B lymphocytes, and a small percentage of T and non-T, non-B lymphocytes have also been reported to interact with Clq. The molecular structure of the Clq receptor is not yet firmly established, and substantial evidence exists for the presence of more than one receptor form.

Biologic effects of Clq receptors that have been proposed based on *in vitro* studies include the opsonization of IC targets with the subsequent "activation" of phagocytosis, promotion of the oxidative burst in the polymorphonuclear cell, enhanced ADCC and cytokine release by macrophages, and immunoglobulin secretion and class switch by B lymphocytes. The endothelial protein has been proposed to serve as a receptor trap for circulating ICs bearing Clq, possibly resulting in the subsequent development of vasculitis. Like many complement receptors, the Clq receptor interacts best with polymers and aggregates of Clq. The portion of Clq that binds cells is within the collagen-like tail in contrast to the globular region, which contains the immunoglobulin binding domain.

Complement Receptor 1 (CR1/CD35)

The C3b receptor was discovered almost 30 years back when bacteria which had been incubated with serum containing specific antibody and active complement were shown

Table 3.2: Complement binding receptors

Receptor	Major ligands	Activity	Cellular distribution
CR1 (CD35)	C3b, C4b	Blocks formation of C3 convertase; binds immune complexes to cells.	Erythrocytes, neutrophils, monocytes, macrophages, eosinophils, follicular dendritic cells, B-cell, certain T-cells.
CR2 (CD21)	C3d, C3dg, iC3b	Part of B-cell coreceptor, binds Epstein-Barr virus.	B-cells, follicular dendritic cells, certain T cells.
CR3 (CD11b/18) CR4 (CD11c/18)	iC3b	Bind cell-adhesion molecules on neutrophils, facilitating their extravasation; bind immune complexes, thereby enhancing their phagocytosis.	Monocytes, macrophages, neutrophils, natural killer cells, certain T-cells.
C3a/C4a receptor	C3a, C4a	Induces degranulation of mast cells and basophils.	Mast cells, basophils, granulocytes.
C5a receptor	C5a	Induces degranulation of mast cells and basophils.	Mast cells, basophils, granulocytes, monocytes, macrophages platelets, endothelial cells.
C1q receptor	C1q	Opsonization of immune complex targets.	Leucocytes, endothelial cells, fibroblasts, platelets, smooth muscle cells and epithelial cells.

to adhere to human erythrocytes. This immune adherence receptor of the erythrocyte was shown subsequently to be specific for C3b in the IC and to reside on the cell types including PMN, monocytes and macrophages, a subset of T lymphocytes, glomerular podocytes and in soluble form in the plasma.

Structure and Molecular Biology of CR1

Human CR1 is a single chain glycoprotein having 1998 (~220 kD) amino acids with complex tri and tetra N-linked oligosaccharides in its mature form. Minor differences of ~ 6kD in apparent molecular weights has been observed between CR1 isolated from erythrocytes and those isolated from neutrophils or T cells of the same individual which is due to differential glycosylation.

A second polymorphism of CR1 was described, in which CR1 isolated from different individuals varied in molecular weight from 160 to 250 kD. Pedigree analysis demonstrated that this polymorphism is regulated by four autosomal co-dominant alleles. The two most common alleles of CR1 having gene frequencies of 0.8 and 0.2 have been named A and B respectively encoding proteins having molecular weights (non-reducing conditions) of 190 and 220 kD respectively. Two rarer alleles, Type C and Type D with molecular weights under non reducing conditions of 160 and 250 kD respectively have also been described. The gene coding for CR1 has been localized in long arm of chromosome 1 in the lq32 region.

Quantitative Expression of CR1 on Cells

Pedigree analysis also revealed that the amount

of expression of each allotype is dependent on a regulatory element that determines the net quantitative expression on erythrocytes. The linkage of this element to the structural gene has also been established. The above observation was further confirmed by Hind III Restriction Fragment Length Polymorphism (RFLP) which proved an association of low and high expression with 6.9 kb and 7.4 kb allelic fragments. The occurrence of a new Hind III site due to a single base change within intron and hence a shorter 6.9 kb fragment was shown associated with low CR1 expression. Various methods have been employed for the determination of E-CR1 like measuring the binding of radiolabelled dimeric C3b, or radiolabelled polyclonal or monoclonal anti-CRI antibodies as well as by flow cytometry. A four-fold stable difference in number of CR1 per erythrocyte has been observed within groups of homozygous and heterozygous individuals indicating existence of additional genetic mechanism which regulate number of E-CR1. Unstimulated phagocytic cells express only 10 to 20% of total cell associated CR1 on the cell membrane. The remaining CR1 is stored in an intracellular pool from where it can be mobilized to the cell surface in a Ca^{++} dependent process on stimulation of the cells. Molecules that induce enhanced expression of CR1 on phagocytic cells include C5a, its stable plasma derivative C5a desArg and tumor necrosis factor (TNF).

Cellular Expression of CRI

In human beings, CRI is expressed on erythrocytes, eosinophils, monocytes/macrophages, B-lymphocytes, a subpopulation of $CD4^{+}$T lymphocytes, dendritic cells, Langerhans cells in the skin and kidney podocytes. A small amount is present in plasma and urine. About 10% of the total pool of CR1 in blood is present on neutrophils and monocytes, while about 90% is present on the red blood cell (RBC).

Biological Functions of CR1

The CR1 acts as a surface regulatory protein and as a complement receptor. Its biological functions are depicted in the **Figure 3.4**.

a. The role of erythrocyte CR1 system in limiting complement-mediated tissue injury:

The CR1 prevents the formation of the alternative pathway convertase C3bBb, because the binding site for CR1 on C3b is close to that for factor B. By binding to CR1, it inhibits the formation of the classical pathway convertase, C4b2b, in a similar fashion. By binding with C3b and C4b, CR1 serves as a cofactor for irreversible cleavage of C3b into iC3b and C3dg and C4b into C4c and C4d by factor I. This complement inhibitory activity of CR1 occurs both when CR1 is bound to the membrane and when present in the soluble form in the plasma. A recombinant soluble form of CR1 (sCR1) is able to reduce infract size in rat after induced myocardial ischemia. Also, soluble CR1 is effective in reducing inflammation and tissue injury in rat after intradermal injection of ICs, and is able to provide protection against complement dependent acute inflammatory lung and dermal injury, and prevent hyperacute rejection of porcine xenograft.

b. Functions of CR1 on erythrocytes: Processing and transport of immunecomplexes:

A physiological function of the complement system is to maintain antigen-antibody complex in solution and to facilitate their elimination. In circulation, C3b bearing IC preferentially bind to CR1 on erythrocytes. The IC, once bound to E-CR1, may also be acted upon by agents present in the plasma, and the altered IC becomes less pathogenic. The ICs that bind less efficiently to E-CR1 showed enhanced nonhepatic, nonsplenic uptake (especially in lungs and kidney). The liver is the main site for removal of C3b bearing IC. Complexes are trapped by Kupffer cells after cleavage of C3b into iC3b or C3dg. The latter fragments have little or no affinity

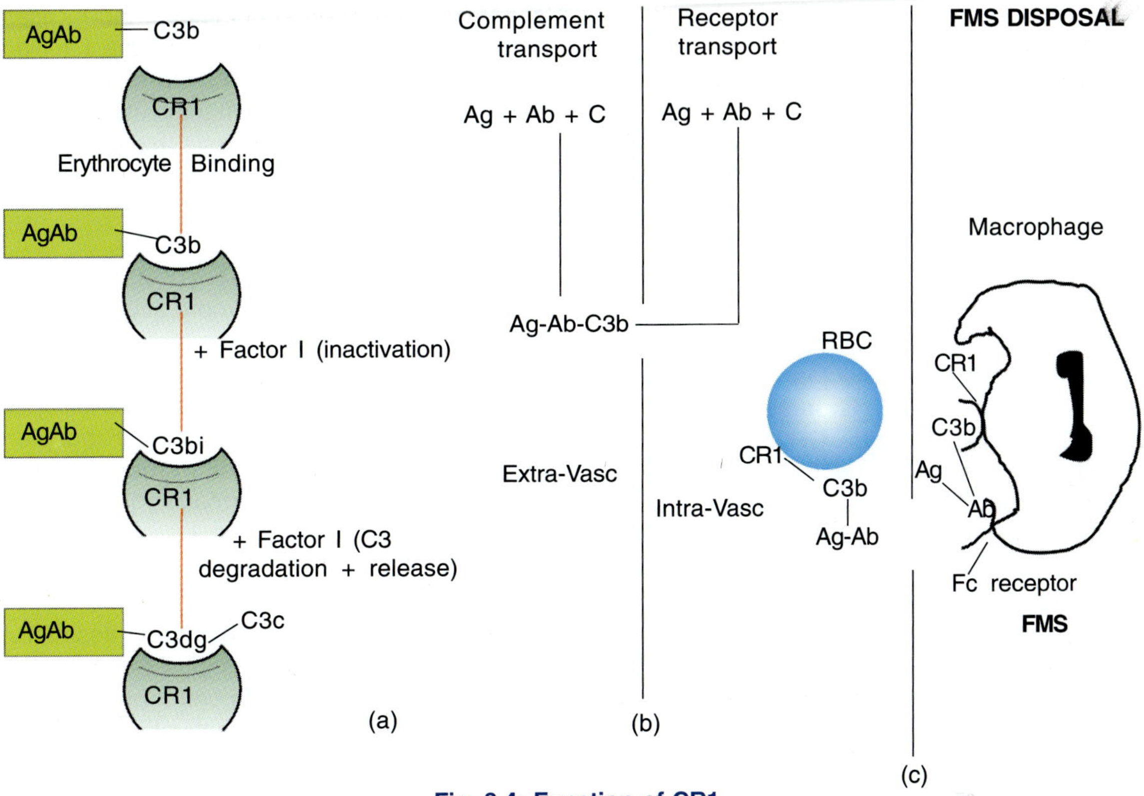

Fig. 3.4: Function of CR1

a. CR1 as a regulatory protein.
b. Role of CR1 in processing and transport of immunecomplexes.
c. Function of CR1 on phagocytic cells.

for CR1. However, they bind to CR3 and CR4 respectively, the two receptors that are present in high density on Kupffer cells. ICs that contain C3dg or C3d may also be trapped by B-cells which express CR2 receptors. In addition, complexes bearing iC3b and C3dg can be trapped by follicular dendritic cells.

c. Functions of CR1 on phagocytic cells:

The CR1 on phagocytic cells may bind soluble polymeric C3b which is covalently fixed to ICs or particles and enhance their phagocytosis. The CR1 and Fc gamma receptors co-operate for phagocytosis of targets that have been coated with suboptimal amounts of IgG. Resting neutrophils and monocytes just bind but do not phagocytize C3b coated particles. The receptors may acquire phagocytic capacity after stimulation of the cells with phorbol ester, T-cell derived lymphokines or co-opsonization of the target with extracellular matrix proteins (i.e. fibronectin, laminin and amyloid P). The crosslinking of the receptors elicits a number of secondary responses in phagocytic cells including neo-synthesis and release of arachidonic acid metabolites, stimulation of oxidative burst and release of toxic oxygen derivatives and release of lysosomal enzymes.

d. Role of CR1 in regulation of immune response:

The stimulation of human monocyte with C3b induces the intracellular production and extracellular release of interleukin I (IL-1) in serum free conditions. It enhances the differentiation of B-cells but does not have any effect on memory responses.

Complement Receptor 2 (CR2/CD21)

CR2 is glycoprotein that binds several degradation products of C3b including C3d, C3dg and C3bi. Unlike CR1, which is present on all types of circulating blood cells, CR2 expression is limited to B-cells and some T-cells. CR2 is also the receptor for Epstein-Barr virus, which accounts for the susceptibility of B-cells to infection by this virus. The interaction between C3d and CR2 occurs subsequent to the cleavage of C3b to C3bi mediated by Factor I and cofactors H, MCP and CR1. CR2 on B-lymphocytes modulates Ag-mlg B-cell activation and promotes antigen processing and presentation of C3d bound targets. The CR2 may act as an interferon receptor and T-cell-CR2 may mediate infection of cells with complement coated human immunodeficiency virus type 1, independently of CD4.

Complement Receptor 3 (CR3, Mac1, CD11b/CD18) and Complement Receptor 4 (CR4)

The CR3 and CR4 bind primarily the C3b degradation product C3bi. These are the members of a family of proteins termed integrins, that are composed of two chains: a chain of variable size and a conserved 95 kD chain. They are found on monocytes, macrophages, neutrophils, Kupffer cells and NK cells. It also possesses lectin like activities as evident by its role as an organizer of cytoskeletal events during adhesive interactions and membrane rearrangement in phagocytosis. CR3 also mediates neutrophil attachment to P-selectin and intercellular adhesion molecule 1 (ICAM-1) proteins on endothelium and facilitate extravasation of neutrophils from the capillary into the tissue spaces during an inflammatory reaction. Binding of complement-coated particles to CR3 triggers phagocytosis by phagocytic cells.

C5a, C3a and C4a Receptors

C5a and C3a are potent anaphylatoxins that are released during complement activation. C4a is also released but has substantially less bioactivity. Receptors for these fragments are present on basophils, mast cells and granulocytes. Binding of C3a, C4a and C5a to its receptors on mast cell or basophil induces cell to degranulate, releasing pharmacologically active mediators.

REGULATION OF COMPLEMENT ACTIVATION

Because of the pro-inflammatory and destructive capabilities of complement, precise control is necessary. Deficiencies of control proteins lead to excessive complement activation, which in turn results in a pathologic state. Control of the complement system is achieved by two primary mechanisms. First, activated components have relatively short half-lives and spontaneously decay. Second, specific proteins assist the regulatory process by proteolytically inactivating components or by disengaging them from their molecular couplings. The net result of such interactions is the prevention of inadvertent complement activation in the host while allowing its appropriate activation against foreign elements.

The complement system is regulated at the critical steps of initiation, C3 and C5 convertase formation, MAC formation and insertion, and by control of its proinflammatory anaphylatoxins.

Complement Regulatory Proteins

The complement pathway is tightly controlled by regulatory proteins acting at a number of sites using different strategies to block activation. The regulatory proteins are found in the fluid phase, on cell membranes and in the matrix. In general, regulatory proteins are to inactivate a specific component irreversibly, to maintain a protein transiently in an inactive form or to dissociate components from multiprotein complex such as the C3 and C5 convertases. These regulatory proteins are best classified on the basis of their primary location (fluid phase, membrane, matrix). However, the sites at which they regulate complement overlap substantially, and some proteins also have both membrane and soluble forms. The regulatory proteins and their functions are listed in **Table 3.3**.

Fluid Phase Regulatory Proteins

C1 esterase inhibitor: C1 esterase inhibitor (C1-INH) is a soluble glycoprotein and a member of the serine proteinase inhibitor (serpin) family. C1INH inhibits the complement proteases C1r and C1s and also inhibits the proteases kallikrein, factor XIa, XIIa and plasmin of the contact and clotting systems. The major complement related role of C1-INH is to inactivate C1r and C1s and thus restrict their effects to the specific site of C1 binding and activation.

Factor I: Factor I (C3b inactivator, C3bINA) was purified as a protein that cleaved and inactivated C3b and C4b. Subsequently, it was found to require cofactors to accomplish this cleavage, to cleave C3b and C4b at specific sites, and to act on the proteins when they are either free in the fluid phase or target bound. Factor I plays the very important role of cleaving both C3b and C4b in a highly regulated fashion into forms of the molecules that cannot act as part of a C5 convertase.

Factor H: Factor H is alternative pathway regulator and have two distinct enzymatic activities to accomplish this role. These activities are acceleration of the normally slow spontaneous decay of Bb from C3b, thus dissociating both the C3 and C5 convertases, and the required cofactor activity for factor I to mediate cleavage of C3b into a hemolytically inactive form, C3bi. Factor H can perform these activities on C3b bound to targets such as bacteria and ICs, or on free, soluble, C3Bb-containing complexes.

C4b-binding protein: C4b-binding protein (C4bp) is a protein with parallel activities as factor H but directed toward C4b and the classical pathway rather than C3b and the alternative pathway. C4bp inactivates C4b by serving as an obligate cofactor for factor I-mediated cleavage and also accelerates the spontaneous decay of C2a from C4b. Therefore, C4bp has both of the functional characteristics of factor H, cofactor activity and decay acceleration, but instead exerts it activities on C4.

S protein (vitronectin): Soluble protein that inhibits the assembly or membrane insertion of the MAC (C5b-9) has also been identified. The two best characterized are proteins and designated SP-40. S protein is postulated to act by incorporation into the C5b-7 complex, thus converting the latter to a hydrophilic, non-membrane-binding and inactive complex.

Many cells have receptors for S protein. This has led to the proposal that it is involved not only in complement regulation but also in the control of platelet and other cell adhesion to sites of inflammation.

SP-40, 40 (clusterin, cytolysis inhibitor): SP-4,40 is a disulfide-linked heterodimer that is derived by proteolytic cleavage of a single chain precursor. It is found free in normal serum and in complement activated serum associated with soluble C5b-9 complexes. SP-40 has same type of complement regulatory activity as S protein.

Carboxypeptidases: Once released, the potent anaphylatoxins C5a and C3a undergo a rapid loss of activity in serum primarily caused by C-terminal cleavage of Arg to make the desArg form. Serum carboxypeptidases perform this cleavage, resulting in protein forms with two to three orders of magnitude less cell stimulating activity.

Table 3.3: Complement regulatory proteins, their structural features and functions

Proteins	Structural features	Ligands	Pathway affected	Functions
Soluble Serum Proteins				
C1 inhibitor	Serine protease inhibitor	C1r,C1s	Classical	– Blocks the ability of C1r and C1s to participate in classical pathway. – Binds to inactive C1 and prevents spontaneous activation. – Also inhibits kallilrein, plasmin and factor XIa, XIIa of coagulation system.
C4b-binding	SCR	C4b	Classical and Lectin	– Accelerates decay of protein (C4bp) classical pathway convertase.
Factor H	SCR	C3b	Alternative	– Accelerates decay of alternative pathway convertase. – Acts as cofactor for factor I mediated cleavage of C3b.
Factor I	Serine protease	C3b, C4b	Classical, alternative and Lectin	– Inactivates C4b and C3b, using C4bp, factor H, CR1 or MCP as cofactor.
S-protein		C5b-7	Terminal	– Binds to C5b-7 and prevents membrane insertion of MAC.
SP-40, 40	Heterodimer	C5b-9	Terminal	– Modulates MAC formation.
Anaphylotoxin inactivator		C3a, C4a, C5a		– Inactivates anaphylatoxin activity of C3a, C4a and 5a by Carboxypeptidase N removal of C-terminal Arg.
Integral Membrane Proteins				
Complement receptor type 1 CR1 (CD35)	SCR	C3b, C4b, iC3b	Classical, alternative and lectin	– Binds IC and promotes their dissolution and phagocytosis.

Contd.

Contd.

				– Accelerates dissolution of classical and alternative C3 convertase.
Membrane cofactor protein (CD46) (MCP)	SCR	C3b, C4b	Classical, alternative and Lectin	– Acts as a cofactor for factor I mediated cleavage of C3b and C5b.
Decay accelerating factor (CD55)	SCR, P1 anchor	C4b2b, C3bBb	Classical, alternative and lectin	– Accelerates dissolution of C3 convertases.
Homologous restriction fragment insertion (HRF20)/C8bp	P1 anchor	C8/C9	Terminal	– Inhibits lysis of bystander cell. – Prevents MAC insertion into lipid bilayer of autologous cells and lysis.
CD59 (membrane inhibitor of reactive lysis)	P1 anchor	C8	Terminal	– Blocks C7, C8 binding to C5b, 6 preventing MAC formation and lysis.

Membrane Bound Regulatory Proteins

Over the last few years, a series of membrane proteins that are capable of blocking the activation of complement at specific points in the pathway have been described. These proteins can effectively inhibit the assembly of functional complement C3 and C5 convertase and the MAC, thereby stopping the cascade. They include CR1, DAF (decay-accelerating factor, CD55) MCP (membrane cofactor protein, CD46), CD59 (MIRL, MACIF, HRF20, P18, Protectin), and HRF/C8bp (homologous restriction factor/C8-binding protein).

CR1: The CR1 protein, apart from being the receptor for C3b fragment has a regulatory role as well. CR1 was observed to increase the dissociation of both convertases, those in the fluid phase or associated with membranes. It has been shown that CR1 can significantly decrease the damage caused by ischaemic injury in liver and heart. Further, the role of CR1 in regulation of C5 convertases has also been proved.

Decay accelerating factor: Human DAF was shown to be an approximately 70-kD glycoprotein with a substantial amount of O-linked sugars. DAF acts by binding C3b or C4b on the cell membrane and markedly increasing the spontaneous decay of both the classical pathway C4b2a and alternative pathway C3bBb complexes. DAF is capable of controlling complement C3 deposition on cell membranes in which it is expressed but not on other cells. DAF is a widely distributed protein that has a glycophosphatidylinositol (GPI) anchor which allows soluble GPI containing forms of DAF to reincorporate into membranes and provide complement resistance. Soluble forms of DAF have been found in urine, tears, and most biologic fluids in which it has been sought.

Membrane cofactor protein: MCP, initially designated gp45-70, acts as a required cofactor for the cleavage of C3 or C4 into their hemolytically inactive forms, C3bi and C4bi. MCP, therefore, plays a similar biologic role as DAF, protection of cells from inadvertent complement deposition.

However, the specific enzymatic activity is different and results in an inactive form of the C3 protein, albeit now capable of binding to its receptors CR2, CR3 and CR4. MCP and DAF play cooperative roles in the inactivation of C3 and C5 convertases. Like DAF, recombinant MCP can protect cells from complement-mediated lysis.

CD59: CD59 is found on erythrocytes, monocytes, granulocytes, platelets, endothelial cells, and many cells of the nervous and reproductive tissues. A soluble form has also been found in urine, seminal plasma, serum and amniotic fluid. CD59 manifests both complement-related and complement-unrelated activities. With regard to complement regulation, CD59 is able to bind C8 in the C5b-8 complex and blocks the effective incorporation of C9. In addition, CD59 is capable of binding C9 already in the MAC and of blocking the subsequent polymerization of C9 and full formation of the transmembrane pore. Other studies have suggested that CD59 can regulate the alternative pathway C3 amplification pathway in addition to blocking the addition of C7 to C5b-6. Therefore, CD59 has a substantial role in control of the lytic formation of the MAC. Despite the sequence and functional similarity of the cytotoxic lymphocytes granule protein perforin with C9, CD59 cannot regulate perforin activities.

Homologous restriction factor: A second membrane protein that has the ability to regulate the assembly of C5b-9 has also been proposed. HRF has been described as a 65kD. GPI-anchored, widely distributed protein. A soluble form has also been identified in urine. The purified protein is reported to block C8 and C9 (but not C7) deposition into membranes, and antibodies to it increase the sensitivity of erythrocytes to reactive lysis substantially.

C3-membrane proteinases: Certain complement-resistant melanoma cell lines have been shown to express a protein, designated p57, with C3b cleaving and inactivating capabilities. This protein has been proposed to mediate complement resistance of these tumors. The molecular identity of this protein and others with this reported type of activity is not known, however.

Matrix Proteins that Regulate Complement Activation

Decorin: Some tissue sites with a preponderance of matrix proteins have also been shown to have a complement inhibitory protein. In the skin, bone, articular cartilage, cornea, and arterial wall adventitia, a dermatan sulphate proteoglycan, designated decorin is found. Purified decorin has been shown to bind Clq with a high affinity at physiologic ionic strength. Decorin can also inhibit complement activation in some types of assays, presumably by binding and altering the activity of Clq. Although other matrix proteins such as fibrinogen, fibrin, fibronectin and laminin have been shown to bind Clq, they have not been reported to block this activity. Therefore, like the fluid phase and cell membranes, complement inhibitors are also present in the matrix.

PATHOGENIC EFFECTS OF COMPLEMENT IN DISEASE

Complement is an important mediator of tissue injury in many diseases. The complement system plays an important role in the amplification of tissue injury following myocardial infarction and burns. The activation of complement by persisting IC which are not removed by the MPS is a second important mechanism by which complement contributes to the pathogenesis of disease. Circumstances where these mechanisms operates are:

1. Where the antigen is an autoantigen.
2. Where there is a continual release of antigen into the tissues or circulation; and
3. Where the antibody response may not efficiently clear the antigen, e.g., low-affinity antibodies.

A third mechanism whereby complement activation contributes to disease is in circumstances of massive systemic complement activation. In these circumstances there is substantial activation of C3 and C5, leading to production of large amounts of the anaphylatoxins.

The other mechanisms whereby complement promotes tissue damage includes:

i. Attraction and activation of inflammatory cells, including neutrophils and monocytes.
ii. Direct damage mediated by insertion of MAC into cell membranes; and
iii. Promotion of accelerated clearance of blood cells from the circulation by the MPS.

The system, which handles the antigen-antibody complexes may fail for various reasons. The most important of them are:

a. **A depletion or deficiency of complement:** A failure of the complement dependent handling of ICs is the most likely cause for IC load in complement deficiencies. Further, there are other specific properties of complement like the role of C3 in immunologic B-cell memory and the induction of immune response. Such immunoregulatory aspects may influence the characteristics of the antibody response that in turn affects the susceptibility to IC disease.

b. **Failure of the ICs to fix the complement:** Even in presence of a normal complement activity, there are instances of insoluble IC formation. Arthus reaction is one such circumstance where the precipitating ICs can induce an inflammatory reaction. In addition, the autoimmune disease like RA and SLE are associated with abnormal ICs. The IgG component in ICs in RA are unglycosylated which renders them incapable to bind to the Fc receptors and eventually their stagnation in the circulation. Another reason for persistence of abnormal complexes would be due to their inability to fix the complement component Clq, such is the case observed in IgA nephropathy where the IgA complexes are unable to fix C3. The third relevant finding is that reaction between circulating antibodies and cell surface antigens can result in IC formation as in Heymann's nephritis. The protective role of complement proves ineffective as it can block Fc-Fc interactions but has little ability to disrupt antigen-antibody interactions.

c. **A depletion, deficiency or blockade of the complement receptors by other ligands:** The CR1 number on the cells has a wide range and is determined by co-dominant alleles as observed by the RFLP of the CR1 gene earlier. In our earlier studies, we have proved a reduction of the E-CR1 in SLE and RA where the loss was attributed to have been acquired in course of the disease. This has been supported by the transfusion studies where the transfused erythrocytes rapidly lost CR1. This defect in CR1 number can also be extended to other cell types especially macrophages of the fixed macrophage system which are responsible for the handling of the ICs. A defect in macrophage CR1 has been reported in patients with biliary cirrhosis, SLE, podocytes in kidney biopsies of SLE and other forms of nephritis.

d. **Reduction of the access of immune complex bearing erythrocytes to the fixed macrophage system and an impairment in macrophage function due to disease:** Subsequent to the transport of ICs to the macrophages, there may be defects in the further processing of these complexes. Such impairment might include a diminished contact between IC bound to erythrocytes and the macrophages of liver and spleen, an alteration in the functional processing by macrophages etc. A reduced contact is possible during the cirrhosis of liver when the liver is bypassed and also during infectious and non-infectious states. Also the role of monocytes derived from blood in IC processing is not very well evident.

It is well understood that blood monocytes undergo a process of differentiation to macrophages on migrating to tissues where they assume functions specific to the tissue. They also undergo an additional maturation or activation under inflammatory conditions. The use of peripheral blood monocytes might prove useful in the context where the availability of tissue macrophages is not possible. The development of functional receptors both (Fc and CR) with the in vitro maturation of monocytes further supported the use of the cultured cells in lieu of tissue macrophages.

GENETIC COMPLEMENT DEFICIENCIES

Genetic complement deficiencies have been reported for each of complement components. Homozygous deficiencies of any of the early components of classical pathway (C1q,C1r, C1s, C4 and C2) exhibit similar symptoms, especially a marked increase in immune complex diseases viz. systemic lupus erythematosus, glomerulonephritis and vasculitis. These deficiencies illustrate the importance of early complement activation/reactions in generating C3b and the critical role of C3b in solubilization and clearance of immune complexes. Moreover, individuals with these complement deficiencies may suffer from recurrent infections by pyogenic (pus forming) bacteria viz. Streptococci and Staphylococci. These organisms are gram positive and hence resistant to lytic effect of membrane attack complex.

Deficiencies in Factor D and Properdin (early components of the alternative pathway) appear to be associated with Neisseria infections but not with immune complex disease.

Patients with C3 deficiencies have the most severe clinical manifestations, emphasizing the central role of C3 in activation of C5 and formation of the membrane attack complex. The majority of patients with C3 deficiency have recurrent bacterial infections and may also have immune complex diseases.

Homozygous deficiencies in the complement components involved in the membrane attack complex (MAC) lead to recurrent meningococcal and gonococcal infections caused by Neisseria species. MAC-deficient individuals normally do not have immune complex disease suggesting that they produce sufficient C3b to clear immune complexes.

Congenital deficiencies of complement regulatory proteins are also known. Deficiency of C1 inhibitor (C1 Inh) gives rise to a condition called hereditary angioedema, which manifests as localized edema of the tissue, which could be in subcutaneous tissue or in the upper respiratory tract or within the bowel. Deficiency of C1 Inh is an autosomal dominant condition with a frequency of 1 in 1000.

LEARNING OBJECTIVES AND SUMMARY

- The complement system comprises a group of approximately 30 serum proteins, several of which exists in inactive forms and forming one of the major defence system of the body.
- There are three pathways to complement activation; the classical, alternative and lectin pathways. Only the classical pathway is triggered by the specific immune response and the mannose binding ligand (MBL) pathway i.e. the lectin pathway and the alternative activation pathway are triggered directly by microbes and their products.
- The three pathways converge in a common sequence of events that leads to generation of a molecular complex (membrane attack complex; MAC) that causes cell lysis. Membrane attack complexes are regulated by proteins in serum and on host cell membrane.
- The classical pathway is initiated and activated by immune complexes wherein antibody binds to a cell target; reactions of IgM and certain IgG subclasses (IgG_1, IgG_2 and IgG_3) activate this pathway.
- Activation of the alternative and lectin pathways is antibody independent. These pathways are initiated by reaction of complement proteins with surface molecules of microorganisms.
- The activation pathways and amplification loop are tightly controlled.
- In addition to its key role in cell lysis, the complement system mediates opsonization of bacteria, activation of inflammation and clearance of immune complexes.

- C5a and C3a cause chemotaxis and mast cell activation. C3b acts as an opsonin. The activated state C3b lasts only a few milliseconds. Therefore C3b deposition will be confined to the immediate vicinity of the activation site. Bound C3b can act as a focus for further complement activation by the alternative pathway, and it can act as an opsonin, i.e., it facilitates binding to phagocytes.
- Interactions of complement proteins and protein fragments with receptors on cells of the immune system control both innate and acquired immune responses.
- Because of its ability to damage the host organism, the complement system requires complex passive and active regulatory mechanisms with involvement of complement receptors and break down products.
- Inherited complement deficiencies lead to clinical consequences ranging from increases in susceptibility to infections to tissue damage caused by immune complexes.

At this time you should know the following:

1. The detailed overview of complement system and its receptors.
2. How it is activated and regulated?
3. What are consequences of their activation?
4. How classical and alternative pathways are different?
5. What is lectin pathway?
6. What is the role of complement in pathophysiology of disease?
7. Different genetic disorders associated.

Further Reading

1. Complement System: Novel roles in health and disease. Edited by Janos Szebeni (2004), Kluwer Academic Publishers Drodrect, Netherlands.
2. Infection and Immunity, Ed. John Playfair and Gregory Bancroft, Third Edition, 2008, Oxford University Press, Oxford.
3. Complement System in the book, "Textbook of Biochemistry and Human Biology Ed. G P Talwar and LM Srivastava Printing 2010, Prentice-Hall of India Pvt. Ltd.
4. Kirsschfink M (1997), Controlling the Complement System in Inflammation; Immunopharmacology 38, 51-62.
5. Makrides SC (1998) Therapeutic inhibition of the Complement System; Pharmacol. Rev 50, 59.
6. Volanakis, JE (1995), Transcriptional regulation of Complement genes, Ann Rev. Immunol 13, 277-305.
7. Muller-Eberhard HJ (1988), Molecular Organization and Function of the Complement System; Ann Rev. Biochem 57, 321.
8. Raju KR, Sivasankar B, Anand, V, Luthra K, Tiwari, SC, Dinda AK, Das N and Srivastava, LM (2001) Use of Complement Receptor 1 (CD 35) assay in the diagnosis and prognosis of Immune Complex Mediated Glomerulopathies, Asian Pacific J. of Allergy and Immunology 19, 23-27.

4

CHAPTER

Antigen

(Dr. Seema Garg seegarg@yahoo.com)

OBJECTIVES

1. To understand the concept of immunogen, antigen, hapten and epitope.
2. To define the chemical nature of immunogens and factors influencing immunogenicity.
3. To compare the structures of T-independent and T-dependent antigens.
4. Molecular features of the antigens recognized by T-cells and B-cells.
5. To describe hapten-carrier conjugates.
6. To introduce the concepts of superantigens, PAMPs and PRRs.

INTRODUCTION

Substances that can be recognized by the T-cell receptors (along with MHC) and the B-cell receptors (Ig) are called the antigens. Nature/molecular configurations and properties of an antigen as well as the immune system of the host, both play an important role in eliciting an immune response. Both T- and B-lymphocytes recognize each antigen differently owing to the presence of different antigen recognition sites on each type of lymphocyte. These sites or receptors recognize the different molecular features of an antigen and a response is generated accordingly. Objective of the present chapter is to elaborate properties and features of antigens in details and the type of immune responses to different types of antigens.

Immunogens and Antigens

Immunogen is a substance which induces a detectable immune response (humoral or cellular). Immunogen stimulates the immune reaction resulting in either production of antibodies or activation of T-cells, finally leading to either the immune response or immune tolerance **(Figure 4.1)**.

Immunogenicity is the ability to induce humoral and/or cell mediated immune response.

Antigens are molecules that interact specifically with the products of immune response generated by an immunogen i.e. with antibodies, B-cell receptors (BCRs), and/or T-cell receptors (TCRs).

Antigenicity is the property that allows a substance to combine specifically with antibodies or TCR, whether or not they are immunogenic. An immunogen can trigger an immune response and acts as an antigen in that immune response. A complete antigen is able to induce antibody formation and produces a specific and observable reaction with the antibody so produced. Thus, all immunogens are antigens but vice versa is not true. Though the two terms are different, these are sometimes used interchangeably. Some small molecules called Haptens are antigenic but lack immunogenicity.

Hapten is a substance that is non-immunogenic but can react with the products

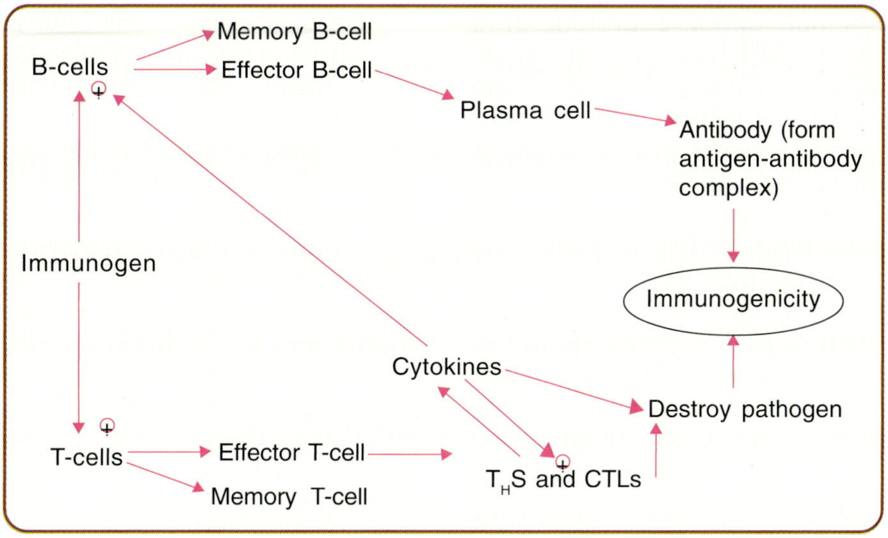

Fig. 4.1: Immune response

of a specific immune response. (The term hapten is derived from the Greek haptein which means 'to fasten'.) Haptens are small molecules which could never induce an immune response when administered by themselves but when coupled to a carrier molecule, they behave as complete antigens and are able to elicit an immune response. Free haptens, however, can react with products of the immune response after such products have been elicited. Small non-protein organic molecules, for example trinitrophenyl (TNP), benzene arsonate, mono- or disaccharides like glucose or lactose, oligopeptide like pentalysine, or even antibiotics like penicillin, can behave as haptens.

Haptens may be complex or simple; while complex haptens are the high molecular weight substances such as partial proteins or protein derivative, capsular polysaccharides (of type II pneumococci) and can precipitate with specific antibodies, simple haptens are of low molecular weights like drugs and are non-precipitating. Moreover, simple haptens can inhibit precipitation of specific antibodies by the corresponding antigens or complex haptens. Complex and simple haptens have been described as polyvalent and univalent respectively, since it is assumed that precipitation requires the antigen to have two or more antibody combining sites.

Immune response is a bodily response to an antigen that occurs when lymphocytes identify the antigenic molecule as foreign and induce the formation of antibodies and lymphocytes capable of reacting with it and rendering it harmless—also called immune reaction.

FACTORS INFLUENCING IMMUNOGENICITY

Several factors affect immunogenicity of a molecule and are categorized as those which are intrinsic to immunogen itself and those extrinsic to immunogen that are related to responder or the biological system.

A. Contribution of the Immunogen

1. **Chemical composition and complexity:** Immunogens can be proteins, polysaccharides, lipids or nucleic acids. While proteins are the most potent immunogens followed by polysaccharides; lipids and nucleic acids act as immunogens when combined with either a protein or a polysaccharide. Owing to their potency,

scientists use either a protein or a polysaccharide to induce the formation of antibodies experimentally. In general, more complex the substance is chemically, more immunogenic it will be. Thus, a homopolymer of an amino acid or a sugar is less immunogenic than a heteropolymer. Similarly, structural organization of molecule also determines its immunogenicity. All the four levels of structural organization of protein contribute to this property. The antigenic determinants are created by the primary sequence of residues in the polymer and/or by the secondary, tertiary or quaternary structure of the molecule.

Lipids typically behave as haptens but elicit immune response as a glycolipid or a lipoprotein. Examples of glycolipid antigens include major blood group antigens. Many antigens from *Mycobacterium* species are identified which are lipoprotein or glycolipids in nature. Tuberculosis Glycolipid Antigens (TBGLs) derived from the cell walls of *Mycobacterium* species is one such lipid which can generate anti-TBGL antibodies. Complete lipid antigens can induce both T-cell and B-cell response. For generation of an antibody by humoral response for commercial and experimental uses, lipids may be conjugated to proteins like Bovine Serum Albumin (BSA) to generate antibodies against lipids like steroids, fatty acid derivatives etc. Blood lipoproteins also act as immunogens and are used to generate monoclonal antibodies. These antibodies are commercially available for quantitative analysis of various lipoproteins and steroids etc.

For the T-cell response lipids must be recognized by T-cells. Lipid antigens are internalized, partially degraded and the fragments are expressed with CD1 molecules (resembling MHC), on the surface of APC.

Demonstration of anti-DNA antibodies in serum of patients suffering from SLE has evoked an interest in nucleic acid behaving as immunogen. The immunologic properties of bacterial DNA result from CpG motifs and may influence the human immune system in several settings. In normal immunity, bacterial DNA can nonspecifically stimulate the immune system by activating B-cell immunoglobulin secretion and cytokine production which activate macrophages and are mitogenic for B-cells **(Figure 4.2)**. Self DNA is differentiated from bacterial DNA since cytosine in bacterial CpG motif is non methylated.

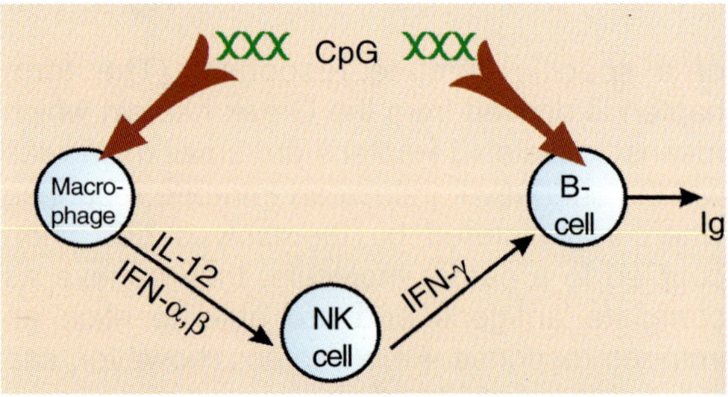

Fig. 4.2: Immune stimulation by DNA (Source: Adapted from Pisetsky D Annals of Internal Medicine 1997; 126: 169-171)

2. **Foreignness:** The immune system normally discriminates between self and non-self such that only foreign molecules are immunogenic. Tolerance to self antigen develops because lymphocytes are exposed to self components during the process of maturation. Loss of tolerance to self antigen can have pathogenic implications (autoimmune diseases). However, certain cells or tissues, from the same individual, when injected evoke an immune response (e.g. corneal and lens tissue, sperm). The reason lies in the fact that these tissues are sequestered away from the developing immune systems/cells.

The antigens to which the immature lymphocytes are not exposed will be recognized as foreign. More foreign the immunogen is (i.e. more the phylogenetic distance between the species), more pronounced the immune response will be. The antigens which are present in some members of a species are termed *Alloantigens or Isoantigens.* The ABO, and Rh blood factors in humans constitute important examples.

3. **Size:** There is not absolute size above which a substance will be immunogenic. However, in general, the larger the molecule the more immunogenic it is likely to be. This is so because larger molecules are more susceptible to phagocytosis. Compounds with high molecular mass (1,00,000 daltons) are highly active but those with low molecular mass (less than 5,000 daltons) show minimal immunogenicity.
4. **Physical form:** In general particulate antigens are more immunogenic than soluble ones because large insoluble molecules are more easily phagocytized. Antigens that are easily phagocytized are generally more immunogenic. This is because for most antigens (T-dependant antigens, see below) the development of an immune response requires that the antigen be phagocytized, processed and presented to helper T-cells by an antigen presenting cell (APC). Different APCs are listed in **Table 4.1**.
5. **Degradability:** Macromolecules that cannot be degraded and processed by APCs are poor immunogens. For example, polymers of D-amino acids are not immunogenic. Proteolytic enzymes can only degrade proteins containing L-amino acids. Once, an immunogen is degraded the peptides are presented on the surface of APCs along with the MHC molecule.

B. Contribution of the Biological System

1. **Genetic factors:** Some substances are immunogenic in one species but not in another. Similarly, some substances are immunogenic in one individual but not in others i.e. responders and non-responders. The species or individuals may possess or lack altered genes that code for the receptors for antigen on B-cells and T-cells or they may not have the MHC gene products needed for the APC to present antigen to the helper T-cells.
2. **Age:** Age can also influence immunogenicity. Usually the very young and the very old have a diminished ability to mount an immune response in response to an immunogen.

C. Method of Administration

1. **Dose:** The dose of administration of an immunogen can influence its immunogenicity. A dose of antigen below the optimal range fails to activate enough lymphocytes so that immune system is unresponsive. A very high dose can result in tolerance. Sometimes a single dose is not sufficient to induce an optimal response. In such cases repeated doses (*Boosters*) are required. A perfect example encountered in clinical practice is vaccination with DPT, hepatitis B etc.

Table 4.1: Antigen presenting cells

Common APC	Other APC	
Dendritic cells	Fibroblasts (skin)	Thymic epithelial cells
Macrophages	Glial cells (Brain)	Thyroid epithelial cells
B-cells	Pancreatic beta cells	Vascular endothelial cells

2. **Route:** In experimental animals an immunogen is usually administered parenterally i.e. intravenously, subcutaneously, intramuscularly, intraperitoneally though sometimes enteral route may also be used (oral polio drops which induces local immunity in human beings). The route of antigen administration can also alter the nature of the response. Generally, the subcutaneous route is better (the antigen first reaches to the local lymph nodes), than the intravenous (the antigen first reaches the spleen), or intramuscular routes.
3. **Adjuvants:** Substances that can enhance the immune response to an immunogen are called adjuvants. In contrast to carrier (used with haptens), adjuvants are not chemically bound to antigens and are not immunogenic. Increase in immune respose by an adjuvant is brought about by prolonging antigen exposure, co-stimulating signals, inducing granuloma formation and nonspecifically stimulating lymphocyte proliferation. The use of adjuvants, however, is often hampered by undesirable side effects such as fever and inflammation. Commonly used adjuvants include salts like alum (aluminum potassium sulfate), and water in oil adjuvants like Freund's incomplete adjuvant and Freund's complete adjuvant.

   Alum causes precipitation of antigen which after injection is released slowly: thus increasing the time of exposure to antigen. In addition precipitate is more readily phagocytized.

   Freund's adjuvant, being an emulsion disperses antigen in small oil droplets which cause slow release of antigen.

   Both adjuvants result in formation of local granuloma which contains activated macrophages resulting in activation of T_H cells also.

EPITOPE

Immune cells do not interact with, or recognize an entire immunogen molecules; instead, lymphocytes recognize discrete sites on the macromolecule called *epitopes*, or *antigenic determinants*. Thus, epitope is the smallest portion of antigenicity which is immunologically active. An epitope physically interacts with a *paratope* (corresponding binding sites) present on secreted antibody or a specific receptor on lymphocytes.The residues which come in contact with paratope are called *contact residues*. Antigens such as bacteria or viruses carry many different types of epitopes, presenting an antigenic mosaic. The presence of the same or similar epitopes on different antigens results in antigenic cross reaction.

Structural Organization of Epitopes

The term epitope was coined by Neils Jerne in 1960, when he proposed that an antigen particle carries several epitopes. Each epitope possesses a specific chemical structure, electrical charge and steric (spatial) configuration. In polysaccharide antigens, short oligosaccharide chain (approx. 1-5 sugar long) at the non-reducing end of polymer or various branched chains constitute an epitope and the rest of the molecule behave as a carrier molecule just as with hapten. Moreover, branched points provide attachment to many antigenic determinants. Structure of epitope of carbohydrate antigen depends on the sequence of carbohydrate and their linkage, rather than their conformation. Epitopes on protein antigens are constituted by primary, secondary, tertiary, and even quaternary structures. A protein may contain many epitopes, however only a few are antigenic in a given species or in a member of a given species. Furthermore, some epitopes may induce stronger immune response than the others and are called *immunodominant*. Protein epitopes consist of 6-8 amino acid residues and are classified as:

1. *Sequential or linear epitope:* A single linear segment of the primary sequence containing 6-8 amino acids (**Figure 4.3A**).

2. *Conformational epitope:* Several discreet amino acid sequences widely separated in the primary structure come together on surface when the protein folds to form native structure (**Figure 4.3B**).

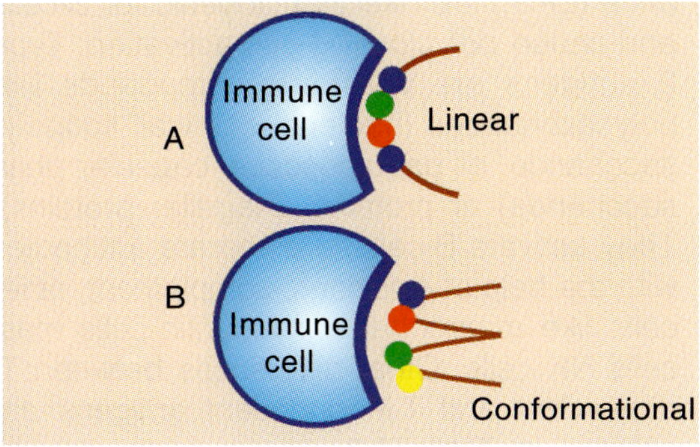

Fig. 4.3: Structure of sequential and conformational epitopes

Whale sperm myoglobin has 5 distinct sequential epitopes shown in **Figure 4.4**. This protein also contains non-sequential or conformational epitopes.

Difference between the two types of epitopes is that while sequential epitope retains its antigenicity, conformational epitope loses its antigenic property after the protein is destroyed by fragmentation or denaturation. A good example of non-sequential epitope is hens' egg white lysozyme in which a loop created by disulfide bridge between cysteine residues at positions 60 and 83 acts as a major antigenic determinant. Opening up of the loop by cleavage of this –S-S- bond results in destruction of antigenic properties.

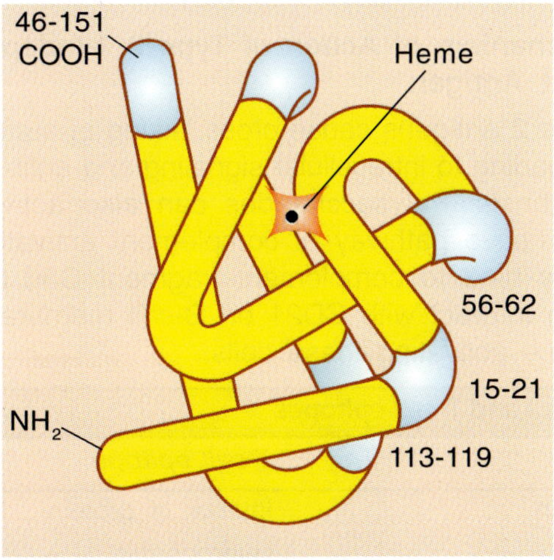

Fig. 4.4: Sperm whale myoglobin showing 5 distinct sequential epitopes
(Source: Adapted from MZ Atassi and AL Kazim, Adv. Exp. Med. Biol 1978; 98:9)

An important factor that may play role in immunogenicity of protein epitopes is their mobility. It has been seen experimentally that more mobile segments are likely to be present on surface and show better binding with antibodies, may be because both the epitope and paratope adopt more complementary confirmation by a two way induced fit. This result applies to short peptide sequential antigenic determinants. However, antibodies to longer peptides bind to less mobile regions of the proteins.

T- and B-lymphocytes recognize different epitopes from same or distinct antigens in different manner.

Properties of B-cell and T-cell Epitopes

Membrane bound antibodies on B-cells recognize soluble antigens and hence the epitopes must be easily accessible sites. The most accessible residues are the ones which are present on the surface and, therefore, amino acids constituting these epitopes are hydrophilic in nature. Often the epitopes are found where the molecule bends or where there is a high degree of segmental mobility [atomic mobility]. B-cell epitope may be either sequential or non-sequential.

In contrast, antigens recognized by T-cells are first processed to small peptides containing epitope. These epitopes are expressed on surface of APC in association with MHC molecules, and then presented to T-cells. The epitope, therefore, is present in the interior of the protein (may be called cryptotope) and consist of hydrophobic amino acid residues. Only oligomeric peptides serve as T-cell epitopes. Epitopes which bind to Class I MHC have an optimal size range of 8-11 amino acids. Epitopes which bind to Class II MHC have an optimal size range from 12-25 amino acids. T-cell epitopes must have two binding regions; one for TCR and the other region which binds to MHC (termed the agretope). Differences between B-cell and T-cell epitopes are listed in **Table 4.2**.

Types of Antigens

Depending on the nature of antigen, B-cell activation occurs by two modes: one dependent upon T_H cells and the other independent of the T_H cells. Thus, antigens can be divided in two classes:

1. Thymus dependent (T dependent).
2. Thymus independent (T independent).

1. T-dependent antigens: Most natural protein are T dependent antigens and B-cells can not respond to these antigens without co-stimulatory signal from T_H cells. Structurally, these antigens are characterized by a few copies of many different antigenic determinants.

These antigens bind to the surface Ig on B-cells and are internalized and processed to smaller peptides, which are then expressed on the surface of B-cell complexed with MHCII and are presented to T-cells. Once these complexes are recognized by T_H cells, they secrete cytokines and start expressing CD40 ligand which interacts with CD40 on B-cells. This T-B interaction and cytokines provide stimulus for B-cell activation.

2. T-independent antigens: T-independent antigens are antigens which can directly stimulate the B-cells to produce antibody without the requirement for T-cell help. These antigens react with B-cell receptors of innate immunity. Most microbial sugars, lipids and certain nucleic acid are T-independent antigens. These are of two types of which type 1 antigens [endotoxin, lipopolysaccharide (LPS)] are directly mitogenic for B-cells and cause *polyclonal* B-cell activation. Type 2 antigens are polymeric compounds like polysaccharides (bacterial cell wall lipopolysaccharide, or pneumococcal capsular polysaccharide) or proteins (Flagellar proteins). They activate B-cells to elaborate antibodies with the help of cytokines, complement, other cells like macrophages, dendritic cells mast cells NK cells. Other differences between T-dependent and T-independent antigens are enlisted in **Table 4.3**.

Mechanism of Action of Type 1 T-independent Antigen

These antigens, like LPS after being transferred by LPS binding protein (LPB) to CD14 are incorporated into cell membrane and interact with protein kinases and cause polyclonal activation of these cells in high concentration. At low concentration LPS stimulates production of antibodies specific for LPS.

Mechanism of Action of Type 2 T-independent Antigen

Type 2 antigens cause cross linking of surface Ig leading to intracellular signaling and antibody synthesis. Polysaccharides can also activate alternative pathway of complement activation. They bind to complement fragment C3d and then interact with CD21 on B-cell membrane, hence activating these cells.

Table 4.2: Comparison of B-cell and T-cell epitopes

Characteristics	*B-cell epitope*	*T-cell epitope*
Site on antigen	Surface of protein	Interior of protein
Nature of amino acids	Hydrophilic	Hydrophobic
No. of aminoacids	6-8	8-15
Type of epitope	Sequential or conformational	Sequential only

Table 4.3: Comparison between T-dependent and T-independent antigens

S. No.	*Property*	*T-dependent*	*T-independent*
1.	Involvement of T-cell	Involved	Not involved
2.	Interaction with antigen	Involves tertiary complex of T-cell receptor, Ag, MHC molecule	Involves binary complex of membrane Ig and Ag
3.	Binding of soluble antigen	No	Yes
4.	Processing by macrophase	Required	Not required
5.	Involvement of MHC molecule	Required to display processed antigen	Not required
6.	Chemical nature of antigen	Mostly proteins but some lipids and glycolipids presented on MHC- like molecule	Type 1 are LPS, Type 2 are polymeric proteins and Polysaccharide
7.	Properties	Repetition of different determinants	Repetition of same determinants
8.	Degradability	Easily degradable	Type 2 have poor degradability
9.	Complement activation	No	Type 2 antigen cause complement activation
10.	B-cell mitogenesis	No	Type 1 is direct mitogen
11.	Generation of memory cells	Yes	No
12.	Polyclonal activation	No	Type 1 antigen cause polyclonal activation in high doses
13.	Effect on antibody production	Full range; IgM, IgG, IgA, IgE	Limited to IgM, IgG3
14.	Immunological memory	Produced	Not produced

HAPTEN-CARRIER CONJUGATES

Hapten-carrier conjugates are immunogenic molecules to which haptens have been covalently attached. The immunogenic molecule is called the carrier. A commonly used carrier is Bovine Serum Albumin (BSA).

Structure: Structurally these conjugates are characterized by having native antigenic determinants of the carrier as well as new determinants created by the hapten (haptenic determinants). Thus, an animal immunized with a hapten carrier conjugate develops three types of antibodies as shown in **Figure 4.5**. In such conjugates the hapten is the immuno-dominant epitope and thus the major fraction of antibodies formed are against the hapten. In such conjugates the type of carrier determines whether the response will be T-independent or T-dependent.

Biomedical importance of such conjugates is that these conjugates can be used to produce hapten specific antibodies. These antibodies are useful for measuring presence of various substances in the body. For example anti HCG antibodies are generated and are used for determination of the pregnancy. However, some drugs like penicillin, sulfonamides, aspirin etc. which are low molecular weight compound can not induce immune response but act as haptens in our body and form conjugates with proteins to produce drug allergies.

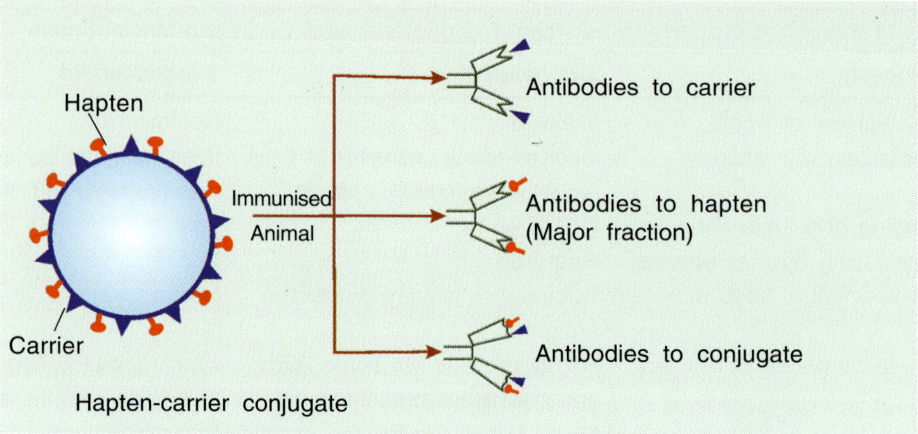

Fig. 4.5: Immune response of hapten carrier conjugate
(Source: Adapted from *Goldsby* RA, Kindt TJ, Osborne BA, Kuby J 2002, In *Immunology, 5th edition,* Kuby J ed., WH Freeman and Company, New York

SUPERANTIGENS

When the immune system encounters a conventional T-dependent antigen, only a small fraction (1 in 10^4-10^5) of the T-cell population is able to recognize the antigen and become activated (monoclonal/oligoclonal response). However, there are some antigens which polyclonally activate a large fraction of the T-cells (upto 25%). These antigens are called superantigens. Microbial superantigens are medium size proteins (Molecular weight 22-29 kDa) characterized by high resistance to proteases and to denaturation by heat. Superantigens are potent activators of $CD4^+$ T-cells and result in release of cytokines (IL-2) which causes massive proliferation of T-lymphocytes. This ultimately leads to further release of variety of cytokines which can have profound effects on the immune system, both acute and long-term. Acute effects include food poisoning and toxic shock syndrome. Long-term effects include autoimmune diseases and immunodeficiency. A number of pathogenic bacteria and viruses have been shown to produce superantigenic proteins which have been implicated in a wide array of human disorders **(Table 4.4)**.

Table 4.4: Human diseases associated with bacterial and viral superantigens

Organism	*Superantigen*	*Disease*
Bacterial		
Staphylococcus aureus	Enterotoxins	Food poisoning
	Toxic shock toxin	Toxic shock syndrome
	Staphylococcal exfoliating toxin	Scalded skin syndrome
Group A streptococci	Pyrogenic exotoxins	Shock
		Rheumatic heart disease
Mycobacterium tuberculosis	Not identified	Tuberculosis
Viral		
HIV	Nef	AIDS
Rabies virus	Nucleocapsid protein	Rabies
Epstein-Barr virus	Not identified	B-cell lymphoma

Examples of superantigens include: Staphylococcal enterotoxins (food poisoning), Staphylococcal toxic shock toxin (toxic shock syndrome), Staphylococcal exfoliating toxins (scalded skin syndrome) and Streptococcal pyrogenic exotoxins (shock). Although the bacterial superantigens are the best studied there are other superantigens associated with viruses and other microorganisms as well.

Superantigens differ from conventional antigens in several ways. Conventional antigens are taken up or are endogenously produced by antigen-presenting cells and are processed into discrete peptides, which are then presented to antigen-specific T-cells *in the antigen-binding groove* of either MHC class I or class II molecules on the surface of the antigen-presenting cell. Superantigens, on the other hand, function as intact molecules and bind outside the antibody binding groove. They bind directly to MHC class II molecules on the surface of antigen-presenting cells and Vβ chain of TCRs **(Figure 4.6)**. Recently, superantigens have been shown to bind to class I MHC antigens also.

The diseases associated with exposure to superantigens are, in part, due to hyper activation of the immune system and subsequent release of biologically active cytokines by activated T-cells. There is excessive uncoordinated release of cytokines, (especially TNF-α), which overloads the body and results in rashes, fever, and can lead to multi-organ failure, coma and death. Superantigens also induce anergy of the T-cells to antigens by undetermined mechanism. A potential benefit from studying these proteins would be to harness their T-cell proliferating abilities by using them to direct T-cells against tumors expressing specific MHC class II antigens. Furthermore, their ability to downregulate the immune response following acute exposure (resulting in anergy and/or deletion of T-cells) could be exploited to eliminate populations of T-cells involved in autoimmune diseases.

Determinants Recognized by the Innate Immune System

Determinants recognized by components of the innate (non-specific) immune system differ from those recognized by the adaptive (specific) immune system. The receptors of adaptive immune system recognize discrete determinants and demonstrate a high degree of specificity, enabling this system to recognize and react to a particular pathogen. In contrast, components of the innate immune system recognize molecular patterns which are shared by many

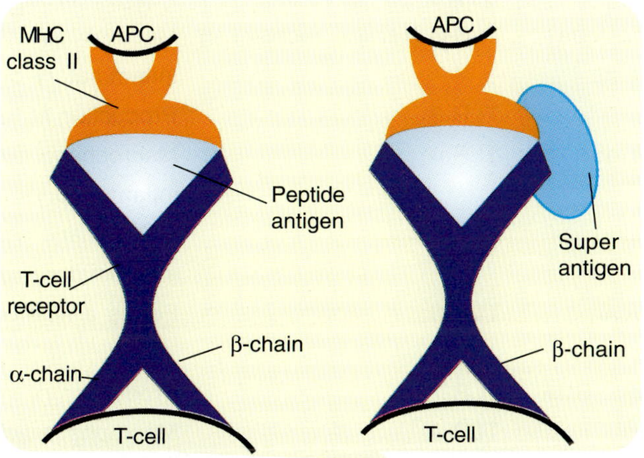

Fig 4.6: Interaction of conventional antigens and superantigens with MHC class II and T-cell receptors (Source: Adapted from Torres BA, Kominsky S, Perrin GQ, Hobeika AC, Johnson HM, Experimental Biology and Medicine 2001, 226: 164-176)

related pathogens but not shared with their host. Thus, they lack a high degree of specificity seen in the adaptive immune system. The broad molecular patterns recognized by the innate immune system have been called PAMPS (pathogen associated molecular patterns) and the receptors for PAMPS are called PRRs (pattern recognition receptors). A particular PRR can recognize a molecular pattern that may be present on a number of different pathogens enabling the receptor to recognize a variety of different pathogens. These receptors also recognize certain endogenous stress signals called DAMPs (danger-associated molecular patterns) like heat-shock proteins and altered membrane phospholipids. Examples of some PAMPs and PRRs are illustrated in **Table 4.5**.

These PRRs are divided into two groups:

1. **Secreted molecules** that circulate in blood and lymph.
2. **Surface receptors** on phagocytic cells like macrophages that bind the pathogen for engulfment.

1. Secreted PRRs

C-reactive protein(CRP), peptidoglycan recognition proteins (PGRs) and mannan-binding lectin (MBL) are all secreted proteins. These circulating proteins bind to the surface of many pathogens leading to activation and fixation of complement resulting in opsonization of the pathogen and its speedy phagocytosis.

2. Membrane associated receptors

These PRRs are divided into 3 classes:

- Toll like receptors (TLRs).
- Scavenger receptors.
- Mannose receptors.

Table 4.5: Important PAMPs and PRRs and their biological actions

PAMP	*PRR*	*Biological consequence of interaction*
Microbial cell wall components	Complement	Opsonization, Complement activation
Mannose-containing carbohydrates	Mannose-binding protein	Opsonization, Complement activation
Polyanions	Scavenger receptors	Phagocytosis
Lipoproteins of Gram$^+$ bacteria Yeast cell wall components	TLR-2 (Toll-like receptor 2)	Macrophage activation, Secretion of inflammatory cytokines
Double stranded RNA	TLR-3	Production of interferon (antiviral)
LPS (lipopolysaccharide of Gram$^-$ bacteria)	TLR-4	Macrophage activation, Secretion of inflammatory cytokines
Flagellin (bacterial flagella)	TLR-5	Macrophage activation, Secretion of inflammatory cytokines
Responds to peptidoglycan and certain lipoproteins	TLR-6	Forms a heterodimer with TLR-2
U-rich single stranded viral RNA	TLR-7	Production of interferon (antiviral)
CpG containing DNA	TLR-9	Macrophage activation, Secretion of inflammatory cytokines

Toll like receptors are transmembrane receptors present on cells like macrophages, and dendritic cells. There are 12 different TLRs that recognize pathogens and enhances phagocytosis. Further, an effector response is initiated leading to activation of NF-κB which turns on many cytokine genes such as those for tumor necrosis factor-alpha (TNF-α);Interleukin-1 (IL-1); and chemokines, which attract white blood cells to the site leading to inflammation at the site.

Scavenger receptors include CD-36, CD-68, and SRB-1.These can bind to bacterial cell wall components such as LPS, peptidoglyans as well as, infected, injured or apoptotic cells and modified lipoproteins.

Mannose receptors on the surface of phagocytes bind mannose-rich glycans, the short carbohydrate chains with the sugar mannose or fucose as the terminal sugar that are commonly found in microbial glycoproteins and glycolipids but are rare in those of humans. Human glycoproteins and glycolipids typically have terminal N-acetylglucosamine and sialic acid groups and thus can be differentiated from microbial components.

At this time you should know the following:

1. How an immunogen is different from an antigen?
2. What are haptens and hapten carrier conjugates and their importance?
3. Factors which affect immunogenicity.
4. Structural and functional properties of T-and B-cell epitopes.
5. What are T-dependent and T-independent antigens?
6. How superantigens are different from other antigens?
7. What are PAMP and PRRs?

Further Reading

1. Goldsby RA, Kindt TJ, Osborne BA, Kuby J 2002. In *Immunology, 5th edition,* Kuby J ed., WH Freeman and Company, New York.
2. Torres BA, Kominsky S, Perrin GQ, Hobeika AC, Johnson HM *Experimental Biology and Medicine* 2001, 226: 164-176.
3. Berzofsky JA and Berkower, 1999, Immunogenicity and antigen structure. In *Fundamental Immunology*, 4th ed., WE Paul, ed., Lippincott-Raven, Philadelphia.

5

CHAPTER

Immunoglobulins: Structure and Functions

(Dr. Alpana Sharma dralpanasharma@gmail.com)

OBJECTIVES

1. To understand the detailed structures of Immunoglobulins.
2. To know the different classes and sub-classes of antibodies and their properties.
3. To explain the various effector functions mediated by different classes of antibodies.

INTRODUCTION

Four peaks (albumin α, β and γ globulin) are seen when plasma or serum glycoproteins are separated by electrophoresis (migration in an electric field) **(Figure 5.1)**. Most of the antibodies are found in gamma globulin fraction, referring to the immunity, hence named immunoglobulin (Ig). Therefore antibody and immunoglobulins are interchangeable terms.

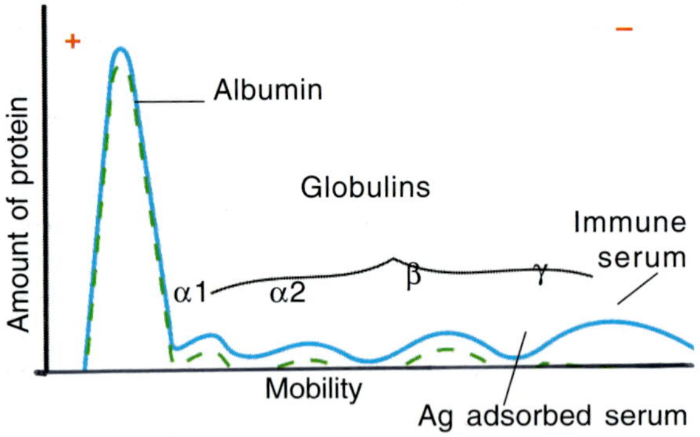

Fig. 5.1: Electrophoretic pattern of serum glycoproteins showing different peaks. Most of the antibodies are in the γ-globulin fraction of serum proteins. Blue line shows the electrophoresis pattern of untreated serum. Green dashed line shows the pattern of serum which was incubated with antigen to remove antibody

Antibodies are glycoprotein molecule that recognize a particular epitope on an antigen and binds specifically to it and finally facilitates the clearance of that antigen. They are present on the B-cell membrane and secreted by plasma cells. Secreted antibodies circulate in the blood where they eliminate/neutralize the antigen by their effector functions such as phagocytosis, antibody dependent cell-mediated cytotoxicity (ADCC) and opsonization etc. The antibodies have unique structural features and motifs and bind to antigen to destroy it effectively.

Antibody Structure

Antibody or immunoglobulins are glycoprotein molecules consisting of 4 polypeptide chains.

- 2 identical heavy (large) chains (H) - molecular weight > 50 kDa.
- 2 identical light (small) chains (L) - molecular weight >25 kDa.

There are two types of light chains kappa (κ) and lambda (λ).

In humans 60% of L chains are kappa and 40% are lambda. Each light chain is bound to a heavy chain by both interchain and intrachain disulphide bonds **(Figure. 5.2)**.

The heavy chains are of 5 types called alpha (α), gamma (γ), delta (δ), epsilon (ε) and mu (μ).

The amino terminal region of light and heavy chain varies greatly in different antibodies. First 110 amino acids from N terminal are quiet variable in amino acid sequence called variable region (v).

V_L – variable light chain

V_H – variable heavy chain

The sequence beyond variable region in all antibodies is relatively constant throughout rest of the molecule and called C- region.

C_L – constant light chain

C_H – constant heavy chain

The carbohydrate moieties are linked to constant region of H–chains.

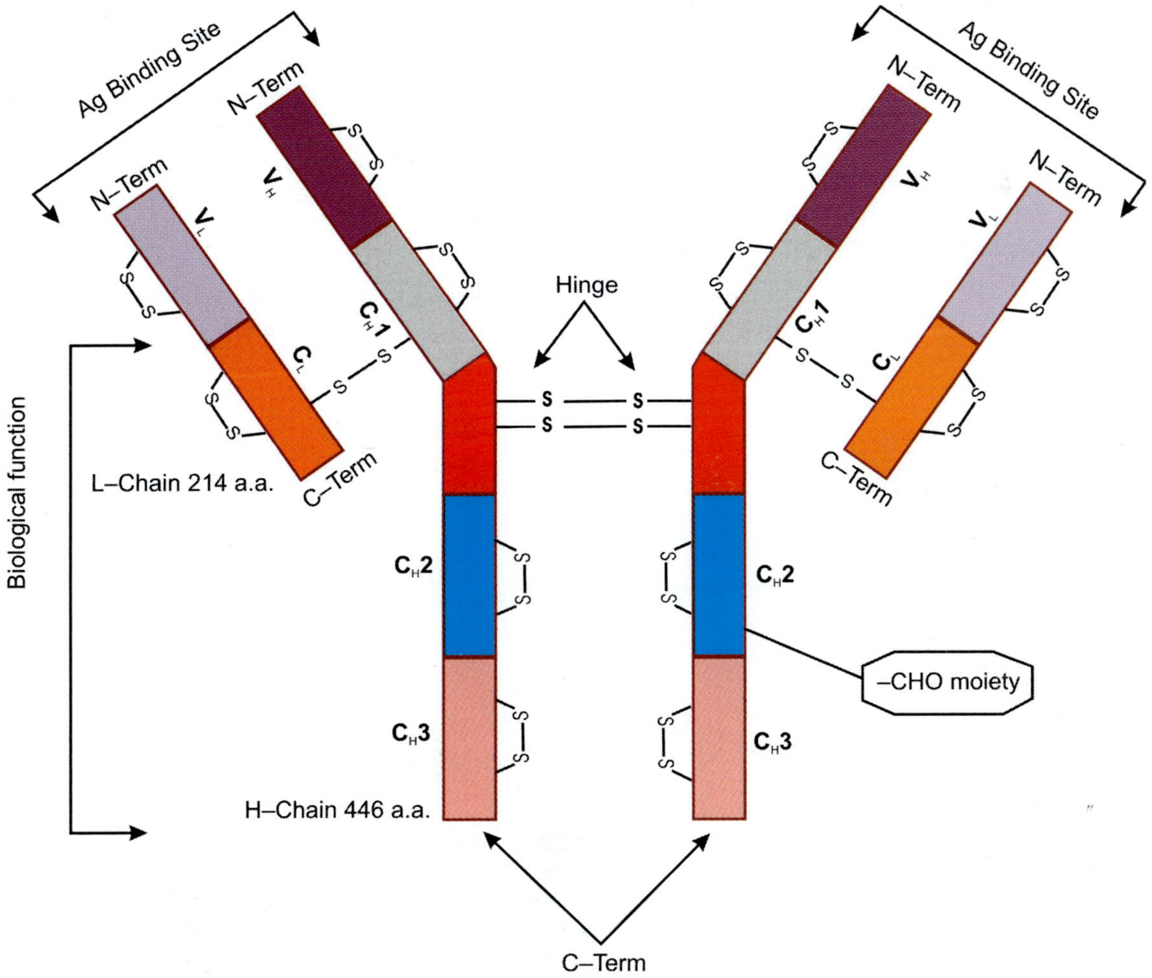

Fig. 5.2: Schematic diagram of immunoglobulin structure illustrating the four chain composition of antibody and various domains comprising each chain

The amino terminal variable region of both light and heavy chains participates in antigen recognition and carboxyl terminal constant region of heavy chains mediate effector functions. The C-region of light chains does not attach to cell membrane and does not participate in its functions.

Enzyme digestion studies reveal some basic antibody structure. A brief digestion of IgG with enzyme papain produced three fragments. Two identical fragments of molecular weight of 45 kDa had antigen binding activity called Fab fragment. The other fragment of 55kDa was crystallizable during cold storage called as Fc fragment.

$$IgG \xrightarrow{\text{Papain}} 2\ Fab + Fc$$

Pepsin digestion generates a single 100 kDa fragment composed of two Fab like fragment $F(ab)_2$ which binds with antigen **(Figure 5.3)**.

$$IgG \xrightarrow{\text{Pepsin}} F(ab)_2 + Fc$$

FINE STRUCTURES OF IMMUNOGLOBULIN

Structure of Ig determined by its primary, secondary, tertiary and quaternary protein structure.

Primary St → Amino acid sequence accounts for variable and constant regions of H and L chains.

Secondary St → Extended polypeptide chain folds back and forth upon itself forming an antiparallel beta pleated sheet.

Tertiary St → Chains are folded into 3° structures of compact globular domains connected to neighboring domains by narrow more exposed areas.

Quaternary St → Finally, globular domains of adjacent H and L chains

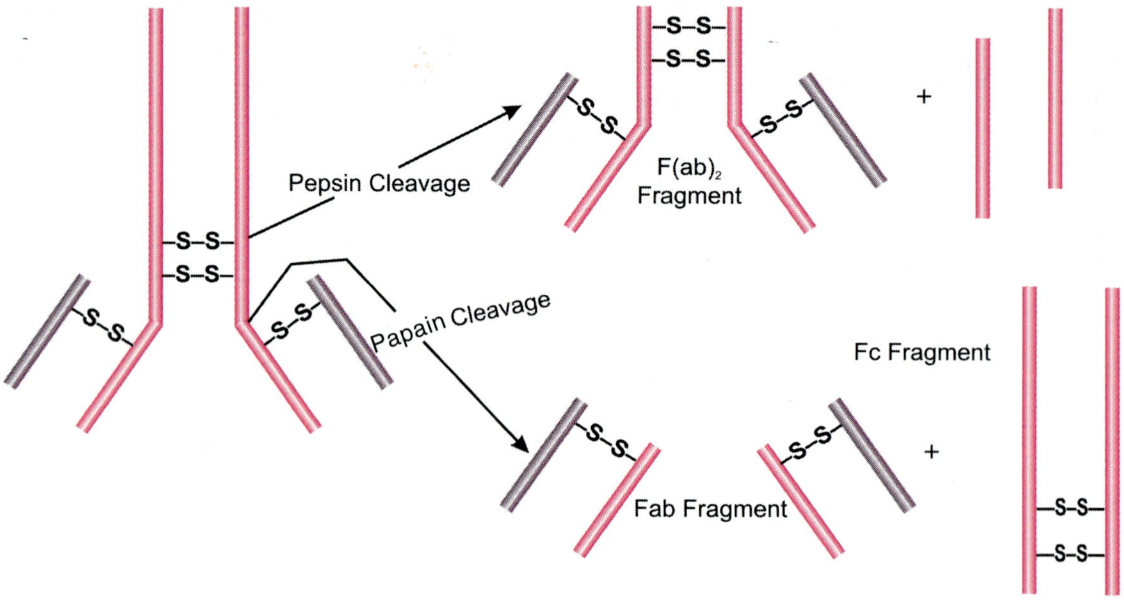

Fig. 5.3: Enzyme digestion of immunoglobulin

interact and form functional domains ⟶ enable the molecule to specifically bind antigen and perform biological effector functions.

Immunoglobulin Domains

Both L and H chains contain several homologous units of about 110 a. a. residues within each unit, an intrachain disulphide bond forms a loop of 60 a. a. called domain **(Figures 5.4 and 5.5).**

L–chain ⟶ 1 variable domain V_L
1 constant domain C_L

H–chain ⟶ 1 variable domain V_H
3 or 4 constant domain depending on the Ig class C_H1, C_H2, C_H3, C_H4.

X-ray crystallographic analysis revealed that Ig domains are folded into a characteristic compact structure known as immunoglobulin fold. Structure of Ig domain is a sandwich of two β-antiparallel pleated sheets stabilized by hydrophobic interactions between them and by disulfide bonds. β-strand with a sheet is stabilized by hydrogen bonds that connect the $-NH_2$ group in one strand with a -COOH group in an adjacent strand and characterized by alternating hydrophobic and hydrophilic amino acids. Variable and constant domains have similar structure except some subtle differences e.g. V-domain slightly longer than C-domain contains an extra pair of β-strands and extra loop sequence connecting this pair of β-strand.

The quaternary structure of immunoglobulin is facilitated by non-covalent interactions between domains across the faces of the β-strand.

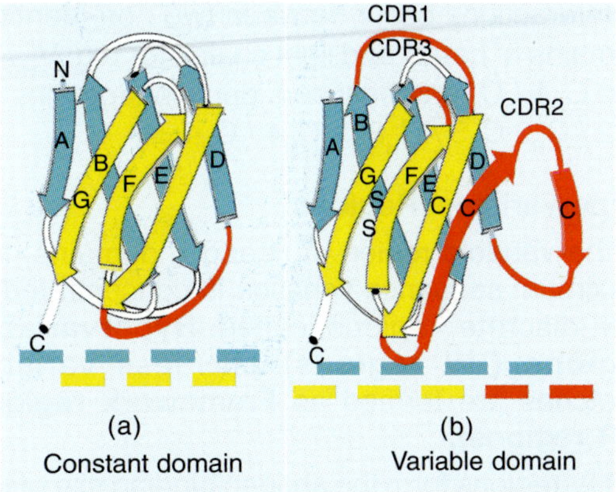

Fig. 5.4: Schematic representation of human immunoglobulin light chain depicting the immunoglobulin-fold structure of its variable and constant domains. Each domain is composed of two antiparallel arrays of β-strands represented by flat arrows, coloured blue and yellow respectively to form two β-pleated sheets, which are held together by hydrophobic interactions and a disulphide bond. The hypervariable regions or CDRs (complementarity-determining regions) in variable domain are shown in red colour

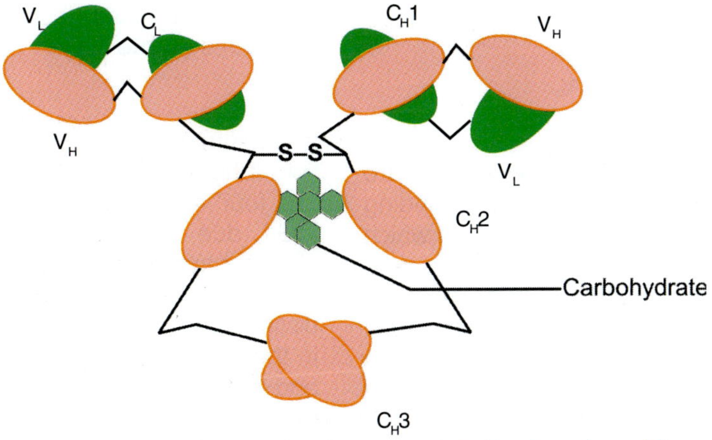

Fig. 5.5: Schematic diagram showing interacting immunoglobulin domains of heavy and light chains

Interactions occur between two non-identical domains of heavy and light chains for e.g. V_H / V_L and C_H1 / C_L and between identical domains as C_H2 / C_H2 C_H3 / C_H3 or C_H4 / C_H4.

Hypervariable Regions

In the variable region of H and L domains, the maximum sequence variation is concentrated in few discrete regions called **Hypervariable regions (HV regions)** and less variable stretches are termed as **Framework regions (FR regions).**

HV regions form the antigen binding site of the antibody molecule and is complementary to the structure of epitope, these HV areas are called **complementarity determining regions (CDRs).**

Each Fab fragment has 6 CDRs (3 in H and 3 in L chain). The wide range of specificity exhibited by antibodies is a function of variations in the length and amino acid composition of 6 CDRs. The framework region acts as a scaffold support to 6 CDR loops in each Fab fragment.

Crystallographic studies suggest that out of 6 CDRs, mainly 4 CDRs make contact with antigen's epitope. In general more residues in H chain CDRs appear to contact with antigen than L-chain CDRs. Average contributions to the overall building interactions are as follows:

H–chain CDR 3	:	29%
H–chain CDR 2	:	23%
L–chain CDR 3	:	21%
H–chain CDR 1	:	10%
L–chain CDR 1	:	9%
L–chain CDR 2	:	4%
Framework regions	:	4%

CDR1 and CDR2 of L and H chains are positioned at the ends of the antigen binding site whereas CDR3 in the central position which has majority of contact with Ag epitope and most variable amongst all. Thus variability in HV regions with significant conformational changes in the loops upon Ag binding enables a given antibody to assume a shape more effectively complementary to that of their epitopes.

Constant Region Domains

C-region domains are associated with various biological functions and determined by amino acid sequence of each domain.

The presence of C_H1 and C_L domains appears to increase the number of stable V_H and V_L interactions that are possible, thus contributing to the overall diversity of antibody molecule.

Hinge Region

An extended amino acid sequence between C_H1 and C_H2 domains is called hinge region. It is rich in proline and cysteine amino acids and is more flexible. Proline residues provide an extended conformation, more susceptible for proteolytic cleavages and cysteine residues form interchain disulfide bonds and holds the two heavy chains together.

The γ, δ and α heavy chains have hinge regions but μ and ε chains lack it, thereby have an additional domain of 110 a. a. (C_H2/C_H2) having hinge like features.

Classes and Subclasses of Antibody

Antibody molecules can be divided into distinct classes and sub classes on the basis of difference in the structure of their heavy chain constant regions. There are five classes of antibody also called isotypes and are named IgG, IgA, IgM, IgD, and IgE.

Each class can also exist in two types with the presence of either kappa or lambda light chains. Each class has different functions and properties (**Table 5.1**).

IgG

It constitutes about 80% of total Ig in circulation. It has longest half life of 23-25 days. There are four sub classes. IgG1, IgG2, IgG3 and IgG4, due to presence of $\gamma1$, $\gamma2$, $\gamma3$ or $\gamma4$ H-chains having subtle differences in sequence of their constant regions. The subclasses are distinguished in characteristics from one another in the size of the hinge region and the number and position of the interchain disulfide bonds between the heavy chains.

Table 5.1: Properties and functions of different classes and subclasses of antibodies

Antibody class	IgG				IgA		IgM*	IgE	IgD
Subclasses / **Property/Activity**	IgG1	IgG2	IgG3	IgG4	IgA1	IgA2			
Heavy chain	γ1	γ2	γ3	γ4	α1	α2	μ	ε	δ
Molecular weight (kDa)	150	150	150	150	150-600	150-600	900	190	150
Serum conc.(mg/ml)	9	3	1	0.5	3	0.5	1.5	0.0003	0.03
Half life (days)	23	23	8	23	6	6	5	2.5	3
Complement activation	+	+/-	++	-	-	-	+++	-	-
Crossing of placenta	+	+/-	+	+	-	-	-	-	-
Membrane-bound Ab (on B-cell)	-	-	-	-	-	-	+	-	+
F_c Receptor binding	++	+/-	++	+	-	-	?	-	-
Induction of mast cell	-	-	-	-	-	-	-	+	-

*IgM pentameric (secreted) and monomer form is membrane bound.

tion. It has longest half life of 23-25 days. There are four sub classes. IgG1, IgG2, IgG3 and IgG4, due to presence of γ1, γ2, γ3 or γ4 H-chains having subtle differences in sequence of their constant regions. The subclasses are distinguished in characteristics from one another in the size of the hinge region and the number and position of the interchain disulfide bonds between the heavy chains.

It provides immunity to newborn because it can readily cross placenta and enter into neonatal circulation. It is potent activator of complement system. Out of all subclasses IgG3 is most efficient. It plays major role in neutralization of toxins because it can easily diffuse into extravascular spaces. IgG3 enhances the phagocytosis of antigen bound to it.

IgA

It constitutes 10-15% of total Ig in serum. Its

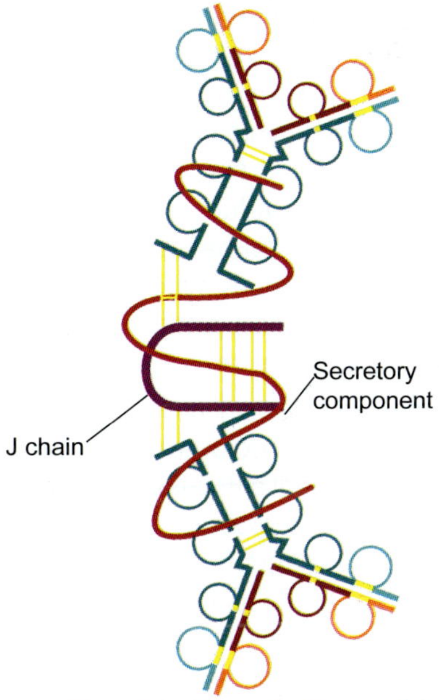

Fig. 5.6: Dimeric form of IgA

present on the serosal surfaces of the epithelial cells. It helps in trapping the pathogen in the lumen by preventing their attachment to the epithelial cell wall. This is done by cross-linking the multivalent antigen with polymeric IgA, and finally the pathogen is eliminated. Secretory IgA provides an important defense mechanism against bacteria such as salmonella, vibrio cholera and viruses such as polio and influenza etc. Breast milk rich in IgA concentration helps to protect the newborn against infection during first month of life.

IgM

It constitutes 8-10% of all immunoglobulins in serum (average serum concentration 1.5 mg/ml). It is the first antibody produced following antigen exposure hence called primary response antibody. IgM is present in both monomeric and pentameric form. The monomeric form is present as membrane bound antibody on B-cell. The pentameric form is secreted by plasma cells. The five monomeric sub units are arranged with their F_C regions in the center of the pentamer and ten antigen binding sites on the periphery of the IgM pentamer molecule. The IgM also has an additional F_C linked polypeptide called J (Joining chain) chain bonded by disulfide linkage to C-terminal cysteine residue of two of the ten μ chains added first before secretions of the pentamer. By virtue of its 10 antigen building sites, serum IgM has a higher valency and efficiency than other isotypes. It possesses greater avidity in binding antigens and many repeating epitopes **(Figure 5.7)**.

IgM activates complement more efficiently than IgG by providing two F_C regions in close proximity required for complement activation. IgM pentamer is also known as macroglobulin with a molecular weight of 900kDa and high sedimentation coefficient (19S). Due to its large size, IgM does not diffuse well and present in very low concentration in extracellular tissue fluids.

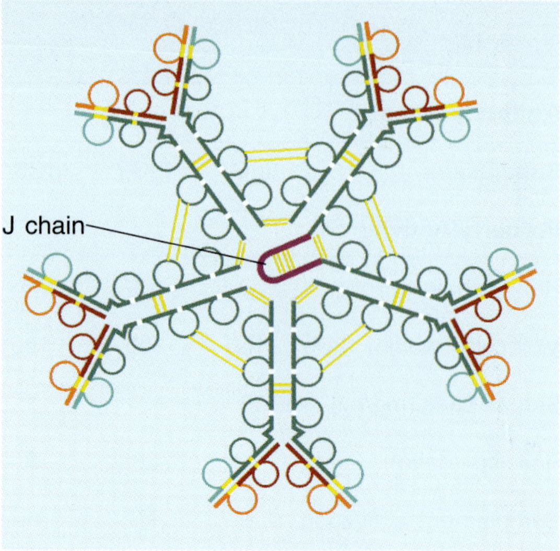

Fig. 5.7: Pentameric form of IgM

IgD

It constitute about 0.2% of total Ig in serum. It is found on mature β-cells together with IgM as major membrane bound immunoglobulin. Its functions are still unknown.

IgE

It is present in extremely low concentration (0.3 μg/ml) but it mediates the important biological function. Immediate hypersensitivity reactions e.g. asthma, hives and anaphylactic shock are mediated by IgE. It is bound to F_C receptors on the basophils and tissue mast cells. Allergen and bound IgE molecule crosslink and induce basophils and mast cells to translocate their granules to plasma membrane and activate degranulation. This leads to release of the pharmacologically active substances like histamine and bradykinin etc.

Antibody-Mediated Functions

An antibody performs mainly two important functions:

1. It recognizes and binds with antigen at its antigen binding sites in variable region.

2. It involves the immune responses by its binding with other cells, tissues or proteins through its F_C region (constant region of heavy chains) and performs the effector functions to eliminate the antigen/pathogen.

The effector functions and functional properties are not same for all classes of immunoglobulins, since, the interactions between heavy chain constant region and serum proteins or cell membrane receptors invoke these responses antibody isotypes differ in these F_C regions.

The major effector functions mediated by antibodies are as follows:

I. Complement activation.
II. Opsonization.
III. Antibody dependent cell-mediated cytotoxicity (ADCC).

Some more functions are based on Ig class:

I. Mucosal immunity.
II. Neonatal immunity.
III. IgE mediated hypersensitivity.

I. Complement Activation

The F_C dependent effector mechanism of humoral immunity is the activation of the classical pathway of the complement system (collection of serum glycoprotein that can perforate cell membrane). Many immunoglobulins and their subclasses activate the complement pathway. IgM and IgG3 are the main antibodies, which activate the complement through the receptors present on their F_C region. The system generates inflammatory mediators and promotes microbial phagocytosis and lysis. It is initiated by the binding of a complement protein called C1q to the F_C portions of antigen complexed IgG or IgM. The $F_C\gamma$ receptor and complement binding sites of antibodies are found within the heavy chain constant domains of the different isotypes **(Figure 5.8)**.

II. Opsonization

The vital effector function of humoral immunity is opsonization. It promotes phagocytosis of antigens by macrophages and neutrophils. All cells (macrophages and neutrophils) have surface receptors for F_C region of Ig molecule that specifically bind antibody coated (opsonized) particles. The process of coating particles for phagocytosis is called opsonization and substances that perform this function including Ig and complement proteins are called specific 'Opsonins' **(Figure 5.9)**.

F_C receptors for different Ig heavy chain isotypes are expressed on different cell types (leukocytes population) and perform diverse functions with variable affinity. The F_C receptor for IgG antibodies is called $F_C\gamma R$.

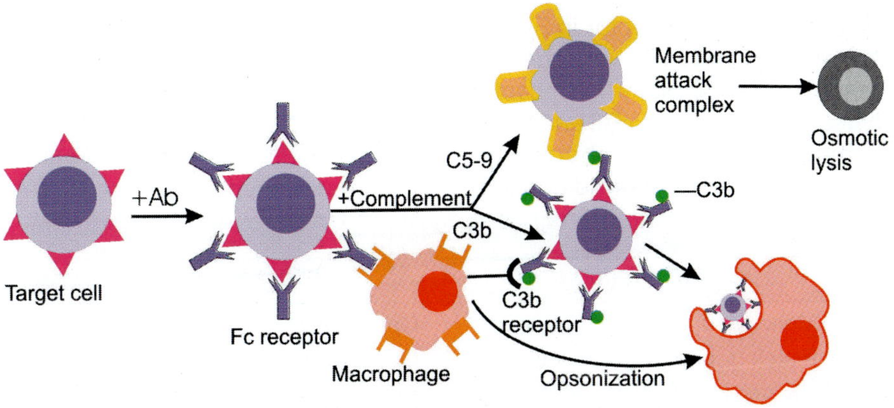

Fig. 5.8: Complement activation by binding of antibodies to the Fc receptors which subsequently leads to phagocytosis or lysis of the target cell

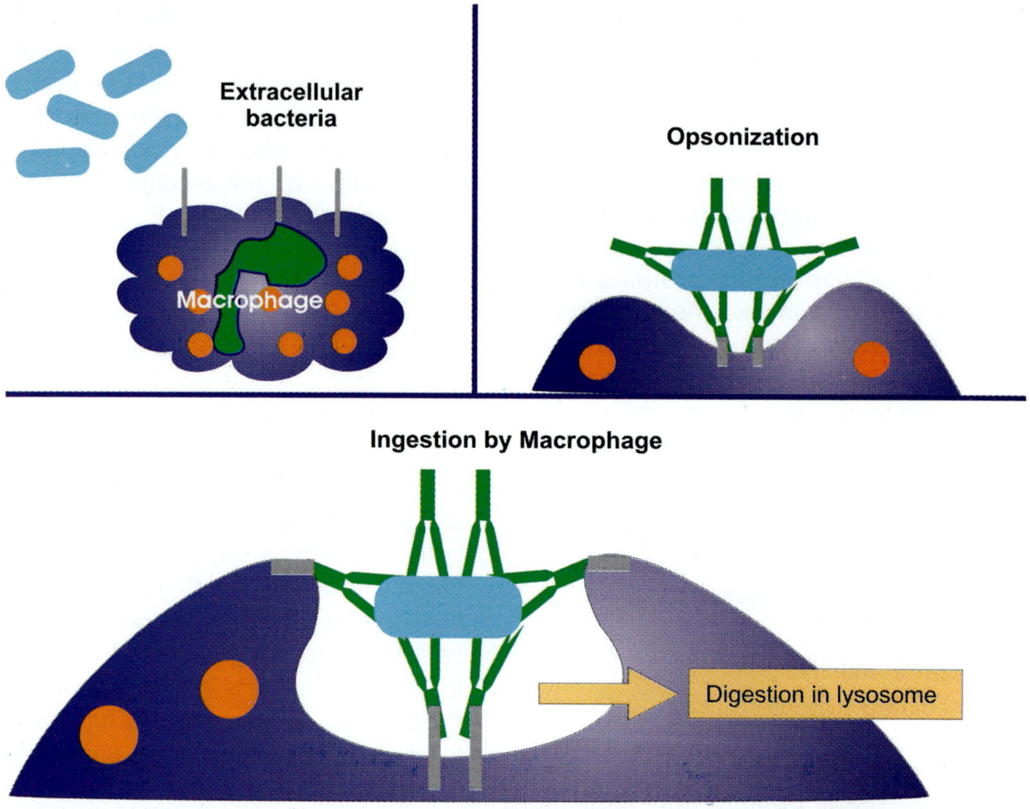

Fig. 5.9: Opsonization. Coating of antibodies on bacterial cell renders it recognizable as foreign by phagocytes such as macrophages and neutrophils which then ingests it and destroy it (Source: http://pathmicro.med.sc.edu/bowers/immune%20cells.htm)

There are 3 types of $F_C\gamma R$ receptors having different affinities for IgG subclasses and expressed on different cell types (**Table 5.2**). Of these, the major high affinity phagocyte receptor is $F_C\gamma R1$, which binds human IgG1 and IgG3 very strongly and activates phagocytosis. Similarly Fcε-receptor also has two types of $F_C\varepsilon R1$ and $F_C\varepsilon RII$ and binds with variable affinity. Inside the phagocyte, pathogen is targeted by enzymatic digestion, oxidative damage and finally killed and eliminated. Then antibody which functions as opsonin enhances phagocytosis manifold for particulate antigens.

III. Antibody Dependent Cell-mediated Cytotoxicity (ADCC)

Many cells have cytotoxic potential and express membrane receptors for the F_C region. Natural

Table 5.2: Features of types/subtypes of F_C receptors

Type	*Tissue distribution*	*Function*	*Binding affinity*
$F_C\gamma R$ I	Monocytes and macrophages	Opsonization	High
$F_C\gamma R$ II	Platelets and B-lymphocytes	Opsonization	Low
$F_C\gamma R$ III	NK cells and phagocytes	ADCC	Low
FcεR I	Basophils and mast cells	Immediate hypersensitivity	High
FcεR II	Granulocytes	ADCC, hypersensitivity	Low

killer (NK) cells and other leukocytes bind to antibody coated cell by F_C receptors and destroy/lyse these cells. This process is called ADCC and was first described as a function of NK cells, which use $F_C\gamma R$ III receptors. A low affinity receptor $F_C\gamma R$ III binds clustered IgG molecules displayed on cell surfaces and does not bind circulating monomeric IgG. Therefore, ADCC occurs only when the target cell is coated with antibody molecule which ultimately activates the NK cells to secrete cytotoxic substances like interferon-γ (IFN-γ) and tumor necrosis factor (TNF), which mediate the lysis and killing of this cell type.

The effector mechanism against some helminthic parasite is a special type of ADCC killing. They can be killed by a basic protein present in the granules of eosinophils involving IgE antibodies. Eosinophils are activated by $F_C\varepsilon RI$ – induced signals and destroy the target cell/parasite by releasing its cytotoxic granular contents **(Figure 5.10)**.

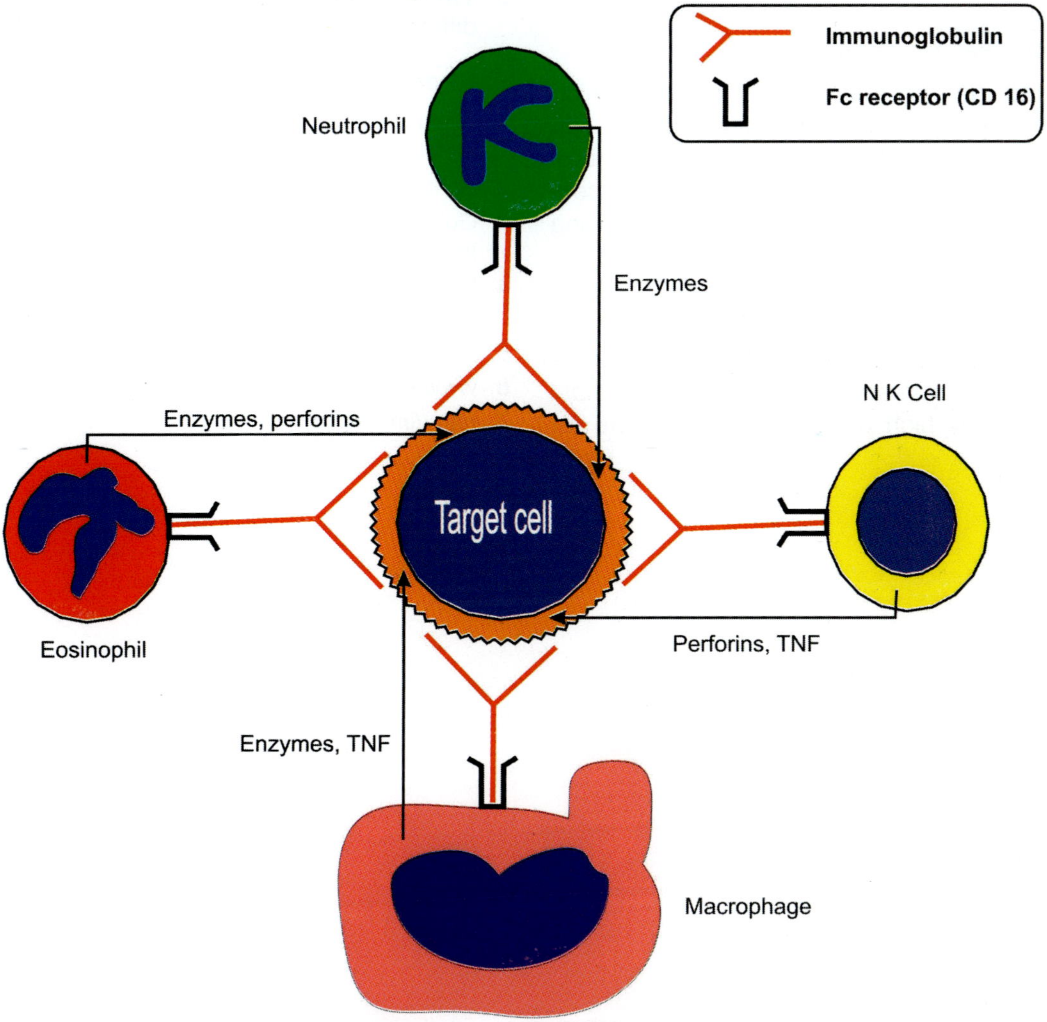

Fig. 5.10: Antibody dependent cell-mediated cytotoxicity. Antibody coated target cells can be killed by NK cells. The process involves the release of cytoplasmic granules containing perforins and enzymes from NK cells

IV. Mucosal Immunity

IgA class predominant in body secretions and is transported across the mucosal surfaces by poly Ig mediated mechanism. It helps in trapping the pathogen in the lumen by preventing their attachment to the epithelial cell wall. The antibody protects the mucosal surfaces by cross-linking the multivalent antigen with polymeric IgA. It supports in neutralization of toxins etc and also initiates ADCC through $F_C\alpha$-receptor.

V. Neonatal Immunity

IgG and IgA are the antibody classes which protect the neonates from infection. IgG can cross the placenta therefore it provides protection immediately after birth. IgA is present in mother's milk, which further helps in providing immunity to newborn in early days.

VI. IgE Mediated Hypersensitivity

IgE antibodies mediate the immediate hypersensitivity reactions. Basophils and mast cells express high affinity $F_C\varepsilon RI$ receptors for IgE. Antigen stimulation leads to cross-linking between bound IgE molecule and F_C receptors and activates basophils and mast cells. These cells induce degranulation and causing release of active substances like histamine and bradykinin etc. that mediate allergic manifestations.

At this time you should know the following:

1. Details of the structure of immunoglobulin.
2. Different classes and subclasses of antibodies, their structure and properties.
3. Various effector functions mediated by different classes of antibodies.

Further Reading

1. Abbas KA and Lichtman HA. Cellular and molecular immunology, fifth edition
2. Roitt I. Essential Immunology, ninth edition.
3. Goldsby AR, Kindt JT, Osborne AB and Kuby J. Immunology, Sixth edition.
4. Murphy K, Travers P and Walport M Janeway's Immunobiology, seventh edition.
5. www.nature.com
6. www.theimmunology.com
7. http://imgt.cines.fr/

6

CHAPTER

Immunoglobulins: Iso-, Allo- and Idiotypes

(Dr. Rashid Ali, Dr. Hasan Kammal and Dr. Rekha Gupta raliamu@yahoo.com)

OBJECTIVES

1. To clearly differentiate between, iso-, allo- and idiotypes and to know how antibodies against these variants are generated.
2. To explain how nine kinds of Igs are found in the sera of all normal individuals?
3. How isotypes are regulated by T-cells?
4. The location of these variants on Ig molecule.
5. To distinguish between private, public, shared, site related and cross reacting idiotopes.
6. Regulatory roles of anti-idiotypic antibodies in immune response.
7. To understand idiotypic specific suppression, regulation by T-helper cells, network theory of immune regulation.
8. Role of idiotopes in autoimmunity.

INTRODUCTION

The antibody molecule is made up of two identical heavy and two identical light chains held together by inter-chain disulfide bonds (**Figure 6.1**). In the human, there are five major types of heavy chains giving five classes of immunoglobulins. These are IgG, IgM, IgE, IgA and IgD. The most abundant Ig in the extra-vascular fluids is IgG. IgA exists mainly as a monomer (basic four-peptide unit) in plasma, however in the seromucous secretions is present as a dimer, linked by a secretory J chain. This antibody is concerned in the defense of external body structures. IgM is basically a pentameric molecule and because of high valency, is a powerful first-line defense against micro-organisms. IgD is largely present on the lymphocyte and probably functions as an antigen receptor. IgE binds firmly to mast cells and its contact with antigens leads to local recruitment of antimicrobial agents. The antibody is also of importance in certain parasitic infections.

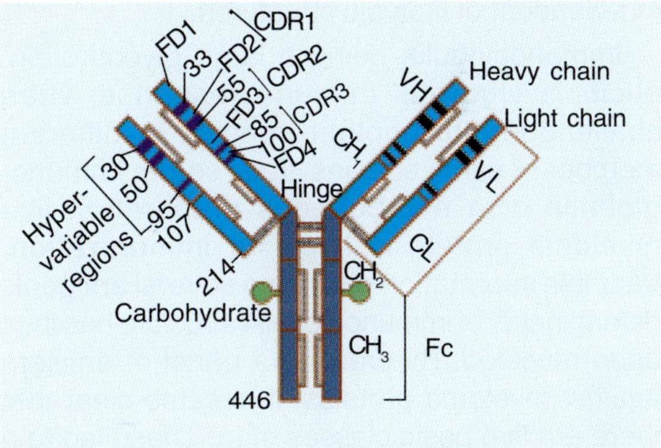

Fig. 6.1: Structure of immunoglobulin showing hypervariable, constant and Fc regions

ISOTYPES

The various classes of immunoglobulins may be differentiated by their amino acid sequence as well as their antigenicity. Antibodies raised in rabbit against human myeloma IgG (homogeneous) if absorbed by mixtures of myelomas of other classes to remove cross reacting antibodies, will recognize IgG and not IgM, IgA, IgE or IgD. All the heavy chain constant region (C_H) structures which give rise to classes and subclasses are expressed together in the serum of a normal subject; they are termed as isotypic variants (**Table 6.1**).

Similarly light chain constant regions (C_L) exist in isotypic form known as κ or λ but never mixed. Thus IgG exist as IgGκ or IgGλ; IgM as IgMκ or IgMλ and so on. It is possible to generate antibodies that recognize isotypic variants. Specific anti-serum can also be raised for individual antibody molecules. These antibodies discriminate between one monoclonal antibody and another, independent of isotypic structures.

Immunoglobulin being a large glycoprotein, elicits a vigorous immune response when challenged into another species or different member of same species. Total serum immunoglobulin or a homogenous preparation like myeloma protein is used for immunization. Valuable information regarding several antigenic determinants of immunoglobulin structure has thus been revealed. By creating a panel of antisera against myeloma proteins, it became clear that there are five basic classes of Ig. These led to a number of subclasses giving nine kinds of immunoglobulins. These nine kinds of immunoglobulins are found in the sera of all normal individuals, thus the term isotype (iso=equal) is used to describe them.

The five isotypes represent the five heavy chain classes. The reactivities that can be split further are the λ and α subclasses. Heterologous anti-isotype sera raised in rabbits against human myeloma protein recognize the epitopes unique to human isotypes. The antisera do not cross react with all human isotypes because of common epitopes between rabbit and human immunoglobulin. Similarly, light chain components can also be identified with anti-isotypic reagents and appropriate sera.

Therefore, reagents can be generated to distinguish between the light chain types and subtypes as well as heavy chain classes and subclasses. Extensive studies of the human myeloma proteins and rabbit immunoglobulin revealed determinants similar to isotype on some individuals and not all members of a species.

Upon antigenic stimulation, B-cell proliferates and differentiates into antibody forming cells (plasma cells) under the influence of T-cells. During this process, B-cell progenies switch from producing one Ig class to another. This phenomenon is called "class switch" or "isotype switch". The process of class switch is essential for the generation of functional diversity like interaction with mast cell or basophils, binding of complements etc. of antibodies of a given specificity. Administration of anti-IgM antibodies during early development in chicks and mice prevent the appearance of not only IgM but all isotypes of Ig, demonstrating that B-cells producing IgG, IgE or IgA isotype have progenitors that first express IgM. The isotype switch is caused by genetic recombination.

Isotype Regulation by T-Cells

The importance of T-cells and their soluble products in regulating isotypes during antigenic stimulation has been well established. Different T-cell subsets induce preferentially IgG or IgE antibody response and distinct T-cell-derived

Table 6.1: Isotypic variation of immunoglobin molecule

Type of variation	*Distribution*	*Variant*	*Location*	*Examples*
ISOTYPIC	All variation present in serum of a normal individual	Classes	C_H	IgM, IgE
		Subclauses	C_H	IgA_1, IgA_2
		Types	C_L	κ, λ
		Subgroup	C_L	λO^{z+}, λO^{z-}
		Subgroup	V_H/V_L	V^{KI} V^{KII} V^{KIII} V^{HI} V^{HII} V^{HIII}

soluble factors may regulate IgE and IgG response. A similar isotype specific regulation by T-cells has also been reported in IgA response. T-cells actually induce class switch in B-cells.

It has been established that T-cells or their products influence isotype expression in the antibody response either by stimulating B-cells that have already undergone the class switch or by actually inducing class switch. Both IL-4, IL-5, B-cell growth and differentiation factors, were also found to influence isotype expression. The following points are in relation to isotype regulation by T-cells.

1. IL-5 acts on LPS-stimulated murine splenic B-cells inducing a three to six fold increase in IgA production without any effect on the biosynthesis of IgG subclasses or IgM.
2. IL-4 induces not only IgG_1 but also IgE production in LPS-stimulated B-cells, whereas it suppresses IgM, IgG_3, IgG_{2a}, and IgG_{2b}. IL-4 has been found to act *in vivo.*
3. IFN-γ was found to induce IgG_{2a} production but inhibits the expression of IgG_3, IgG_1, IgG_{2b}, and IgE in LPS-stimulated murine splenic B-cells.

These results indicate that IL-4 and IFN-γ act as reciprocal regulatory elements in the expression of Ig isotype. These T-cell-derived regulatory factors, were reported to be generated by different T-cell subsets. Type I helper T-cell (T_H1) produces IL-2 and IFN-λ, while type II helper T-cells (T_H2) produces IL-4 and IL-5.

Therefore, antigenic stimulation leading to the activation of T_H1 cells results in the preferential synthesis of IgG_{2a}, whereas the stimulation of T_H2 cells results in the production of IgG_1, IgE and IgA (**Figure 6.2**).

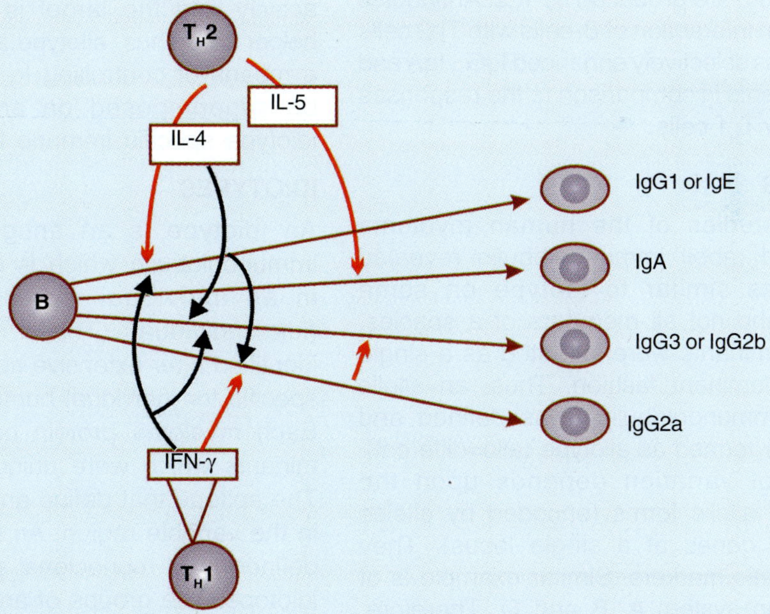

Fig. 6.2: Isotype regulation of T-cells. Red arrow indicates positive effects and Black arrow indicates negative effects on each isotype production, respectively
(Source: Fundamental Immunology, second edition, 1989 (Ed. W. Paul), Raven Press, New York, Page 405)

Isotype Regulation by T-Helper Cells

Some of the lymphokines produced by T-helper cells are known to have selective activities on the induction of specific classes or subclasses of Ig response. It might, therefore, be expected that those T-helper cells (T_H1 versus T_H2) which produce certain of these lymphokines, might preferentially induce responses of certain Ig isotypes. These are as follows:

1. IL-4 selectively promotes IgG_1 responses in anti-μ-activated B-cells and enhances the IgG_1 and IgE responses while inhibiting the IgG_{2a}, IgG_{2b}, IgG_3 and IgM responses induced by LPS.
2. IL-5 has been shown to preferentially enhance IgA polyclonal B-cell response to LPS.
3. IFN-λ has been reported to enhance IgG_{2a} and to decrease IgG_{2b}, IgG_1 and IgG_3 responses to LPS.

IL-4 and IL-5 are produced by T_H2. Antibodies resulting from interaction of B-cells with Th2 cells would express selectively enhanced IgG_1, IgA and IgE components in comparison to the responses supported by T_H1 cells.

ALLOTYPES

Extensive studies of the human myeloma proteins and rabbit immunoglobulin revealed determinants similar to isotype on some individuals and not all members of a species. These determinants were inherited as a single autosomal dominant fashion. Thus, an allelic marker of immunoglobulins was defined and subsequently termed as allotype (allo=different). This type of variation depends upon the existence of allelic forms (encoded by alleles or alternate genes at a single locus). They provide genetic markers. Similar example is of blood antigen system A, B and O. Therefore, Ig heavy chain differs in the expression of their allotypic group. Typical allotypes are the G_m specificities of IgG (G_m=marker of IgG). Allotypes are more restricted than isotypes. Several allotype determinants have been resolved to the level of polymorphic amino acid interchanges that define them. In **Table 6.2**, the position and identity of the amino acids involved in the allotypic determinants have been indicated. As stated earlier, an allotype is a determinant found in several, but not every members of a species.

The genetic recombination events that lead to the construction of an active H or L chain gene occur only on one of the two allelic chromosomes. Thus, most B-cells and antibody secreting cells produce L and H chains of only one of the two alternative allotypic forms that are specified by their allelic genes. The phenomenon is known as allelic exclusion.

Allotype Specific Suppression

In utero exposure of certain strains of mice to anti-allotypic antibody leads to a specific suppression of that allotype after birth. This is the result of allotype specific T suppressor cell activity and the target is allotype specific T-helper cell. Thus, allotype and isotype represent a means of controlling Ig production and may be superimposed on antigen specific and idiotype specific immune regulation.

IDIOTYPES

An idiotype is an antigenic marker of an immunoglobulin which is generally found only in an individual member of the species (idio=individual). These markers have been identified after extensive absorptions of antisera specific for individual human myeloma protein. Each myeloma protein bore antigenic determinants which were unique to that myeloma. The epitope that define an idiotype are located in the variable region. An idiotypic determinant defined by a monoclonal antibody is called an idiotope. The groups of antibodies produced in response to an antigen have a common feature of recognizing the eliciting antigen. An antiserum against this original antiserum will therefore primarily recognize the variable regions of these expanded, antigen-reactive clones. This anti-

Table 6.2: List of human allotypes

	Type	Class	Allotype	Alphameric	Numeric	Position(s)	Amino acid(s)
Light chains	Kappa		Km1			153, 191	val, leu
			Km2			153, 191	ala, leu
			Km3			153, 191	ala, val
Heavy chains		IgG1	G1m	a	1	356, 358	asp, leu
				f	3	214, 219	arg, ser
				x	2	431	gly
		IgG2	G2m	n	13		
		IgG3	G3m	b0	11		
				b1	5	296, 436	phe, phe
				b3	13		
				b4	14		
				b5	10	419, 422	gln, ile
				c3	6		
				c5	24		
				g	21	291, 296	leu, tyr
				g5	28	419, 422	glu, ile
				s	15		
				t	16		
				u	26		
				v	27	422	ile
		IgA2	A2m	1			
				2		411, 428	tyr, glu
		IgE	Em	1		458, 467	ile, ala

Where it is known, the position of the amino acids involved in the allotypic determinants have been indicated.

(Source: Fundamental Immunology, second edition, 1989 (Ed. W. Paul), Raven Press, New York, P-230)

idiotypic antiserum can be thought of as the "fingerprint" of an individual's immune response to a given antigen.

Conventionally, the antibodies are distinguished by the antigens with which they bind. Another way of distinguishing antibodies serologically involves an analysis of their idiotypes. An idiotype is the collection of antigenic determinants on an antibody, usually associated with the hypervariable regions, recognized by other antigen-specific receptors either antibody (the anti-idiotype) or T-cell receptors.

It is possible to generate antibodies that recognize isotypic and allotypic variants. Specific anti-serum can also be raised for individual antibody molecules. These antibodies discriminate between one monoclonal antibody and another, independent of isotypic or allotypic structures. Such anti-sera define the individual determinant characteristic of each antibody, collectively termed as idiotypes (**Figure 6.3**).

Depending on the manner of preparation, anti-idiotypes may be polyclonal that is directed at a group of idiotopes, or monoclonal and directed against a single idiotype. Idiotypes are thus serologically defined determinants present on the Fab regions of immunoglobulins. They may represent amino acid sequences located on light (L) or heavy (H) chains alone or in combination (conformational determinants).

Anti-idiotypes which recognize one antibody and no other are said to recognize private idiotypes. Therefore, each antibody has a unique structure. A public or cross reacting idiotypes

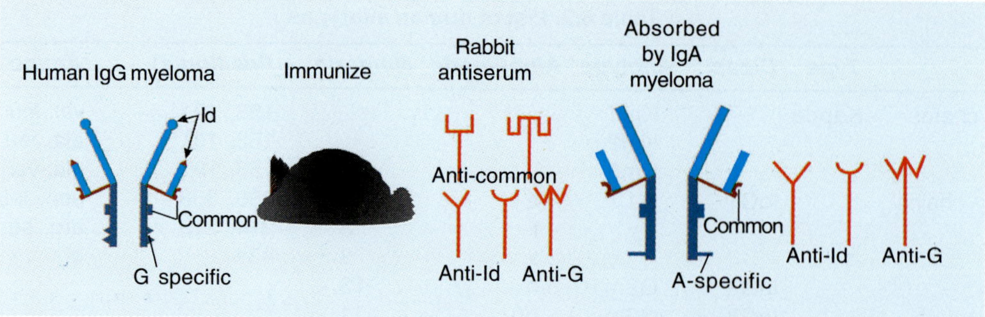

Fig. 6.3: Use of monoclonal myeloma proteins to produce antibodies specific for different Ig structures. Rabbit antibodies against human IgG myeloma are absorbed out with myelomas of those classes leaving other antibodies reacting with class-specific G and variable region-specific structure (idiotype=Id) on the original molecule. Further absorption with other IgG myelomas will remove the common IgG-specific antibodies having antiserum directed to idiotypic determinants alone

share idiotypes and recognize antibody molecules of closely similar amino acid structure.

In an inbred species the immune response of each individual is very similar. Comparison of the immune responses of several inbred strains to the same antigen has revealed that while most strains will respond with their own particular predominant idiotype, minor components of the response may be idiotypically identical to the response of other strains.

Thus idiotype is not necessarily unique to the individual. These shared idiotypes are known as cross-reactive idiotopes. Shared idiotopes generally represent the use of one or more common variable region gene segment. Anti-idiotypic antibodies can be demonstrated in the sera of normal individuals and may have some regulatory role in the nature of the immune response. An anti-idiotypic antibody may regulate the expression of the corresponding idiotype, and hence the nature of immune response, is the central concept of the network theory of immune regulation.

The H and L chain regions because of their structural uniqueness, can themselves act as antigenic determinants. Such immunoglobulin V region antigenic determinants are designated idiotopes and the collection of idiotopes on any antibody molecule is its idiotype. Idiotopes can be constructed of conformations on H or L chain V regions only or, as seems to be true in a majority of cases, of contributions from both chains. Some idiotopes are closely related to the antigen-combining sites and the occupation of the site by antigen prevents anti-idiotope antibody from binding to the immunoglobulin. Such idiotopes are designated "site related" idiotopes. Other idiotopes appear to be less closely related to the combining site. T-cells and antibodies specific for idiotopes may play an important role in the regulation of immune system. An influential theory, the network theory of the immune response, has proposed that they may be the critical regulatory elements of the immune system.

Anti-idiotype serums are useful reagents for identifying same V region on different heavy chains and on different cells, which in turn identify specific immune complexes in patient's serum. These reagents are also useful:

1. In the recognition of V_L type amyloid in subjects excreting Bence-Jones proteins.
2. For the detection of residual monoclonal protein after therapy.
3. For selecting lymphocytes with certain surface receptors.

Idiotypes are historically defined by anti-idiotype antibodies raised by immunizing allogeneic or xenogeneic animals with purified antibodies or their fragments. Depending on the manner of production, anti-idiotypes may be polyclonal, that is directed at a group of idiotypes, or monoclonal and directed against a single idiotype. Idiotypes are thus serologically defined determinants present on the Fab regions of immunoglobulins. They may represent amino acid sequences located on light (L) or heavy (H) chains alone or in combination (conformational determinants). The variable (V) sequences of the Fab region are subdivided into three hypervariable segments which are concerned with antigen binding and designated complementarily determining regions (CDR-1, 2 and 3) with intervening framework sequences **(Figure 6.1)**. Immunoglobulin V genes encode all framework and CDR-1 and 2 sequences of both L and H chains. However, in L chain only 2/3 of CDR-3 is encoded by V genes, the remainder being encoded by the J (junctional) genes. The entire H chain CDR-3 is encoded by the D (diversity) and J genes.

Anti-idiotypes which react only with the immunizing immunoglobulin define restricted or private idiotypes. Sharing of cross-reactive idiotypes (CRI) between antibodies of the same and different specificities from different individuals may reflect common amino acid sequences within framework regions or CDR. Occasionally anti-idiotypes define apparent cross-reactive idiotypes on antibodies throughout many species. This cross-reactivity on antibodies of identical antigen specificity may not be due to common amino acid sequences within the antibody V regions. In some cases, the tertiary structure of the anti-idiotypes happens to resemble that of the antigen and such anti-idiotypes are said to carry the 'internal image' of the antigen.

Idiotype Specific Suppression

In a number of systems, it appears that immune response can be idiotype-specific rather than antigen-specific. It has been observed that antibody responses to certain antigens are characterized by dominant idiotypes. The *in vivo* administration of anti-idiotype antibody led to a specific suppression of the corresponding idiotype in subsequent responses of treated mice to antigenic challenge. This suppression was idiotype specific. The decreased idiotype responsiveness was associated with the presence of idiotype-specific T suppressor cells.

The ability of T-cell suppression to regulate the immune response based on idiotype as well as antigen specificity is well documented. Idiotypes and anti-idiotypes having complementing specificities may interact in regulatory pathways.

Idiotype Regulation by T-Helper Cells

T-cell dependent antibody responses show dominance of a specific idiotype, suggesting that an idiotype specific T-helper cell plays a critical role in immunity. A number of studies in experimental animals showed dominance of a specific idiotype. In certain conditions, experimental evidence has been presented suggesting that an idiotype specific T-helper cell plays a critical role. It has been observed that for an optimal idiotype-positive secondary antibody response requires idiotypic specific T-helper cells in addition to carrier specific T-helper cells (**Table 6.3**).

Immunoglobulins contain both common and individual antigenic determinants. Heterologous antisera produced by immunization with one monoclonal Ig and extensively absorbed with other antibodies of the same light and heavy chain isotype will react with only the immunizing immunoglobulin. The antigen recognized by such sera is defined as idiotope(s) which are recognizing variable regions of immunizing Ig. Diversity of variable regions and by somatic mutations results in the expression of large number of potential idiotopes.

Idiotopes defines a collection of light and/or heavy chain V region associated structures. Idiotopes can involve any part of the exposed V regions. Thus shared idiotopes was evolved. An idiotype is a collection of idiotopes as mapped by monoclonal anti-idiotypic antibodies. Conventional anti-idiotypic antibodies are made by:

Table 6.3: Role of Iidiotype specific T-helper cells in idiotype regulation

T-helper cells		Hapten specific antibody response	Idiotype dominant antibody response
Carrier specific	Idiotype specific		
+	–	Yes	No
–	+	No	No
+	+	Yes	Yes

The indicated population of T-helper cells were cultured with B-cells, and the resulting cells were assayed both for total hapten specific antibody and for expression of dominant idiotype.

(Source: Fundamental Immunology, 2nd Ed., 1989 (Ed. W. Paul), Raven Press, New York, P-598)

1. Intraspecies or interspecies immunization with a purified antigen specific of antibodies or monoclonal antibody.
2. The resulting antiserum is then extensively absorbed against similar molecules with the same constant region to remove antibodies with anti-C_HC_L specificities.

These antisera can detect a range of topographies and idiotypes on different molecules. A given V region can be mapped serologically by the use of monoclonal anti-idiotypic antibodies.

Idiotypes and anti-idiotypic antibodies are extremely useful tools in the functional analysis and delineation of V regions expressed by B-cells and in serum antibody responses. They have also been used in studies on inheritance of genetic markers on Ig V genes, mapping of V genes, and many aspects of the regulation of V gene expression.

Network Theory

The participation of anti-idiotypic antibodies in immune network may be vital to the normal development and function of the humoral immune system. Others are potentially dangerous and at least some of them are functionally silenced in the form of tolerance.

It was proposed that immune system is regulated internally via idiotype recognition because of extreme heterogeneity of variable region of Igs having:

a. Expressed a nominal antigen binding site.
b. By virtue of the antigenic determinants expressed on the variable regions (idiotypes).
c. The ability to recognize other antibody molecules e.g. anti-idiotypic antibody.

Because of apparently unlimited potential of Ig V gene diversity, the idiotope repertoire must mimic the large universe of naturally occurring nonself external and self antigen epitopes. The idiotopes has been termed as internal images of antigens.

The overall idea by the network theory was that the immune system is in a state of equilibrium in that anti-idiotypic antibodies held antigen-induced antibody in check and introduction of antigen would interrupt these interactions in a mutually interactive way, stimulating antibody production which in turn would interrupt these interactions, stimulating antigen-induced antibody which in turn suppressed anti-idiotypic antibody, permitting the growth and differentiation of respective B-cell and secretion of anti-induced antibody (**Figure 6.4**). The theory does not account for T- and B-cells interactions. Also their subsets alter the concept of network interactions.

Idiotype-Directed Regulation of Immune System

It has been well established that administration of anti-idiotypic antibodies in small quantities, especially in the neonatal period, leads to the severe and chronic suppression of that particular idiotype. The suppression has been observed with both heterologous and monoclonal anti-

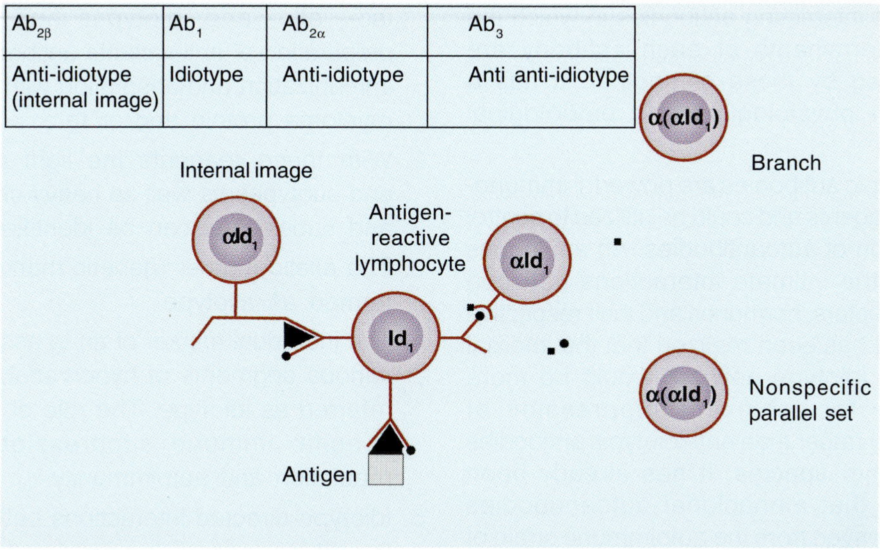

Fig. 6.4: Idiotype network in which antigen receptor on one lymphocyte reciprocally recognizes an idiotype on the receptor of another. T helper, T suppressor and B-lymphocytes interact through idiotype-anti-idiotype reactions producing either stimulation or suppression. One of the anti-idiotypic set $Ab_{2\beta}$ may bear an idiotype of similar shape to the antigen (internal image). The same idiotype (O) may be shared by receptors of different specificity, the non-specific parallel set so that the anti-(anti-Id) does not necessarily bind the original antigen

idiotypic antibodies. This neonatal treatment with anti-idiotypic antibodies leads to a permanent loss of clones of B-cell expressing that particular idiotype, thus regulating the immune system. The extent of loss depends on the amount of cross-reactivity of such anti-idiotypic antibodies.

Idiotype Interactions

The repertoire of B-cells is said to be complete because of the considerable diversity of B cell V regions, generated by combinational diversity and somatic mutation. Completeness means that all Igs or receptor can potentially react with one or many other complementary idiotype-bearing structures. Because of the extent of this diversity it is probable that idiotypes can be shared between different antibodies generated in response to different antigenic determinants. It has been proposed that certain idiotypes are determined possibly by framework regions that are shared by otherwise structurally disparate regions. Such idiotypes have been designated as regulatory idiotypes. Regulatory idiotypes on Ig molecule of seven different specificities have been reported. Perhaps the greatest apparent degree of idiotypic interactions occurs early during B cell development. B-cell interactions occurring through idiotypes occur early in development and have a long lasting effect on the diversity of the B-cell repertoire that is established in adult.

Autoimmunity and Idiotypes

Antinuclear antibodies (ANA) entail a large group of autoantibodies that bind certain nuclear antigens. The ANA test is a useful test for many autoimmune diseases and the presence of a specific binding pattern directs secondary testing for specific antibodies associated with the suspected disease. Idiotypes are the antigenic constitution of the variable region of an antibody, and they are recognized by anti-idiotypic antibodies. The idiotype network is composed of interacting antibodies in which the idiotype determinants of each antibody are complemented by those of another. It has a role in both physiological and pathological conditions.

Anti-idiotypic antibodies are powerful immunosuppressive agents and could be utilized to control the production of autoantibodies. An analogous example is the intimate interactions between hormone receptors, hormones and their respective antibodies. It has been realized that the internal elements of idiotype network would be more appropriate for achieving suppression of autoimmunity rather than anti-idiotypic antibodies raised in other species. It has already been established that monoclonal autoantibodies (idiotypes) derived from the autoimmune strain of mice offered a much better control of autoimmune process than anti-idiotypic antibodies from xenogeneic species. In a number of autoimmune diseases success has been achieved by employing idiotype network.

The difference between iso-, allo- and idiotypes is clearly depicted in **Figure 6.5**.

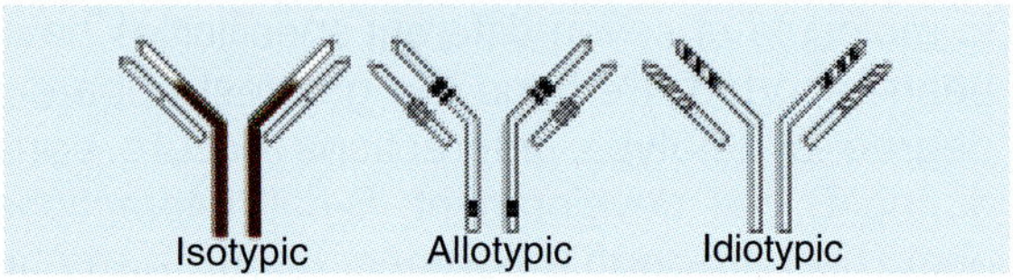

Fig. 6.5: Distinction between isotypic, allotypic and idiotypic sites

At this time you should know the following:

1. A clear distinction between immunoglobulin iso-, allo- and idiotypes and method of preparation of anti-variants antibodies through immunization and absorption with appropriate myeloma protein and or Ig.
2. With these reagents the light chain types and subtypes as well as heavy chain classes and subclasses can be identified.
3. The allelic marker (genetic marker) of Igs is termed as allotype.
4. The individual marker of an Ig associated with various segments of hypervariable region is referred as idiotype. The role of idiotypes in specific immune suppression, immune regulation and autoimmunity.
5. Idiotype-directed interactions between T-and B-cell receptors occur for the normal development and repertoire of these cells. The interactions play key role in certain diseases. *In vivo* interactions may be more complex and diversified.

Further Reading

- William Paul (Ed.), Fundamental Immunology, second edition, 1989, Raven Press, New York.
- HH Fudenberg and others (Eds.), Basic Immunogenetics, third edition, 1984, Oxford University Press Oxford.
- DM Weir (Ed), Handbook of Experimental Immunology, Vol.3: Genetics and molecular Immunology, 1986, Black well scientific, London.
- Ivan Roitt and others (Eds), Immunology, 1985, Gower Medical Publishing, New York.

7

CHAPTER

Immunoglobulins—Genetics

(Dr. Alpana Sharma dralpanasharma@gmail.com)

OBJECTIVES

- To understand the compatible genetic model of immunoglobulins with its structure and function.
- To know the multigene organization of Ig genes.
- To describe antibody diversity, its mechanism and responsible factors.
- To elucidate the possible mechanism of class switching.
- To understand expression of membrane bound antibody (mAb), secreted antibody (sAb) and simultaneous expression of IgM and IgD.

INTRODUCTION

The organization and expression of immunoglobulin genes is the best example of the genetic basis for the combination of constancy and tremendous variation in a single protein molecule. Ig genes have unique organization and differ from the classical genetic model. Therefore, the accepted genetic model should be compatible and fulfill all properties and features of Ig structure and function e.g.:

1. The N-terminal having variable region in heavy and light chains while constant region is at C-terminal.
2. Existence of different classes and subclasses of antibodies having same variable region with different H-chain constant region.
3. Tremendous diversity of antibody specificity.

Dreyer and Bennett (1965) theoretically proposed "two gene model" for Ig which was later proved experimentally by Tonegawa and Hazumi in 1975 and got Nobel prize in 1987 for this work. They suggested the following facts:

1. Two separate genes encode a single Ig heavy or light chain. One gene for variable (V) region and the other for constant (C) region.
2. These two genes, somehow, reorganize and come together and finally translate into a single immunoglobulin H or L chain.
3. There exists hundreds or thousands of genes for V-region while only one C-region gene for each class or subclass of the antibody.

To prove this hypothesis, Tonegawa and Hazumi selected DNA from embryonic cells and adult myeloma cells. DNA was digested using various restriction endonucleases to generate different DNA fragments. Later, these fragments were separated by size and analyzed with a radiolabelled mRNA probe. The embryonic DNA showed two different restriction fragments, whereas adult myeloma cell DNA produced only one fragment with the same probe. They suggested that during differentiation of lymphocytes from embryonic state to fully differentiated plasma cell (myeloma cells), the organization of genes takes place. In the embryonic cell variable and constant region genes are separated by large intervening

DNA sequences (showing 2 restriction fragments). During differentiation, the intervening stretches of DNA are spliced off and thereby variable and constant regions come closer.

Multigene Organization of Ig Genes

The germline organizations of Ig genes are characterized by spatial segregation of sequences that must be joined together to produce functional genes coding for antigen receptor proteins.

Sequencing and cloning studies have revealed the greater complexity of Ig genes.

In the germ-line DNA sequences, following informations were revealed:

1. Multigene organizations of Ig genes:

   Three separate multigene families (loci) encode all Ig genes:

   1 heavy chain, 1 Ig κ light chain and 1 Ig λ light chain.
2. Each multigene family is present on different chromosomes.
3. Within each locus, the sets of each type of gene segments are separated from one another by noncoding stretches of DNA (introns).

During B-cell maturation, these gene segments are rearranged and brought together to form functional Ig genes. The organization of Ig genes is essentially in the same way in all mammals, although their chromosomal locations and the number and sequence of different gene segments may vary.

Immunoglobulin Multigene Families

Ig H chain and L chain genes are organized into clusters called gene families. These genes are located on different chromosomes for H and L-chains (**Table 7.1**).

Light Chain Genes

Each light chain (κ or λ) is encoded by three gene segments V, J and C, two coding sequences in the variable region and one coding sequence in the constant region.

V : Variable gene segment.

J : Joining gene segment.

C : Constant gene segment.

Each V_L-gene segment is preceded by a short sequence at 5' called leader sequence (L).

In both the light chains (κ or λ).

- V gene codes for 1-95 amino acids.
- J gene codes for 96-108 amino acids.
- C gene codes for 109-214 amino acids.

The genes for κ chains are labeled as $V_κ$, $J_κ$ and $C_κ$ and located on chromosome 2, whereas $V_λ$, $J_λ$ and $C_λ$ genes are for lambda light chains and located on chromosome 22.

The number of functional genes coding Ig light chains (κ or λ) variable and constant regions vary.

Kappa light chain genes are as follows:

$V_κ$: 40

$J_κ$: 5

$C_κ$: 1

The functional gene segments in lambda light chain are as follows:

Table 7.1: Functional L-chain and H-chain genes of immunoglobulin

Genes	*L-chain*		*H-chain*
	Kappa L-chain	*Lambda L-chain*	
Variable (V)	$V_κ ≈ 40$	$V_λ ≈ 31$	$V_H ≈ 51$
Diversity (D)	–	–	$D_H ≈ 27$
Joining (J)	$J_κ ≈ 5$	$J_λ ≈ 5$	$J_H ≈ 6$
Constant (C)	$C_κ$ - 1	$C_λ$ - 5	C_H - 9

V_λ : 31
J_λ : 4
C_λ : 7

In addition to these gene segments human λ-light chain, contain many nonfunctional pseudogenes for variable, joining and constant gene segments.

There are intervening non-coding DNA sequences between different gene segments of both the chains.

Heavy Chain Genes

Leroy Hood proposed the various gene segments which encode for Ig heavy chain. Each H-chain is encoded by four genes which are located on chromosome 14.

The variable region is coded by three genes:

V_H : Variable gene segment encodes for 1 to 94 amino acids.

D_H : Diversity gene segment encodes for 95 to 97 amino acids.

J_H : Joining gene segment encodes for 98 to 113 amino acids.

They elucidated that a third germ-line gene segment must join with the V_H and J_H gene segments to encode the entire variable region of the H-chain. This gene segment was designated D or diversity gene segment codes for 3 amino acids with CDR3 and provides major contribution to antibody diversity. All gene segments are joined together with the non-coding sequences in a germ-line DNA.

H-chain germ line DNA contains the following genes:

V_H : 51
D_H : 27
J_H : 6
C_H : 9

There are series of constant gene segments encoding for the constant region of an Ig heavy chain isotypes. In humans, the C_H gene segments are arranged sequentially in the fixed order:

C_μ, C_δ, C_γ, Cε and C_α

This order is related to the sequential expression of the Ig classes in the course of B-cell development and the initial IgM response of a B-cell to its first encounter with an antigen (**Figure 7.1**).

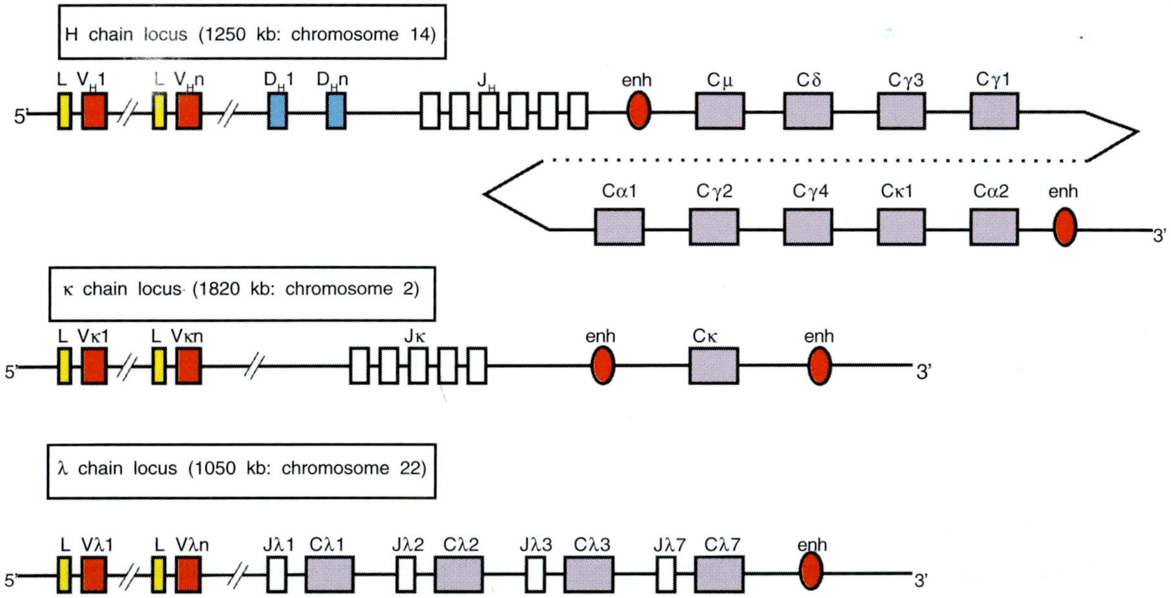

Fig. 7.1: Germ line organization of human immunoglobulin genes. Schematic representation of gene segments which are indicated as follows: L, leader; V, variable; D, diversity; J, joining; C, constant; enh, enhancer. Pseudogenes are not shown for simplicity

Immunoglobulin Gene Rearrangement

In germ-line DNA, Ig genes are not just transcribed and translated into H or L-chains until they are shuffled. During B-cell maturation in the bone marrow, some of these gene segments are randomly shuffled and reorganized by a dynamic genetic system and generate thousands of combinations.

Firstly the H-chain genes rearrange followed by L-chain gene rearrangement.

Light Chain Gene Rearrangement

Variable region of L-chains (κ or λ) have two gene segments: V and J. For the expression of both κ or λ light chains any of V_κ genes can combine with any of the Jκ genes.

As shown in (**Figure 7.2**) in a rearranged κ or λ L-chains, the order of gene segments from 5'-3' end are as follows:

A promoter sequence; a short leader sequence (L); a noncoding intron; a joined VJ gene segment, then a second non-coding sequence and finally joining of constant region gene segments, C_λ for λ-light chain and C_κ for κ-light chain. Finally, the non-coding sequences/introns are spliced off to produce a complete functional V_κ, J_κ, C_κ gene for kappa chain and V_λ J_λ C_λ for lambda light chain.

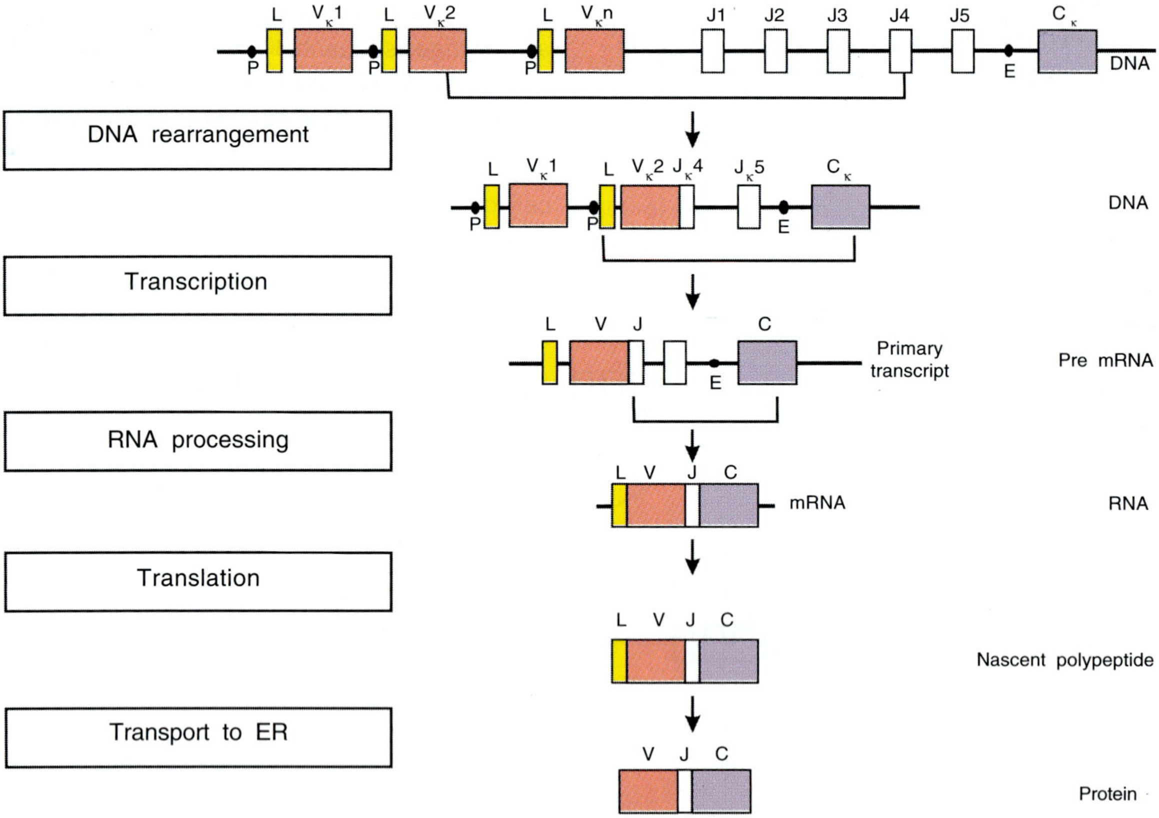

Fig. 7.2: Rearrangement of κ light chain gene segment and RNA processing events required to generate a κ chain protein

Heavy Chain Gene Rearrangement

As shown in (**Figure 7.3**) H-chain gene rearrangement starts in variable region. Here a diversity gene segment is also present in between V and J gene segments. Rearrangement in variable region first begins with the joining of diversity gene segment with joining (J) gene segment. Any of the D_H segment can combine with any of the functional J_H with the removal of intron in between them. This occurs early in the bone marrow in lymphoid precursor cells even before commitment to become B-cell. After D_H J_H joining any of the V_H gene segment can join with any of the joined D_H J_H gene segment, finally generating V_H D_H J_H gene segment in variable region. The sequence of the rearranged genes in V-region from 5'-3'end is as follows:

5'promoter sequence-leader sequence–intron-V_H D_H J_H segment-non-coding introns at 3'end followed by constant region sequences.

After accomplishing the rearrangement of VDJ segment in variable region, the RNA polymerase binds to promoter sequence and transcribes the entire H-chain variable region genes including introns.

Antibody Diversity

One of the important structure-function relationships to antigen recognition is antibody diversity. An individual is capable of making an enormous number of structurally distinct antibodies, each with a distinct specificity. The presence of large number of antibodies that bind different antigens is called ***antibody diversity***, and the total collection of antibodies with different specificities is called the ***antibody repertoire***. This diversity is mainly of genetic origin where recombination of different gene segments plays important role. The genetic mechanisms that can generate such large antibody repertoire occur exclusively in lymphocytes.

Mechanism of Antibody Diversity

Various mechanisms/factors responsible for total antibody diversity are as follows:

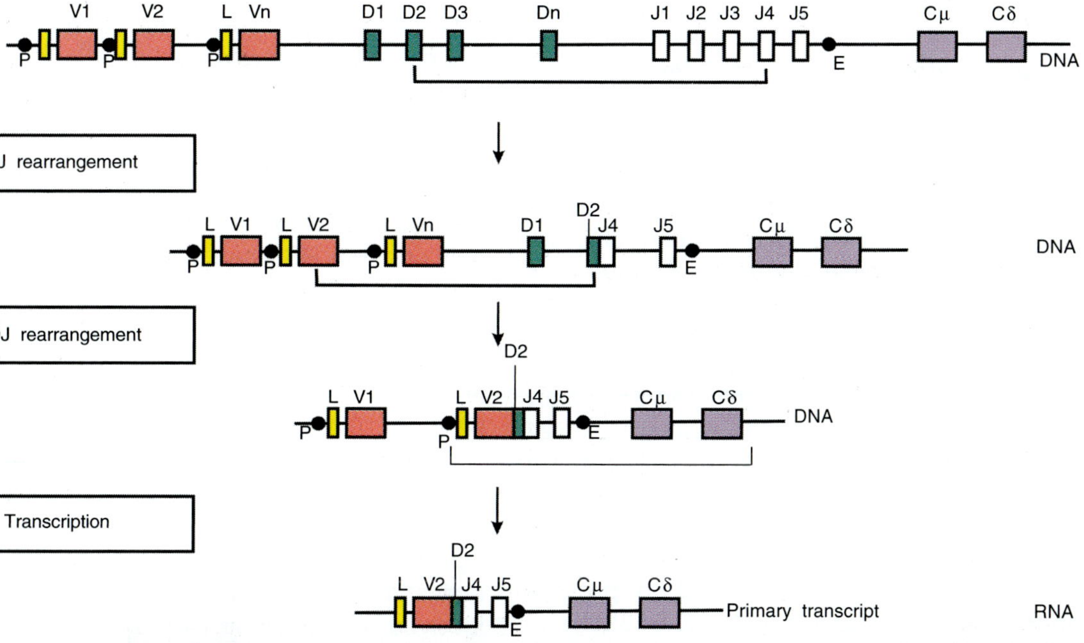

Fig. 7.3: Rearrangement of heavy chain gene segments and generation of heavy chain primary transcript

1. Multigene organization of immunoglobulin chain.
2. Combinatorial joining of different gene segments.
3. Junctional flexibility.
4. P-region nucleotide additions.
5. N-region nucleotide additions.
6. Somatic hypermutation.
7. Combinatorial association of light and heavy chains.

1. Multigene Organization of Ig Chains

As discussed earlier, in germ-line DNA sequence, 3 separate multigene families encode all Ig genes.

In a study, approximately 51 V_H, 27 D_H and 6 J_H functional genes for variable region of H-chain and 40V_κ, 5J_κ for kappa light chain and 31 V_λ, 4J_λ functional genes for variable lambda light chain were reported in a human germ-line DNA. In addition to these functional gene segments there are many pseudogenes.

The presence of enormous multiple germ-line V, D and J gene segments contribute to the diversity of the antigen binding sites in antibodies.

2. Combinatorial Joining of Different Gene Segments

The random rearrangement of the multiple copies of V, D and J gene segments further provides antibody diversity. Many different variable regions can be made by selecting different combinations of these segments. For human κ light chains, approximately 40 functional V_κ and 5 J_κ gene segments can provide 200 different V_κ regions. Similarly for λ light chains, 31 V_λ genes and 4 J_λ gene segments can potentially yield 124 possible V_λ regions. As a result 324 different light chains can be formed. For heavy chains in humans, any J_H segment can join with any D_H segment, further this joined D_HJ_H gene segment can combine with any of the functional 51V_H gene segment to provide enormous combinations (51×27×6=8260) to provide considerable amount of diversity.

3. Junctional Flexibility

Multiple copies of different gene segments join randomly and rearranged into many unique combinations. This combination is specifically guided by some specific conserved sequences present at the junctions or at 5' and 3' end of different gene segments.

Mechanisms of V-region DNA rearrangements: DNA sequencing studies showed two closely related conserved sequences known as *recombination signal sequences (RSS)* flanking each germ-line V, D and J gene segments and on both sides of each D gene segment. These sequences function as signals for recombination and rearrangement of genes. Each RSS contains a conserved palindromic-heptamer (7-bp) and a conserved AT-rich nonamer (9-bp) sequence separated by an intervening sequence of 12 or 23 base pairs (**Figure 7.4**). The intervening 12 base pair sequences are called one-turn RSS and 23 bp sequences called two-turn RSS (12 bp and 23 bp correspond to one turn and two turns of the DNA helix).

In κ light chain, V_κ signal sequence has one turn spacer and J_κ has two turn spacer. In λ light chain this order is reversed, that is V_λ has two turn RSS and J_λ has one turn RSS. On the other hand, heavy chain DNA has two turn RSS on both V_H and J_H gene segments but D_H gene segment has one turn RSS on both sides (5' and 3' end). There is a definite joining rule for these sequences; only one turn RSS can join with two-turn signal sequences. This rule confirms the proper joining order and ensures that similar gene segments should not join with each other e.g., D_H, J_H join first then only it joins with V_H. Similarly V_L segment joins to J_L not with J_H segment (**Figure 7.4**).

The recombination of different gene segments between RSS and coding sequences is catalyzed by enzymes called recombinases, named by David Baltimore and products of recombination-activating genes 1 and 2 (RAG1 and RAG2), involved in recombination of VDJ gene segments. The enzyme terminal-deoxynucleotidyl transferase

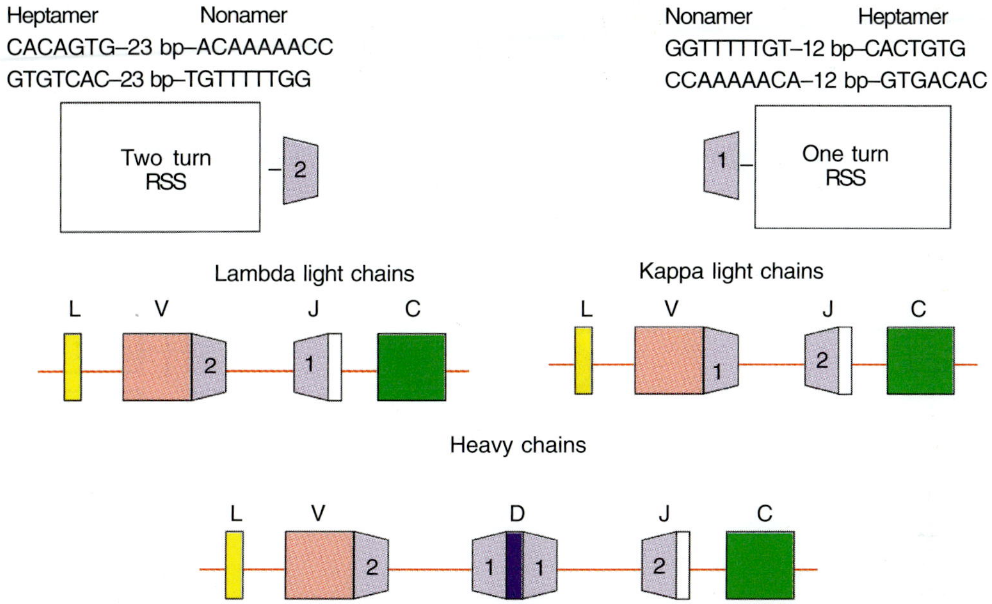

Fig. 7.4: Nucleotide sequence of recombination signal sequences and their location in immunoglobulin DNA

(TdT) has also shown to be involved in recombination of gene segments. Recombinases (RAG1 and RAG2 encoded proteins) mediated joining occurs either by ***deletion*** or ***inversion***. Recombination of V and J gene segments may occur by deletion of intervening DNA and ligation of the V and J segments, when they are in same orientation. When the V gene is in opposite orientation, the recombination occurs by inversion of the intervening DNA followed by ligation of adjacent gene segments. In this the intervening DNA is not removed but retained on the chromosome (**Figure 7.5**).

Recombination involves both the joining of RSS to form a signal joint and joining of coding sequences to form a coding joint. Signal sequences are always joined precisely but coding sequences are often joined imprecisely. The joining of coding sequences may lead to deletion or frame shift mutation. If such a mutation produces a stop codon, then immunoglobulin chain synthesis stops. This is called ***nonproductive arrangement***. At other times, imprecise joining leads to change in amino acid sequence but synthesis of Ig chain continues. This is called ***productive rearrangement***.

Therefore, junctional flexibility leads to productive combination and many other nonproductive rearrangements. Productive combinations encode alternative amino acid at each coding joint, thereby increasing antibody diversity. The variations in amino acid sequence due to junctional flexibility lie in the CDR3 region of third hypervariable region of H-chain and L-chain DNA of Ig and contribute significant role in binding antigen by antibody molecule.

4. P-nucleotide Addition

In both heavy and light chains, the diversity of CDR3 is significantly increased by the addition and deletion of nucleotides in the formation of junctions between gene segments. The added nucleotides are called P-nucleotides because they make up palindromic sequences added to the ends of the gene segments. Following the initial single strand DNA cleavage at the junctions of coding and signal sequences, the nucleotides at the end of coding sequence form hairpin loop structure. After the formation of hairpin loop, the action of recombinases

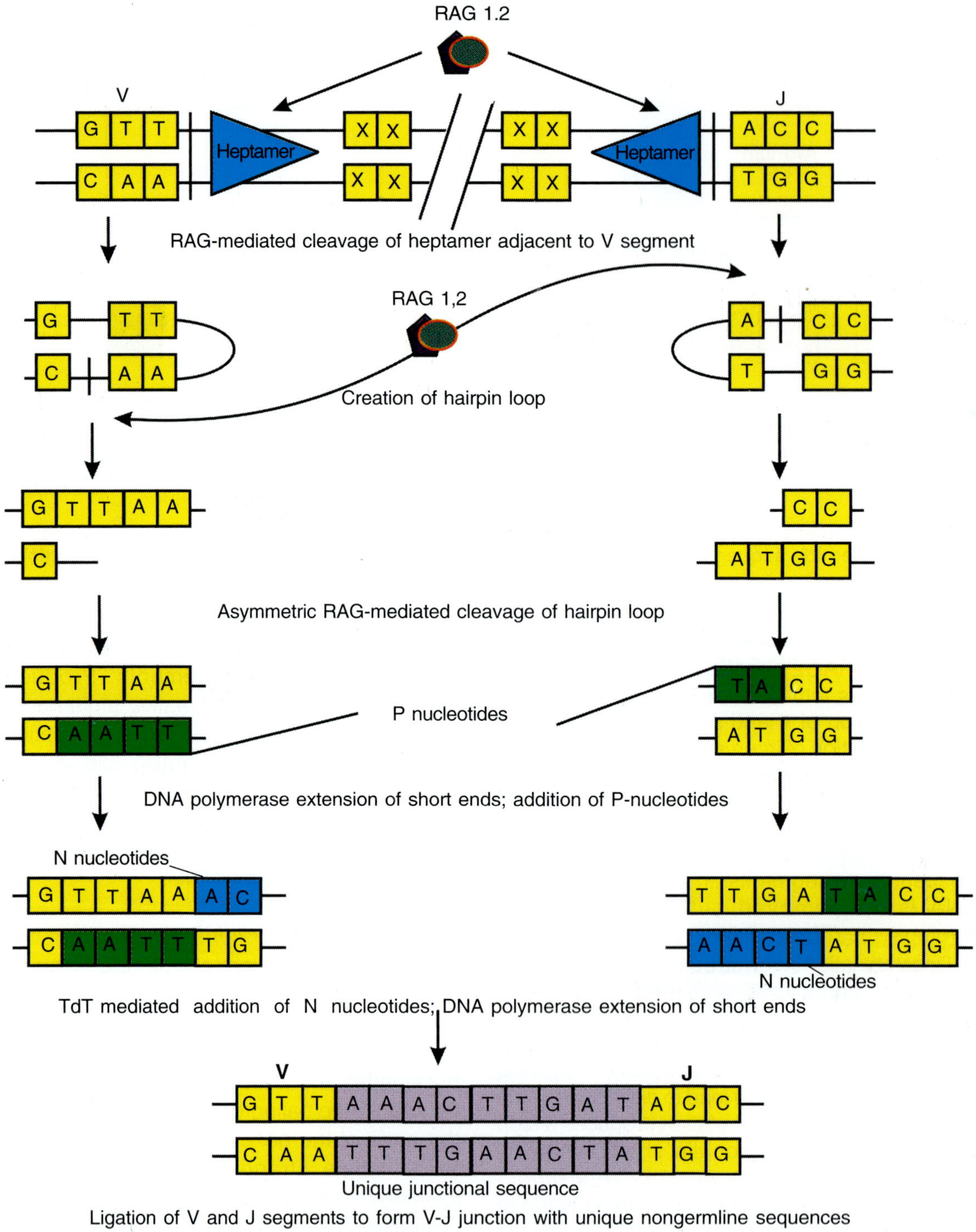

Fig. 7.5: Depiction of the process of recombination of immunoglobulin gene segments and generation of novel sequences previously not present in germline by addition of P- and N-nucleotides

catalyzes a single stranded cleavage at a random point within the coding sequence but near the original point at which the hairpin was first formed. When this cleavage occurs at a different point from the initial break, a single stranded tail is formed from a few nucleotides of the coding sequence plus the complementary nucleotides from the other DNA strand. The addition of complementary nucleotides by repair enzymes generate palindromic sequences (P-nucleotides) in the coding joint which leads to variation in the amino acid sequence of the CDR3 region, further adding to antibody diversity as shown in **Figure 7.5**.

5. Addition of N-nucleotides

Short stretch of amino acid sequences not encoded by V, D or J gene segments. These gene segments are called N-nucleotides because they are non-template-encoded. They are added by the enzyme terminal deoxy-nucleotidyl transferase (TdT) to single strand ends of the coding DNA after hairpin cleavage during joining of segments. After the addition of 15 to 20 nucleotides by this enzyme, the two single stranded stretches at the ends of the gene segments form base pairs over a short region. N-nucleotides are found especially in the V-D and D-J junctions of the assembled H-chain gene, they are less common in light-chain genes because TdT is maximally expressed during the period in B-cell development. H-chain diversity generated by N-region nucleotides is localized in the CDR3 of the H-chain genes (**Figure 7.5**).

Nucleotides can also be deleted at gene segment junctions. This is accomplished by exonucleases, which is not yet identified, although it is very uncommon.

6. Somatic Hypermutation

An additional mechanism that generates antibody diversity throughout the V region and that operates on B-cells in peripheral lymphoid organs after assembly of functional immuno-globulin genes. This process called **somatic hypermutation** introduces bases by point mutation (substitution) into the V-region of the rearranged heavy and light chain genes at a very high rate (10^{-3} per base pair per generation) giving rise to mutant B-cell receptors on the surface of the B-cells. The mutation rate is million fold higher than spontaneous mutation rate in other genes hence known as hyper-mutation. Somatic hypermutations within the CDRs of V_H and V_L gene sequences influence the overall affinity for antigen. The mechanism is still poorly defined.

7. Association of Heavy and Light Chains

Combinatorial association of H and L-chains variable region to form the antigen binding site of an immunoglobulin contributes further to generate antibody diversity.

If we calculate approximately then:

1.6×10^4 H-chain genes

1.2×10^3 L-chain genes

Minimum number of combinations of H and L-chains ~1.9×10^7.

However specificity and diversity is higher i.e. significant number of nucleotide sequences are introduced by junctional flexibility, addition of P and N-nucleotides and somatic hypermutations (**Table 7.2**).

Table 7.2: Overall antibody diversity in humans due to combinatorial joining of different gene segments and H and L-chains

Joining of germline gene segments	*Possible no. of combination*
Heavy chain	V D J
V-D-J joining	$51 \times 27 \times 6 = 8262$
Light chain	
1. *Kappa chain*	V_κ J_κ
V_κ - J_κ joining	$40 \times 5 = 200$
2. *Lambda chain*	V_λ J_λ
V_λ - J_λ joining	30 X 4 = 120
Association of H and L chains possible combination	8262 (200+120) = 2.64×10^6

The combination of all these sources of diversity generates a vast repertoire of antibody specificity from a relatively limited number of genes.

Few studies estimated that antibody diversity might be as high as 10^{11}, but their some mechanisms are not known yet.

Class Switching

On antigen stimulation, H-chain VDJ unit can join with any of constant heavy gene segment and express the particular antibody class. This process called–***class switching***. Exact mechanism is unclear but evidence suggests that DNA flanking regions / sequences located at 2-3 kb upstream of each constant H-chain gene segment (C_H) except C_δ called ***switch sites*** (SS). They are composed of multiple copies of short repeated sequences (GAGCT and TGGGG). Class specific recombinases bind to switch sites and facilitate recombination. Therefore, expression of particular antibody class depends upon specificity of recombinase proteins expressed. Class switching depends upon the interplay of 3 factors.

i. Switch regions / sites (short repeat sequences).
ii. A switch recombinase.
iii. Cytokine signals (IL-4).

Some cytokines (IL-4) act as switch factor inducing class switching from C_μ to $C_\gamma 1$ or C_ε. It dictates the isotype to which the B-cell switches. In some cases, IL-4 has been observed to induce class switching in a successive manner C_μ to $C_\gamma 1$ and then $C_\gamma 1$ to C_ε. During class switching C_μ to $C_\gamma 1$ a circular excision product is generated containing C_μ together with 5' end of $S_\gamma 1$ (switch region of $_\gamma 1$) and 3' end of S_μ (switch region of μ) (**Figure 7.6**).

Expression of Membrane Bound Antibody (mAb) and Secreted Antibody (sAb)

Differential RNA processing at post transcriptional level is responsible for expression of membrane bound antibody (mAb) and secreted antibody (sAb).

Mature B-cell expresses IgM and IgD antibodies on its surface. However, secreted antibodies are also produced during generation of immune responses. The mAb and sAb differ in their C-terminal domains of H-chain. The sAb has a hydrophilic C-domain of about 20 amino acids, whereas mAb has 40 amino acids in its C-domain. Differential RNA processing is based on C_μ gene. This gene has four exons $C_\mu 1$, $C_\mu 2$, $C_\mu 3$ and $C_\mu 4$ encoding the four constant region domains of H-chain. The $C_\mu 4$ exon also has a specific sequence called secreted ('s') site at its 3' end encodes a 13 amino acid long hydrophilic region of sIgM. The 3' end has two more exons called M1 and M2. M1 exon encodes 26 amino acid long transmembrane domain and M2 encodes the cytoplasmic tail of 3 amino acids. The primary transcript of this gene shows two polyadenylation sites—polyA1 at 3' end of $C_\mu 4$ exon and polyA2 at 3' end of M2 exon. The differential cleavage at site A1 produces mRNA of secreted antibody and at site A2 produces mRNA of membrane bound antibody (**Figure 7.7**).

The mature naïve B-cell produces membrane bound antibody while the antigen activated and differentiated B-cell (plasma cells) produces secreted antibody. The mechanism is still unclear as same for simultaneous expression of IgM and IgD.

Simultaneous Expression of IgM and IgD

Rearranged heavy-chain genes in mature B-cells transcribed to produce primary transcripts containing both C_μ and C_δ gene segments. These gene segments are present close together, only 5 kb apart. The switch sites between them are lacking. Therefore, it permits entire VDJ C_μ C_δ region to be transcribed into a single primary RNA transcript containing four poly A sites. Sites 1 and 2 are associated with C_μ and sites 3 and 4 are located in the C_δ gene segment. Further, RNA processing may lead to the expression of membrane bound form of that particular class of antibody i.e. IgM or IgD (**Figure 7.8**).

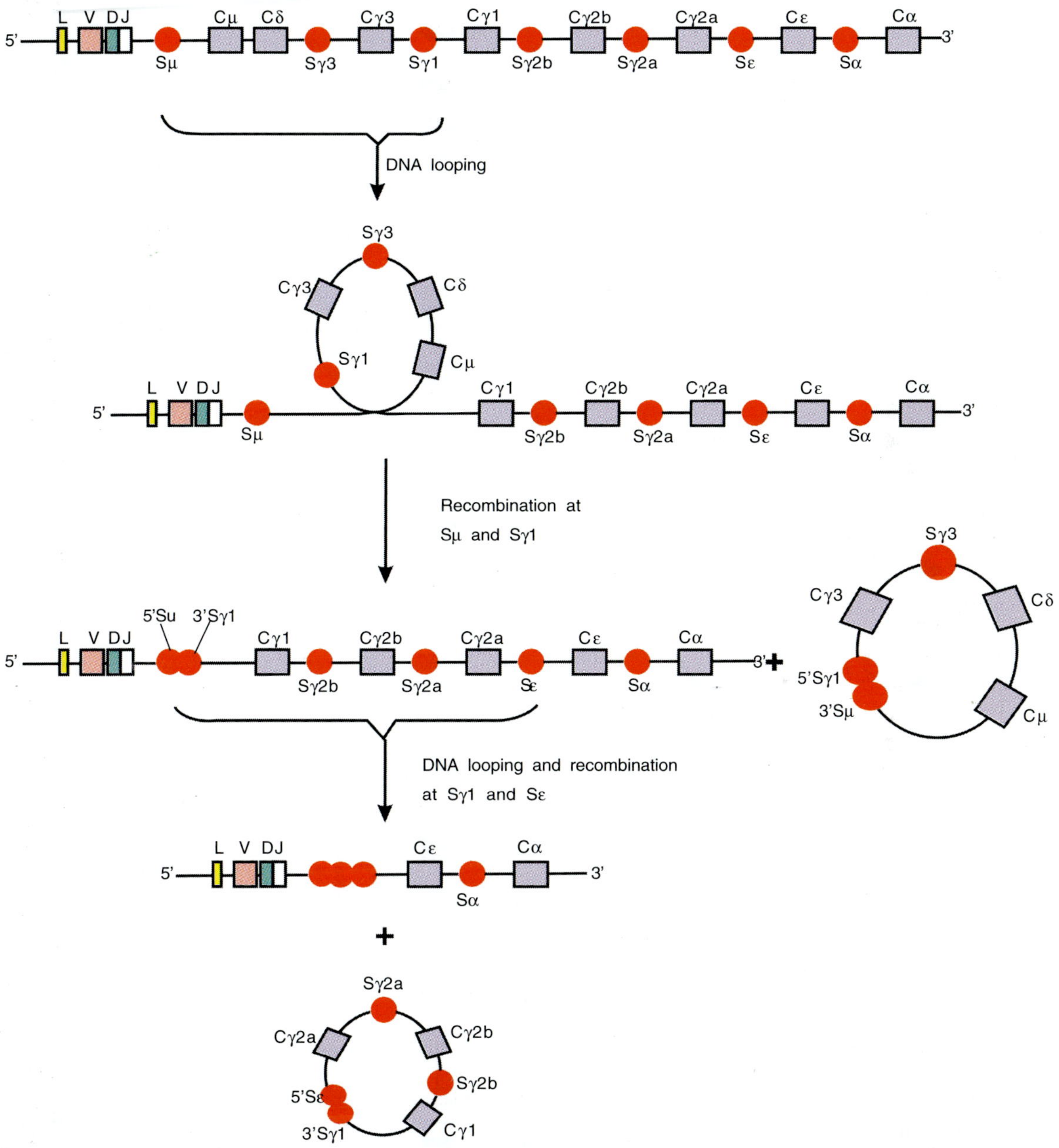

Fig. 7.6: Proposed mechanism for class switching induced by IL-4 in rearranged heavy chain genes. A switch site is located upstream from each C_H segment except C_δ. Circular excision products containing portions of switch sites are generated when sequential class switching occurs from C_μ to Cγ1 to Cε

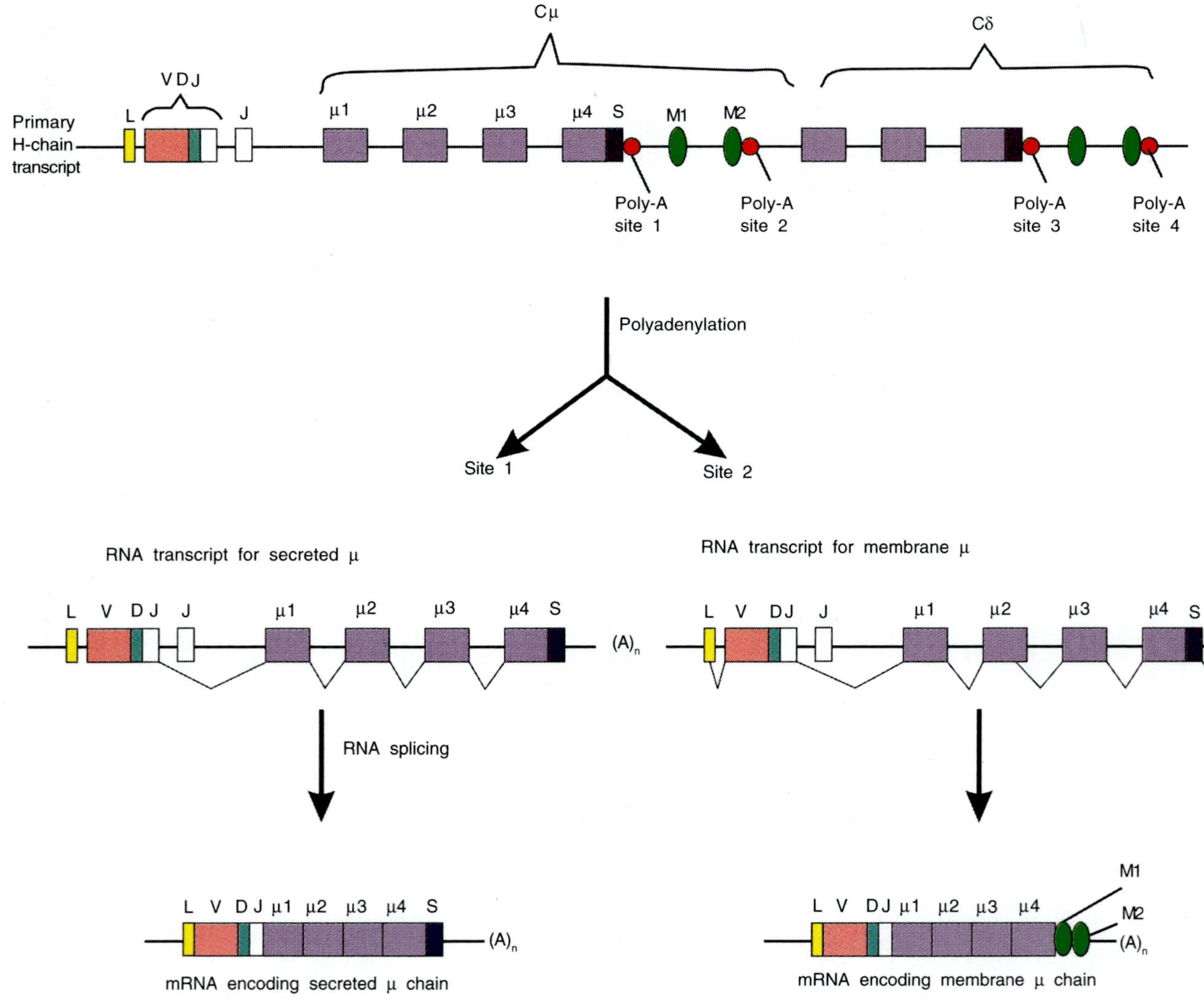

Fig. 7.7: Expression of membrane bound antibody (mAb) and secreted antibody (sAb) by alternative RNA processing. Structure of the primary transcript of a rearranged heavy-chain gene showing various poly-A sites. Polyadenylation followed by splicing generates mRNA encoding either secreted or membrane μ chains

At this time you should know the following:

1. Details of the compatible genetic model of immunoglobulins with its structure and function.
2. The multigene organization of Ig genes.
3. Antibody diversity, its mechanism and responsible factors.
4. The possible mechanism of class switching.
5. Expression of membrane bound antibody (mAb) and secreted antibody (sAb) and simultaneous expression of IgM and IgD.

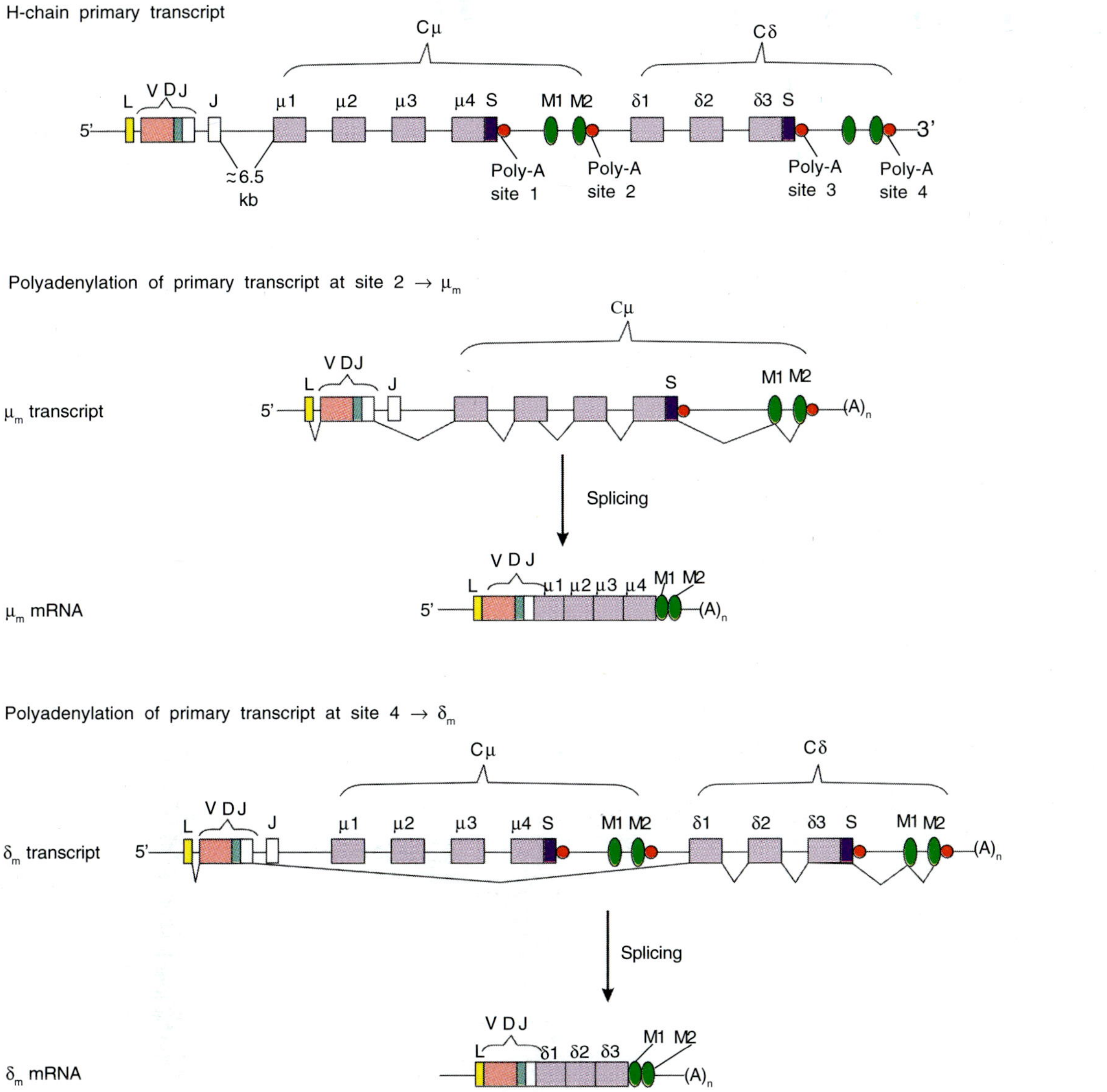

Fig. 7.8: Expression of membrane forms of μ and δ heavy chains by alternative RNA processing

Further Reading

1. Abbas KA and Lichtman HA. Cellular and molecular immunology, fifth edition.
2. Roitt I. Essential Immunology, ninth edition.
3. Goldsby AR, Kindt JT, Osborne AB and Kuby J. Immunology, sixth edition.
4. Murphy K, Travers P and Walport M. Janeway's Immunobiology, seventh edition.
5. www.nature.com
6. www.theimmunology.com
7. http://imgt.cines.fr/

8 CHAPTER

Antigen-Antibody Reactions

(Dr. Nalini Gupta *nalini203@gmail.com*)

OBJECTIVES

1. To show the nature of antigen-antibody (Ag-Ab) reactions.
2. To compare antibody affinity and avidity.
3. To understand the basis for antibody specificity and cross reactivity.
4. To discuss the principles of tests used for antigen/antibody reactions.

Introduction

A variety of immunologic assays used are as follows[1]:

- Assays to detect the minimal level of antibody or antigen for a diagnosis of disease.
- Assays to monitor the degree of a humoral response.
- Assays to identify molecules of biological or medical importance.
- Assays to understand the structural relationships between molecules based on cross-reactivity of antibodies.[1]

Antigen and Antibodies Reactions

- *In vivo* – form basis of antibody mediated immunity in infectious diseases, autoimmune diseases and tissue injury in hypersensitivity.
- *In vitro* – plays role in diagnosing infections.

  To monitor the levels of humoral immune response.

  To identify molecules of biological or medical interest.

Therefore, these reactions can be used for detection and quantification of either antigen or antibody.

Mechanisms for Binding of Antigen and Antibody

Strong antigen-antibody interaction will depend upon a close fit between them and it requires a high degree of complimentarity (basis of specificity) of shapes between the paratope (antibody-binding site) and the epitope (antigenic site).

- Lock and Key Concept: The concept of antigen-antibody reaction is one of a key (*i.e.* the antigen) which fits into a lock (*i.e.* the antibody).

  Combining site of an antibody is located in the Fab portion of the molecule and is constructed from the hyper-variable regions of the heavy and light chains. The antigenic determinant nestles in a cleft formed by the combining site of the antibody.

Physical Forces Binding Antigen to Antibody

- Non-covalent Bonds: These bonds hold the antigen in the antibody combining site and are all non-covalent in nature. Majority of the antigen-antibody interactions involve a strong coulombic attraction between oppositely charged ionic groupings. Other forces responsible are mostly short-range ones such as van der Waals forces, hydrophobic forces and hydrophobic bonds.

AFFINITY

Strength of the total non-covalent interactions between a single antigen-binding site on an antibody and a single epitope is the affinity of the antibody for that epitope. That is, affinity is quantitative measure of binding strength between antibody and an epitope on antigen.

Therefore, it represents the combined strength of all non-covalent interactions.

Interaction between Ag and Ab can be expressed as:

$$Ag + Ab \underset{k_{-1}}{\overset{k_1}{\rightleftharpoons}} Ag{:}Ab$$

Association constant $= k_a = k_1/k_{-1}$

$$\text{At equilibrium } k_a = \frac{[Ag{:}Ab]}{[Ag]\ [Ab]}$$

Dissociation constant $= k_d = 1/k_a$

Where k_1 is the forward (association) rate constant and k_{-1} is the reverse (dissociation) rate constant.

Association constant $(K_a) = k_1/k_{-1}$, a measure of affinity.

At equilibrium, K_a can be calculated from the ratio of the molar concentration of bound Ag-Ab complex to the molar concentrations of unbound antigen and antibody.[2]

Dissociation constant K_d is the reciprocal of K_a

K_d is a quantitative indicator of the stability of an Ag-Ab complex; very stable complexes have very low value of K_d and less stable ones have higher values.[2]

Strength of Ag-Ab Interactions

The association constant, K_a can be determined by equilibrium dialysis or by various newer methods.

Equilibrium Dialysis[2]

- This procedure uses dialysis chamber, which contains two equal compartments separated by semi-permeable membrane **(Figure 8.1)**.

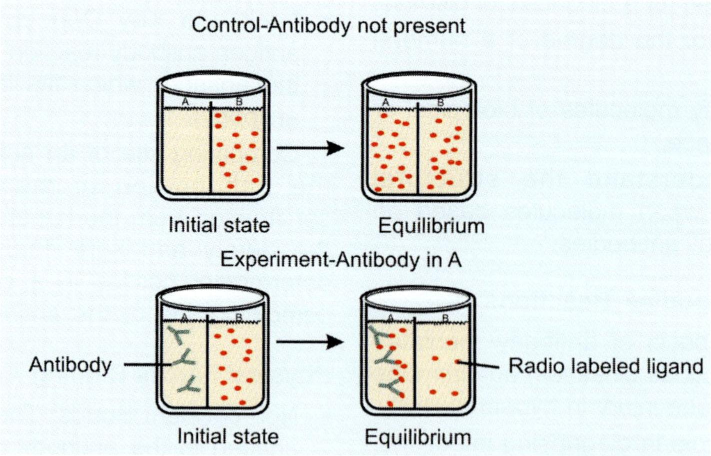

Fig. 8.1: Showing antibody affinity by equilibrium dialysis

- Antibody placed in one compartment and a radioactively labeled ligand, which is small enough to pass through the semi-permeable membrane is placed in other compartment.
- In absence of antibody, ligand added to compartment B equilibrates on both sides of the membrane.
- In presence of antibody, part of labeled ligand binds to antibody at equilibrium and unbound ligand is equally distributed in both compartments.
- The difference in ligand concentration in two compartments will represent concentration of bound ligand (i.e. concentration of Ag-Ab complex).
- Higher the affinity, more ligand is bound.[2]

Equilibrium Equation[2]

- Since the total concentration of the antibody in the equilibrium dialysis chamber is known, the equilibrium equation can also be re-written as:

$$K_a = \frac{[Ag{:}Ab]}{[Ag][Ab]} = \frac{r}{c(n-r)} \longrightarrow \frac{r}{c} = K_a n - K_a r$$

r=the ratio of the concentrations of bound ligand to total Ab.

c=the concentration of free ligand.

n=the number of antigen binding sites on the Ab.

This expression is rearranged to give the Scatchard equation:

$$\frac{r}{c} = k_a n - k_a r$$

Antibody Avidity is a measure of the overall strength of binding of an antigen with many antigenic determinants and multivalent antibodies. It refers to the overall strength of binding between multivalent antigens and antibodies.

Cross-reactivity

Cross-reactions can arise because the cross-reacting antigen shares an epitope in common with the immunizing antigen or because it has an epitope which is similar in structure to one on the immunizing antigen (multispecificity).[3]

- Cross-reactivity forms a basis of blood group antibodies.
- S*treptococcus pyogenes* expresses cell wall proteins called M-Antigen which cross-reacts with several myocardial and skeletal muscle proteins.
- Some vaccines exhibit cross-reactivity e.g. Vaccinia Virus (Cow Pox) and Variola Virus (Small Pox).

Tests for Antigen and Antibody Reactions

Precipitation Reactions

- Interaction between an antibody (precipitins) and a soluble antigen in aqueous solution forms a lattice that eventually will develop into a visible precipitate. Antibodies that aggregate soluble antigens are called *precipitins*.[2]
  a. For the formation of antigen-antibody precipitate, antigen must be bivalent or polyvalent i.e. it must have at least two copies of the same epitope or have different epitopes that react with different antibody present in polyclonal anti-sera.[2]

Stages

a. The stage of sensitization – not visible, reversible (within few minutes).

b. The stage of reaction – visible, irreversible (takes a day or two).

Mechanism for Precipitation Reactions

Marrack's lattice hypothesis: When a multivalent antigen is mixed with bivalent antibody in equal proportions, a complex lattice is formed, which consists of alternative units of antigen and antibody.

Zone Phenomenon (Figure 8.2)

- Prozone phenomenon: Antibody excess.
- Zone of equivalence: Antigen and antibody in equal proportion.
- Post zone phenomenon: Antigen excess.

Precipitation Reaction in Fluids

- First introduced by Kraus in 1897.
- It can provide information such as:
  a. Potency of different batches of anti-sera by measuring the amount of precipitating antibody in an anti-serum.
  b. Proof of antigen-antibody reactions.
  c. Relative heterogeneity system.
- A **quantitative precipitation reaction** is performed by placing constant amount of antibody in a series of tubes and then adding increasing amounts of antigen to the tubes. After overnight incubation, precipitate will form which is weighed. This method can be used to measure the amount of antibody in a sample of interest. All the antigen added is complexed in the precipitate with all antibody available (equivalence zone) and the antibody content would be the difference between the weight of the Ag-Ab complex and weight of the antigen.

Precipitation Reaction in Gels

- Immune precipitates (ppt) can form not only in solutions but also in agar matrix.[2] These immunodiffusion reactions are used:
  a. To see relative concentration of antigen/antibody.
  b. To compare antigen.
  c. To see the relative purity of antigen.
- Types of immunodiffusion reactions:
  a. Single diffusion in one dimension (Oudin Procedure).

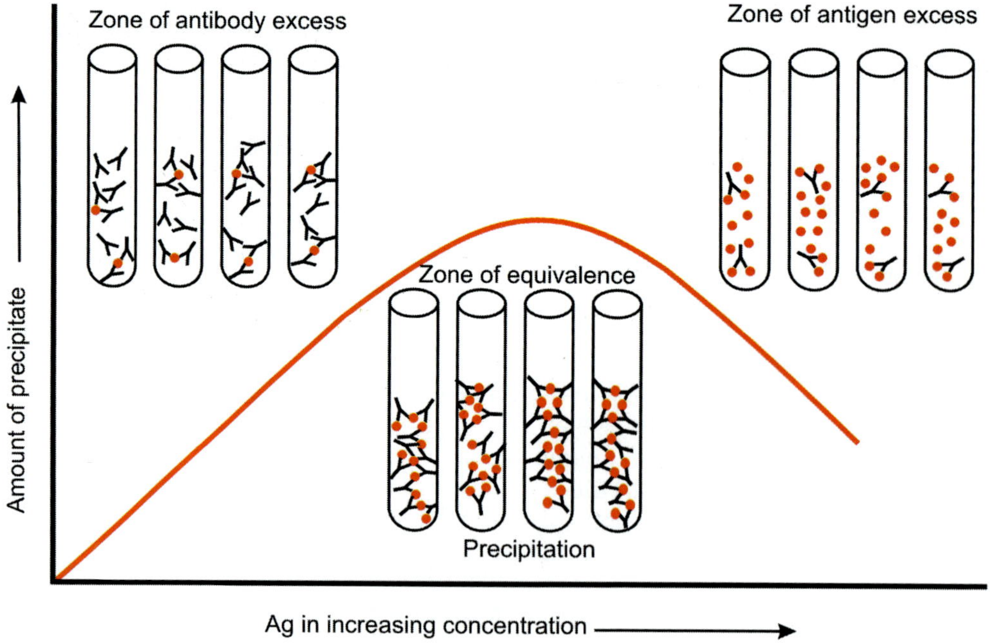

Fig. 8.2: Showing zone phenomenon

b. Double diffusion in one dimension (Oakley Fulthorpe Procedure).
c. Single diffusion in two dimension (Radial immunodiffusion).
d. Double diffusion in one dimension (Ouchterlony procedure).

- Single and double diffusion:
  a. In single diffusion either antigen or antibody is allowed to diffuse.
  b. In double diffusion, both the reactants are free to move towards each other.

Single Diffusion in One Dimension[1] (Figure 8.3)

- Was first introduced by Oudin from France in 1946.
- 1.5% solution of agar with a suitable dilution of an antiserum is taken in a glass tube or glass slide. Fluid antigen is then poured over the gel.
- As antigen diffuses down, a precipitate (ppt) is formed at the zone of equivalence.
- The molecular weight, shape and concentration of the antigen will influence the diffusion co-efficient and thus the rate of migration of antigen.
- By standardizing system with known concentrations of antigen and antibody, an unknown solution of antigen or antibody can be quantitated.[1]

Double Diffusion in One Dimension (Figure 8.3)

- A clear neutral agar zone is laid between the antigen and the antibody mixed agar. This technique can be useful for establishing the multiple Ag-Ab systems in complex reagents.[1]

Single Diffusion in Two Dimensions/Single Radial Immunodiffusion (Mancini)[2]: In this Modified Oudins Method, antibody is incorporated into the agar gel and then, different dilutions of the antigen are placed in holes punched into the agar. Antigen, then diffuses into the gel, it reacts with the antibody and when the equivalence point is reached a ring of precipitation is formed **(Figures 8.3 and 8.4)**.

This test is commonly used for the quantitation of immunoglobulin, complement etc.

Double Diffusion in Two Dimensions (Ouchterlony Double Diffusion)[1] (Figures 8.3 and 8.4)

- Plain gel is taken in a plate.
- Antigen and antibody are placed in separate wells cut in an agar plate.
- Antigen and antibody both diffuse and will form line of precipitate.
- Band form away from the well containing relatively excess amount of antigen or antibody.

By this technique, multiple wells in an agar plate can allow the demonstration of antigenic relationships among multiple antigens or antisera.

The rate of diffusion varies inversely with the molecular weight and therefore, the precipitin line is mainly concave to the well containing the reactant of high molecular weight, be it an antigen or an antibody.[1]

1. **Reactions of identity:** Smooth arc is formed when antigen present in peripheral wells are similar.
2. **Reaction of partial identity:** Line of precipitation is formed with a spur when cross reacting antigen are present.
3. **Reactions of non-identity:** Two separate arcs crossing each other when dissimilar antigen.

Immunoelectrophoresis[1] (Precipitation Reactions in Gel in an Electric Field)

- The technique combines an initial electrophoretic separation of proteins followed by immunodiffusion, which results in precipitation arcs.

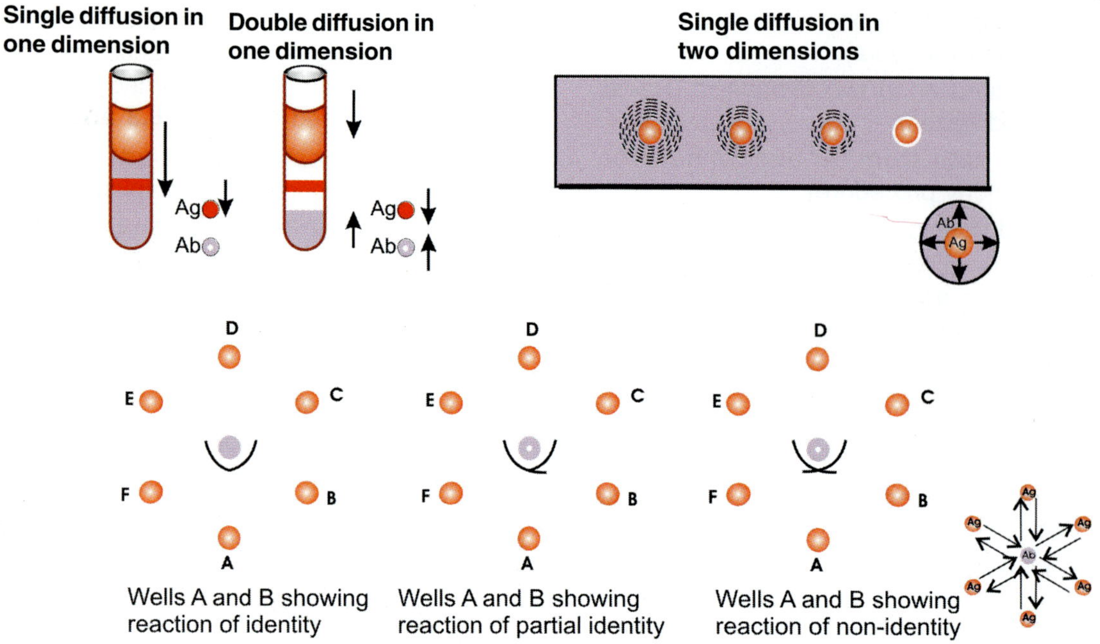

Fig. 8.3: Showing various immunodiffusion tests

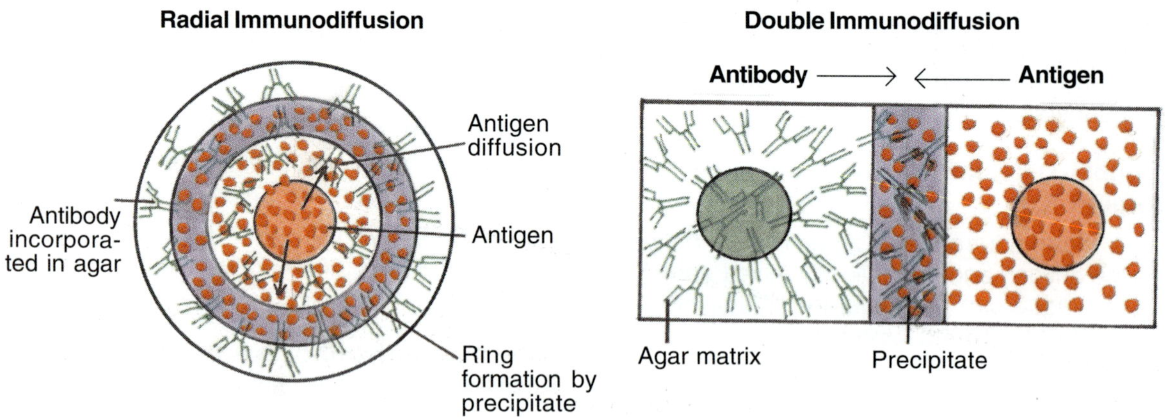

Fig. 8.4: Showing radial immunodiffusion and double immunodiffusion in a gel

- **Electroimmunodiffusion:** The diffusion is faster by applying constant electric current.
- **Application:** Detects the presence or absence of proteins in the serum (Immunodeficiency and Immunoproliferative disorders).

Electrodiffusion

- It is similar to immunodiffusion, but the antigen-antibody diffusion is enhanced by electric current.
- Two most common types are:

A. One Dimensional Double Electroimmunodiffusion (CIEP) Countercurrent Electrophoresis (Figure 8.5)

This is used for antigens and antibodies that can migrate in opposite directions in the electric fields. Wells are punched about 1 cm apart in an agar gel. Antigen and antibody solutions are placed in the wells towards cathode and anode sites respectively. Electric field is then applied electrophoresing both antigens and antibodies from separate wells. The antigen will migrate towards antibody and antibody will migrate towards antigen. A precipitin band will form in between the two wells.

The major advantage is its speed.

- This is 10 times more sensitive than double diffusion.
- Used for the diagnosis of number of infectious diseases.

B. One Dimensional Single Electroimmunodiffusion (Laurell's Rocket immunoelectrophoresis)[1]

In this technique, radial immunodiffusion and electrophoresis has been combined to quantitate negatively charged antigen rapidly.

- Gel with antiserum taken on a slide.
- Sample of antigen is placed in a well.
- Electrophoresis of antigen into the antibody containing agarose is done.
- The resultant pattern of immunoprecipitation will resemble a spike or rocket.
- Height of the resulting rocket shape zone is proportional to the Ag concentration.
- This technique is faster than radial diffusion method and sensitivity being 0.2 to 0.5 microgram per ml of proteins.[1]

AGGLUTINATION REACTIONS

- **Agglutination/Hemagglutination:** Here, the antigen is particulate and the reaction of an antibody with the antigen can be detected by agglutination (clumping) of the antigen.
- When the antigen is an RBC, the term hemagglutination is used.

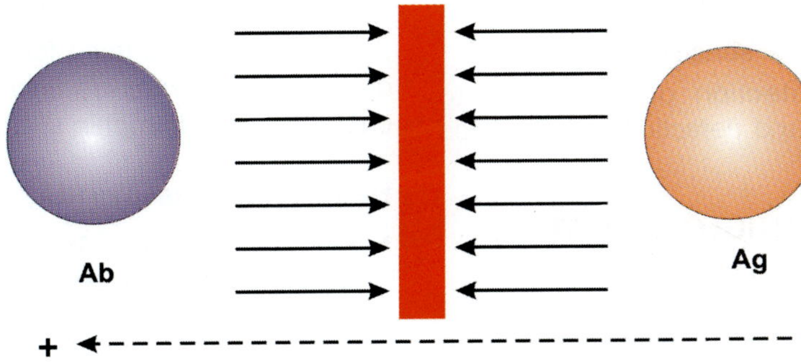

Fig. 8.5: Showing counter immunoelectrophoresis

- Antibodies that agglutinate particulate antigens are called agglutinins.

Qualitative Agglutination Test

Agglutination tests are used in a qualitative manner to assay for the presence of an antigen or an antibody.

- Antibody is mixed with the particulate antigen and a positive test is indicated by the agglutination of the particulate antigen.[4]
- It is used to determine blood types or antibodies to blood group antigens.

Quantitative Agglutination Test

- Agglutination tests are also used to quantitate the level of antibodies to particulate antigens.
- Here, serial dilutions of a sample are tested for antibody and then a fixed number of red blood cells or bacteria or other such particulate antigen is added and the maximum dilution is determined which gives agglutination. Titer is the maximum dilution that gives visible agglutination.
- Can be used to assess bacterial infections.

Passive Agglutination Test

- For identification of antibodies to soluble antigens, they are attached to the surface of various types of particles like RBC (hemagglutination test), polysterene, mineral colloid (bentonite).
- It is relatively more sensitive.
- Applications: Detection of antibodies to soluble antigens and detection of antibodies to viral antigens.[1]

COOMB'S TEST (ANTIGLOBULIN TEST)

Direct Coomb's Test

- Sensitization of RBCs with incomplete antibodies takes place *in vivo* as in case of haemolytic disease of newborn (HDN) due to Rh incompatibility. So, when washed RBCs from such patient are mixed with antiglobulin, agglutination occurs.[5]

Indirect Coomb's Test

- Sensitization of RBCs with incomplete antibodies is performed *in vitro.*
- Rh-positive RBCs are mixed with the serum to be tested for Rh-antibodies and after a short incubation and washing, antiglobulin is added.
- If the test serum was containing anti-Rh antibodies, agglutination will take place.
- Coomb's test is used for demonstrating non-agglutinating blocking antibodies in brucellosis.[5]

Hemagglutination Inhibition

- Here, the agglutination test is modified in order to measure soluble antigens.[1]
- We measure the ability of soluble antigen to inhibit the agglutination of antigen-coated RBCs by antibodies.[1]
- In this test, a fixed amount of antibodies to the unknown antigen is mixed with a fixed amount of RBCs coated with the antigen. If the sample contains the antigen, the soluble antigen will compete with the antigen coated on the RBCs for binding to antibodies, thus inhibiting the agglutination of the RBCs.
- By serial dilution of the sample, we can quantitate the amount of antigen in an unknown sample by its titer.

This assay was used for pregnancy tests to determine, if a woman's urine contained human chorionic gonadotrophin (HCG).[1]

Radioimmunoassay (RIA)[1]

- One of the most sensitive techniques to detect antigen or antibody.
- First developed by S. Aberson and Roselyn Yalow in 1960 to determine levels of insulin-anti insulin complexes in diabetics.[1]
- **Principle:** The test involves competitive binding of radio-labeled antigen and unlabeled antigen to a high affinity antibody.

- **Method**
  1. Ag is generally labeled with γ-ray-emitting iodine (^{125}I) or a beta emitting isotope such as tritium (^{3}H).
  2. Labeled antigen is then mixed with antibody at a concentration that just saturates antigen binding sites of antibody molecules and then increasing amount of unlabeled antigen are added.
  3. Both labeled and unlabeled antigens will compete for binding sites.
  4. There is decrease in amount of radioactive antigen bound, with increasing concentration. Therefore, this decrease is proportional to the amount of unlabeled antigen added.
  5. To detect, the amount of bound labeled Ag-Ab complexes are precipitated to separate it from free antigen and radioactivity as precipitate is measured.

Solid Phase Radioimmunoassay

It eliminates the need for the second antiserum (Anti-Ab).

Uses: To measure hormones, proteins, serum, vitamins and drugs[1]:

1. To detect hepatitis virus or viral Ag in blood.
2. To detect concentration of < 0.001 microgram/ml.

Enzyme Linked Immunosorbent Assay (ELISA)

Principle is similar to RIA but it depends on an enzyme label.

- Described by Enguall and Perlmann in 1972.[1]
- **Principle:** An enzyme conjugated with an antibody reacts with a colorless substrate to generate a colored reaction.
- Substrate is called chromogenic substrate.
- **Enzymes Used:** Horse radish peroxidase, alkaline phosphatase and beta-galactosidase.

  It is sensitive, safer, economical and allows qualitative detection as well as quantitative measurement of either antigen or antibody.
- **Variants of ELISA[2] (Figure 8.6)**
  1. Indirect ELISA – detects antibody.
  2. Sandwich ELISA – detects antigen, the most common version of the ELISA[6].
  3. Competitive ELISA – detects antigen.

ELISA

- **Chemiluminescence:** Measurement of light by chemiluminescence during certain chemical reactions is a convenient and highly sensitive alternative to absorbance measurements in ELISA assays.
- **Advantage:** Under ideal conditions as little as $5X10^{-18}$ moles of target antigen can be detected by this method.

ELISPOT ASSAY[2]

The normal ELISA assay is modified to measure antibody production at the single-cell level.[7] This assay can be used for quantitative determination of the number of cells in a population that are producing antibody specific for a given antigen or an antigen for which one has a specific antibody.[2]

- Wells or plates are coated with the antibody against the antigen to be determined.
- Suspension of cell population, which is considered to secrete the antigen is layered on the well and incubated.
- Most of the antigen secreted by particular cell reacts with nearby well bound antibody.
- Then, well is washed and enzyme labeled specific antibody specific to antigen is added.
- Chromogenic substrate is added.
- Colored product precipitates and forms a spot only on the areas where antigen secreting cells were deposited.
- By counting the number of cells, we can determine how many antigen secreting cells were present in added cell suspension.

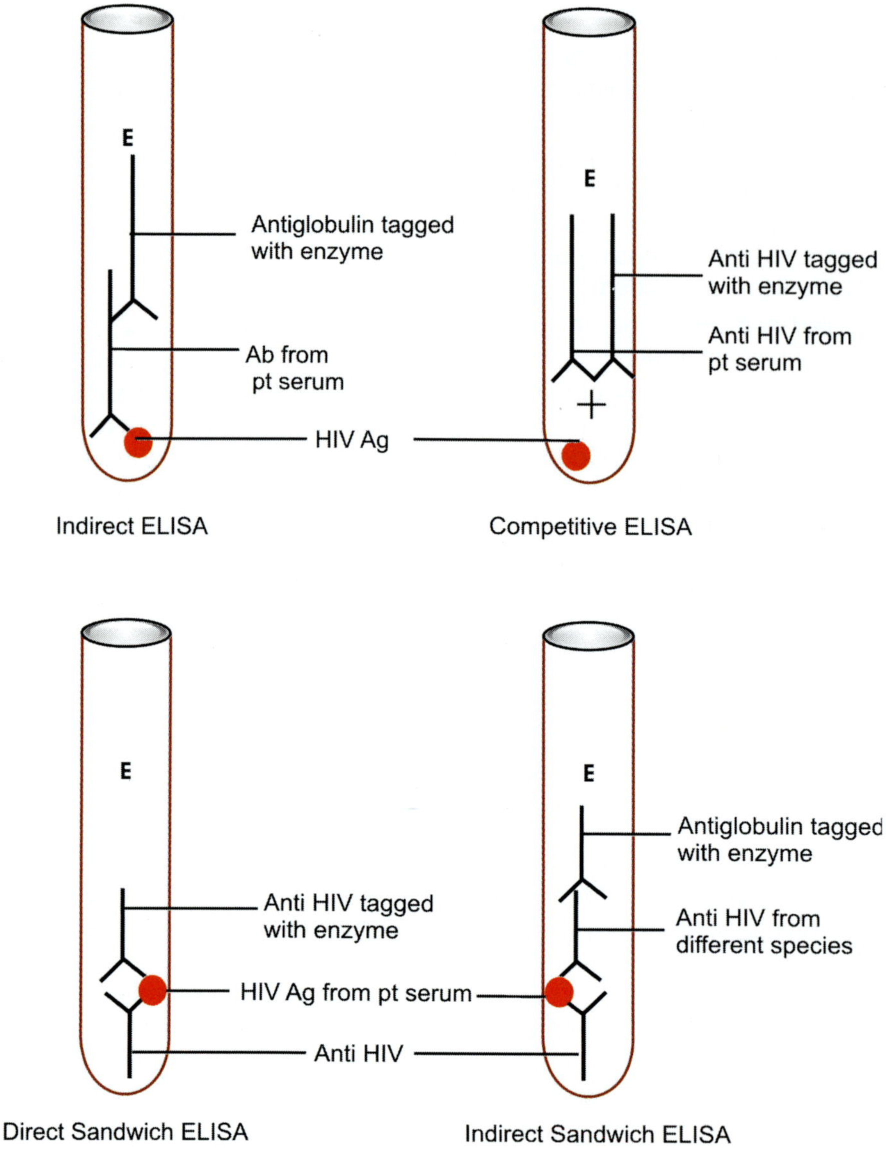

Fig. 8.6: Variants of enzyme linked immunosorbent assay (ELISA)

Western Blot

- To identify specific protein in a complex mixture of proteins.[2]
- Protein mixture is therefore, electrophoretically separated on SDS polyacrylamide gel (SDS PAGE).
- The protein bands are then transferred to a nitrocellulose membrane by capillary action.
- Individual protein bands are then identified by finding the nitrocellulose membrane with radiolabeled or enzyme linked antibody specific to the protein of interest.

- Ag-Ab complex recognized by autoradiography/chromogenic substitute chemiluminiscent.
- Can also identify specific antibody in a mixture **(Figure 8.7)**.
- **Application:** Confirmatory test for Human Immunodeficiency Virus (HIV).[2]

Immunoprecipitation[2]

- It provides a sensitive assay to detect the presence of a particular antigen in a given cell or tissue type.[2]

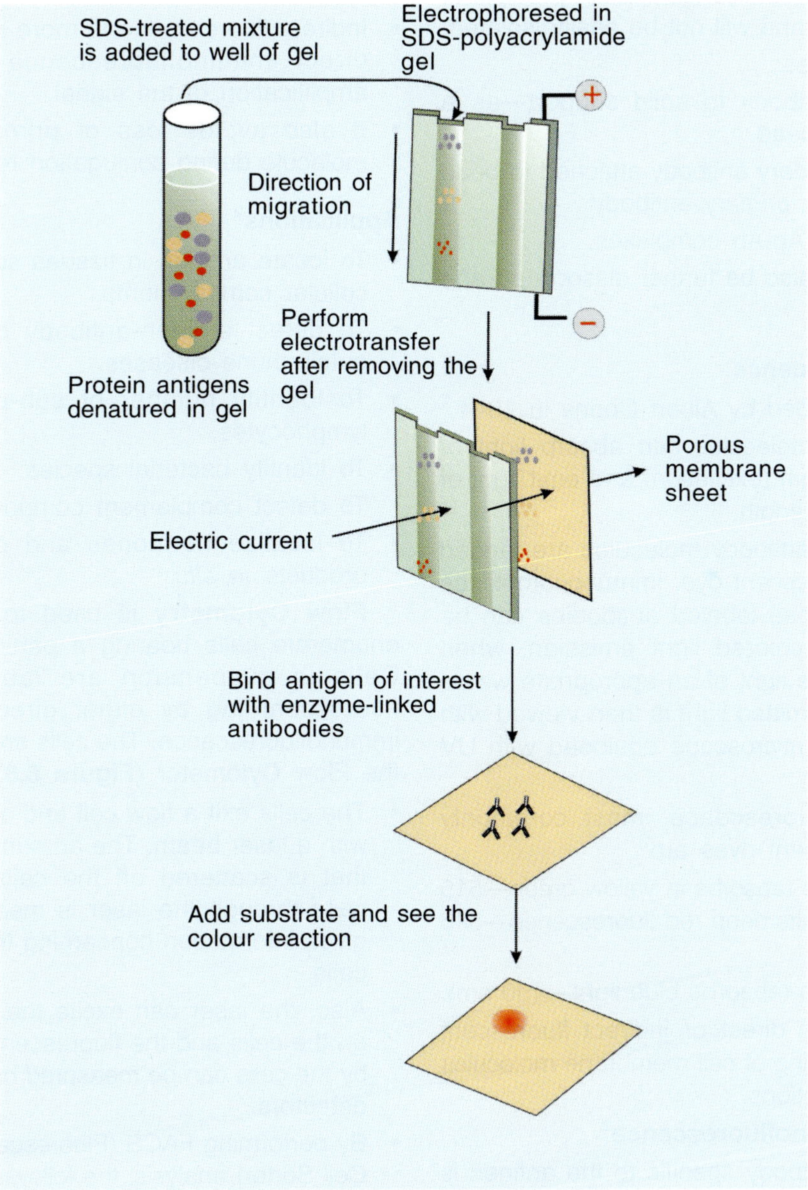

Fig. 8.7: Showing western blotting

- It can allow the isolation of antigen of interest.
- An extract produced by disruption of cells/ tissues mixed with antibody against antigen (to be determined) to form Ag-Ab complex that will precipitate.
- If antigen is in low concentration, precipitate is very small and will not be easily isolated.
- In these cases:
  - Attach antibody to solid support—as a synthetic bead.
  - Add secondary antibody attached to bead specific for primary antibody.
- Collection of Ag-Ab complexes.
- Antigen can also be further dissociated and studied.

Immunofluorescence

- It was described by Albert Coons in 1944.[2]
- Fluorescent molecules can absorb light of one wavelength (excitation) and emit light of another wavelength.
- **Principle:** If antibody molecules are tagged with the fluorescent dye, immunocomplexes containing these labeled antibodies can be detected by colored light emission, when excited by the light of an appropriate wavelength. The emitted light is then viewed with fluorescence microscope equipped with UV light source.[2]
- In immunofluorescence, most commonly used fluorescent dyes are[2]:
  - Rhodamine (absorbs in yellow green—515 nm and emits deep red fluorescence—546 nm).
  - Fluorescein (absorbs blue light—490 nm).
- There can be direct or indirect fluorescent antibody staining of cell membrane molecules or tissue sections.
- **Direct Immunofluorescence[2]**

  Here, the antibody specific to the antigen is directly tagged with the fluorochrome.

Indirect Immunofluorescence[2]

- Here, the antibody specific for the antigen is unlabeled and a second anti-immunoglobulin antibody directed toward the first antibody is tagged with the fluorochrome.

Uses

- Indirect fluorescence is more sensitive than direct immunofluorescence as there is amplification of the signal.
- It also avoids loss of primary antibody molecule during conjugation reduction.

Applications[2]

- To locate antigen in tissues section or sub-cellular compartments.
- To detect antigen-antibody complexes in autoimmune diseases.
- To identify number of sub-population of lymphocytes.
- To identify bacterial species.
- To detect complement components.
- To localize hormones and other cellular products *in situ*.

Flow Cytometry is used to identify and enumerate cells bearing a particular antigen. Cells in suspension are labeled with a fluorescent tag by either direct or indirect immunofluorescence. The cells are analyzed on the Flow Cytometer **(Figure 8.8).[2]**

- The cells exit a flow cell and are illuminated with a laser beam. The amount of laser light that is scattered off the cells, when they pass through the laser is measured, which gives information concerning the size of the cells.
- Also, the laser can excite the fluorochrome on the cells and the fluorescent light emitted by the cells can be measured by one or more detectors.
- By performing FACS (Fluorescence Activated Cell Sorter) analysis, the following information can be obtained[2]:

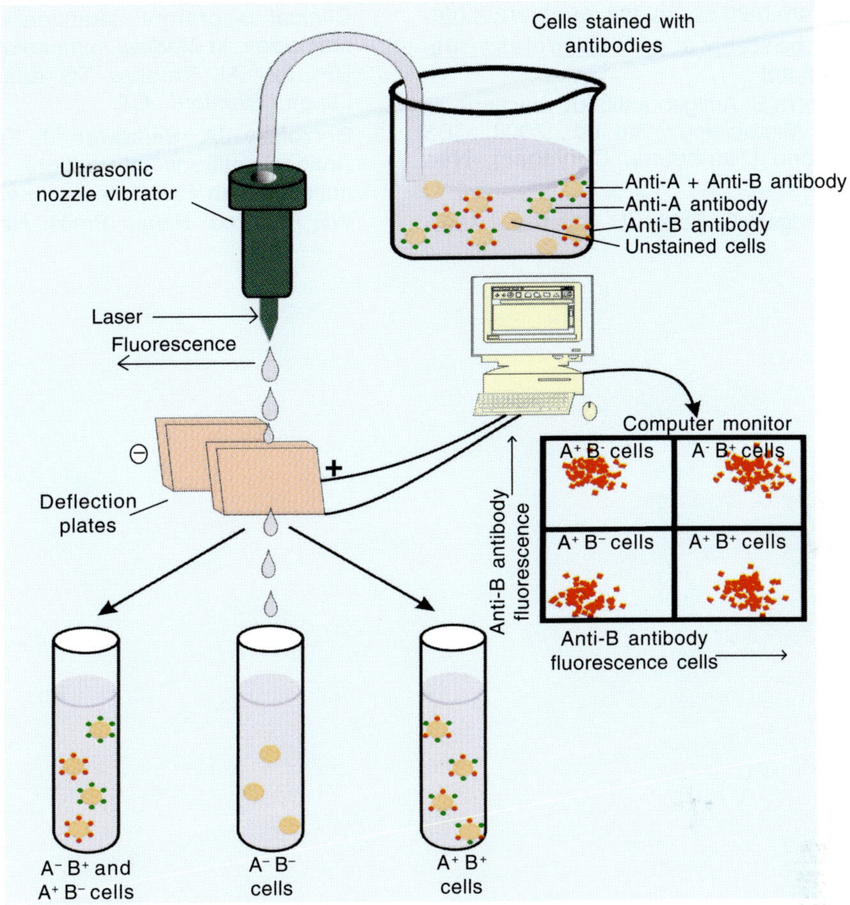

Fig. 8.8: Showing flowcytometry

- The number of cells expressing target antigen as an absolute member and also as percentage of cells passing the beam.
- Distribution of cells according to antigen densities as determined by fluorescence intensities.
- The size of the cells by analyzing light scattering.

At this time you should know the following:

1. The nature of antigen-antibody (Ag-Ab) reactions.
2. Antibody affinity and avidity.
3. The basis for antibody specificity and cross-reactivity.
4. The principles of tests used for antigen/antibody reactions.

References

1. Chakarvarthy AK 2006. Antigen- Antibody Reaction and Diagnostic Procedures. In *Immunology and Immunotechnology,* 1st ed., Chakarvarthy AK ed., Oxford University Press, New Delhi, pp 205-239.
2. Goldsby RA, Kindt TJ, Osborne BA, Kuby J 2003. Antigen-Antibody Interactions: Principles and Applications. In *Immunology,* 5th ed., Osborne B, Goldsby RA, Kindt T eds., W H Freeman, New York, pp 137-160.

3. http://pathmicro.med.sc.edu/mayer/ab-ag-rx.htm
4. http://www.postech.ac.kr/life/vi/class-file/chapter%206.ppt
5. Arora DR, Arora B. Antigen antibody reactions. In Textbook of Microbiology, 3rd ed., 2008; CBS Publishers and Distributors, Daryaganj, New Delhi.
6. Stites DP, Rodgers C, Folds JD, Schmitz J 1997. Clinical laboratory detection of antigens and antibodies. In *Medical Immunology,* 9th ed., Stites DP, Terr AI, Parslow TG eds., Appelton and Lange, Stamford, CT.
7. Berzofsky JA, Berkower IJ, Epstein SL 1991. Antigen-antibody interactions and monoclonal antibodies. In *Fundamental Immunology,* 3rd ed., WE Paul, ed. Raven Press, New York.

9

CHAPTER

Biogenesis of Antibodies

(Dr. Vinod Singh, Dr. Parul Tripathi, Dr. Ranjana Singh and Dr. R K Singh
vsingh3@rediff.com)

TEACHING OBJECTIVE

1. To describe general characteristics of the specific immune response.
2. To compare and contrast primary and secondary antibody responses.
3. To describe the molecular events involved in class switching and membrane immunoglobulin expression.

INTRODUCTION

Humoral immunity is mediated by antibodies, which are produced by cells of the B lymphocyte lineage. The physiologic function of antibodies is to neutralize and eliminate the antigen that induced their formation. The elimination of different antigens or microbes requires several effector mechanisms, which are dependent on distinct classes, or isotypes, of antibodies. The humoral immune system has the capacity to respond to different types of antigens by producing different classes of antibodies. For example, the antibody response to bacteria with polysaccharide rich capsules consists largely of immunoglobulin (Ig) M, which activates the complement system, leading to opsonization and phagocytosis of the bacteria; the response to many viruses consists of high-affinity IgG antibodies, which blocks virus entry into host cells and also promotes phagocytosis by macrophages; and the systemic response to many helminthic parasites is mainly IgE, which participates in eosinophil-mediated killing of the helminthes. The humoral immune response is also different at various anatomic sites. For instance, mucosal lymphoid tissues are uniquely adapted to produce high levels of IgA in response to the same antigens that stimulate other antibody isotypes in non-mucosal lymphoid tissues.

Production of all these varied classes of antibodies is initiated by the interaction of antigens with a small number of mature IgM and IgD expressing B lymphocytes specific for each antigen. Mature antigen-responsive B lymphocytes develop in the bone marrow prior to antigenic stimulation. Such cells enter into peripheral lymphoid tissues, which are the sites of interaction with foreign antigens. An antigen binds to the membrane IgM and IgD on specific B-cells and initiates a series of responses that lead to two principal changes in that clone of B-cells: proliferation, resulting in expansion of the clone, and differentiation, resulting in the progeny of the membrane Ig-expressing, antigen-responsive B-cells actively secreting antibodies of different heavy chain isotypes or becoming memory cells. The analysis of humoral immune responses is, in essence, an analysis of the growth and differentiation of B lymphocytes that occur following specific antigenic stimulation. Cellular basis of the humoral immune response, in particular the stimuli that induce B-cell growth and differentiation and the patterns of responses of B lymphocytes.

General Features of Humoral Immune Responses

The earliest studies of specific immunity were devoted to analyses of antibody responses. As a result, until the 1960s, much of our knowledge of the immune system was based on our understanding of humoral immunity. The most important general properties of antibody responses are the following:

Protein antigens do not induce antibody responses in the absence of T lymphocytes, for instance, in T-cell-deficient individuals. For this reason, proteins are classified as "thymus-dependent" or "T-dependent" antigens. The T-cells that are required for antibody production in response to protein antigens are called helper T-cells. As we shall see later in this chapter, a great role of T-cells in antibody responses is the basis of the concept that naive B-cells, which have not been previously exposed to antigen, require two distinct types of signals for their proliferation and differentiation. One type of signal is provided by the antigen, which interacts with membrane Ig molecules on specific B-cells. Helper T lymphocytes and their secreted products provide the second type of signal. The "two-signal" requirement for lymphocyte activation applies to T lymphocytes as well, because antigen specific helper and cytolytic T lymphocytes also need other stimuli, in addition to antigens, for their full growth and differentiation.

Non-protein antigens like polysaccharides and lipids induce antibody responses without a requirement for antigen-specific helper T lymphocytes. Therefore, polysaccharide and lipid antigens are called "thymus-independent" or "T-independent (TI)".

Antibody responses to T- independent antigens consist mainly of low affinity IgM and some IgG antibodies, with little memory cell generation. In contrast, helper T-cell-dependent responses to protein antigens are much more specialized, with different Ig isotypes, relatively high affinity antibodies and long live memory. The reason for this difference is that heavy chain isotype switching, affinity maturation and memory cell generation are all stimulated by T-helper cells and their products, and only protein antigens activate helper T-cells.

Primary and secondary antibody responses to protein antigens differ qualitatively (**Table 9.1**). Primary responses results from the activation of previously unstimulated B-cells, whereas secondary responses are due to stimulation of expanded clones of memory B-cells.

Signal Transduction by the B Lymphocyte Antigen Receptor Complex

The activation of B-lymphocytes is initiated by the binding of antigen to membrane Ig molecules on specific B-cells. This antigen-membrane Ig interaction can lead to two responses. First, the B lymphocyte antigen receptor delivers biochemical signals to the cells that initiate the

Table 9.1: Features of primary and secondary antibody responses

	Primary response	*Secondary response*
Lag after immunization	Usually 5-10 days	Usually 1-3 days
Peak response	Smaller	Larger
Antibody isotype	Usually IgM>IgG	Relative increase in IgG and, under certain situations, in IgA or IgE
Antibody affinity	Lower average affinity, more variable	Higher average affinity ("affinity maturation")
Induced by	All immunogens	Only protein antigens
Required immunization	Relatively high doses of antigens, optimally with adjuvants (for protein antigens)	Low doses of antigens, adjuvants may not be necessary

process of lymphocyte into endosomal vesicles, and if it is a protein, it is processed and peptides are presented on the B-cell surface for recognition by helper T-cells. Signal transduction by membrane Ig molecules requires the bringing together of two or more of these molecules on a B-cell by an antigen (or experimentally by an anti-Ig antibody) that is able to cross-link Ig molecules. Membrane IgM and IgD, the antigen receptors of resting, mature B-cells, have short cytoplasmic tails consisting of only three amino acids (lysine, valine and lysine).

These tails are too small to transduce signals generated by the clustering of Ig. Signaling via Ig is actually tansduced by two other molecules, called Igα and Igβ, which are members of the Ig super family and are expressed in mature B-cells noncovalently associated with membrane Ig. Igα and Igβ are also required for the surface expression of membrane Ig molecules and, together with membrane Ig, form the B lymphocyte antigen receptor complex. Thus, Igα and Igβ serve the same functions in B-cells as the CD3 and proteins do in T lymphocytes. As might be predicted from this functional similarity, Igα and Ig β contain in their cytoplasmic domains tyrosine-rich motifs (immunoreceptor tyrosine-based activation motifs, or ITAMs) that are also found in CD3 and are known, by mutational analysis, to be required for signal transduction.

The early functional responses to antigen-mediated cross-linking of the B-cell receptor complex are the following:

1. Entry of previously resting cells into the G1 stage of the cell cycle, accompanied by an increase in cell size and cytoplasmic ribonucleic acid (RNA), and increased numbers of biosynthetic organelles, such as ribosome.
2. Increased expression of class II molecules and co stimulators, first B7-2 and later B7-1, because of which antigen stimulated B-cells acquire the capacity to activate helper T lymphocytes; and
3. Increased expression of receptors for several T-cells-derived cytokines, thus enhancing the ability of the antigen specific B lymphocytes to respond to T-cell help. These responses are the result of several intracellular biochemical pathways that are known to be triggered by legation of membrane Ig molecules, similar to receptor-induced signals in T lymphocytes.
   1. Within minutes after cross-linking of membrane Ig, the tyrosines in the ITAMs of Igα and Igβ are phosphorylated, probably by the acton of src family kinases such as lyn, blk, and fyn. The non-src kinase syk then binds to the phosphotyrosine residues of Igα and Igβ, which provide docking sites for the SH2 domains of syk. Thus, syk is the B-cell equivalent of ZAP-70 in T lymphocytes. Syk needs to be phosphorylated by kinases or by syk phosphorylating itself. Mice in which syk is knocked out show a block in B-cell maturation at the pre-B stage, because the enzyme also tansduces signals from the antigen receptor that are required for B-cell development.
   2. The activated kinases may in turn activate numerous substrates. One of these is the γ1 isoform of phosphatidylinositol phospholipase C, which breaks down membrane phosphatidylinositol bisphosphate to generate inositol trisphosphate (IP3) and diacyl-glycerol (DAG). IP_3 mobilizes ionic Ca^{2+} from intracellular stores, leading to a rapid elevation of cytoplasmic Ca^{2+}, which may be augmented by an influx of Ca^{2+}, from the extracellular milieu. In the presence of Ca^{2+}, DAG activates some isoforms of protein kinase C (PKC), and PKC in turn phosphorylates other proteins on serine/theronine residues.
   3. The Ras protein is also activated by Ig cross-linking, and this is associated with activation of kinases of the mitogen-activated protein kinase family, as in T-cells.
   4. A consequence of protein kinase activation is the activaton of various transcription

factors, which induce new gene expression in antigen-stimulated B lymphocytes. Some of the transcription factors that are known to be activated by antigen receptor-mediated signal tansduction in B-cells are c-Fos, JunB, NFkB, and c-Myc.

As in other lymphocytes, many steps in these signaling cascades are incompletely understood. The same pathways are utilized by membrane IgM and IgD on naive B-cells and by other Ig heavy chains on B-cells that have undergone isotype switching, because all these membrane isotypes appear to associate with Igα and Igβ. Also, other surface molecules augment or inhibit signals tansduced by the antigen receptors. These molecules include the type 2-complement receptor (CR2, or CD21) and the B-cell Fc receptor, Fcγ RIIB. The physiologic significance and mechanisms of these regulatory interactions are discussed later in the chapter.

The importance of signaling by the B-cell receptor complex for subsequent proliferation and differentiation of the cells may vary with the nature of the antigen. Many globular protein antigens may not express more than one identical epitope per molecule in their native conformation, in which case they cannot simultaneously bind to and cross-link two Ig molecules. However, even proteins may cross-link antigen receptors if they form aggregates, e.g., as a result of the binding of "natural antibodies" or complement components. Moreover, protein antigens recruit T-cell help, and helper T-cells and their products are capable of inducing B lymphocyte proliferation and differentiation by themselves. This is suggested by the finding that peptide antigens or monovalent anti-Ig antibodies, which cannot cross-link membrane Ig, can induce B-cell responses in the presence of specific helper T-cells. Therefore, protein antigens may only need to trigger minimal signals by the B-cell receptor complex in order to generate humoral immune responses. In such responses, a major function of membrane Ig may be to bind and internalize the antigen for subsequent presentation to helper T-cells. In contrast, most T-independent antigens, such as polysaccharides and glycolipids, are polymeric, i.e., they contain multiple identical epitopes on each molecule. Therefore, such antigens effectively cross-link B-cell antigen receptors and initiate responses even though they are not recognized by helper T lymphocytes. Signaling by the B-cell antigen receptor may also contribute to enhanced survival of the B-cells by blocking various pathways of apoptosis.

After antigen binding has initiated B lymphocyte activation, the subsequent proliferation and differentiation of the cells are stimulated by their interaction with helper T-cells.

Mechanisms of Helper T Lymphocyte-Dependent Antibody Responses

Antibody responses to protein antigens require recognition of the antigen by helper T-cells and cooperation between the antigen-specific B and T lymphocytes. The helper function of T lymphocytes was discovered by experiments in the late 1960s, even before the classification of lymphocytes into T and B-cell subsets was established. Several in vitro experiments have shown that B-cells would proliferate and differentiate in response to protein antigens only if helper T lymphocytes were also present. Subsequent studies have established that most helper T-cells are CD4+ CD8- and class II MHC-restricted in their recognition of foreign protein antigens. Both helper T-cells and B-cell are stimulated by primary immunization, and both are responsible for enhanced antibody production in secondary responses.

Helper T-cell-dependent antibody responses to protein antigens consist of distinct steps. Each step ensures that antigen-specific B and T lymphocytes interact and function in a bidirectional manner to stimulate one another. The T-B-cell interaction is called a "cognate" interaction because it is dependent on the specific recognition of antigen and several other surface molecules on the two interacting cells. The mechanism underlying most of the phases of T-dependent B-cell activation are now understood in quite precise biochemical terms.

Presentation of Protein Antigens by B Lymphocytes to Helper T-Cells

Antigen-specific B lymphocytes bind the native antigen to membrane Ig molecules, internalize and process it in endosomal vesicles, and present on their surface peptide fragments of the antigen complexes to class II MHC molecules.

Thus, the B-cells themselves function as antigen presenting cells (APCs). The peptide - MHC complexes can then be recognized by specific $CD4^+$ helper T lymphocytes.

Our current understanding of antigen presentation by B lymphocytes, and its role in the development of humoral immune responses, evolved from studies aimed at anlayzing antibody responses to hapten-carrier conjugates. Haptens, such as dinitrophenol, are small chemicals that can be bound by B-cell membrane Ig and by self created antibodies but are not immunogenic by themselves. If, however, the haptens are coupled to proteins, which serve as carriers, the conjugates are able to induce antibody responses against the haptens. There are three important characteristics of anti-hapten antibody responses stimulated by hapten-protein conjugates. First, such responses require co-operation between hapten-specific B-cells and protein (carrier) specific helper T-cells. Second, in order to stimulate a response, the hapten and carrier portions have to be physically linked and cannot be administered separately. Third, the interaction is class II MHC-restricted; i.e., the helper T-cells cooperate only with B lymphocytes that express class II MHC molecules recognized as self by the T-cells. The same characteristic applies not only to hapten-protein conjugates but to all protein antigens in which one intrinsic determinant is recognized by B-cells (and is, therefore, analogous to the hapten) and another determinant is recognized by helper T-cells (and is analogous to the carrier).

The explanations for these features of antibody responses to protein antigens and hapten protein conjugates became clear when it was appreciated that B lymphocytes are extremely efficient APCs. Hapten-specific B-cells bind the antigen via the hapten determinant and present peptides derived from the carrier protein to carrier specific helper T lymphocytes. Thus, the two cooperating lymphocytes recognize different epitopes of the same complex antigen. The hapten is responsible for efficient carrier uptake, explaining why hapten and carrier must be physically linked. The requirement for MHC-associated antigen presentation for Tcell-B cell interactions.

At the same time that antigen is being processed and presented, the B lymphocytes have been activated by membrane Ig cross-linking. One of the consequences of activation is the enhanced expression of costimulators, including B7 molecules, on the B-cells. Helper T-cells can then recognize peptide-MHC complexes (signal 1 for T-cells) and costimulators (signal 2) and are stimulated to perform their effector function, which is to promote B-cell growth and differentiation. As we shall see later, this activation of B-cells results from stimuli generated by physical contact with helper T-cells and by cytokines secreted by the T-cells.

In any humoral immune response, B-cells specific for the antigen that initiates the response are preferentially activated as compared with bystander cells that are not specific for the antigen. There are several reasons for this. First, only B-cells expressing specific membrane Ig molecules that bind the antigen receive the first signal for activation. Second, antigen-specific B-cells are able to present the antigen at 10^4 to 10^{6-} fold lower concentrations than all other APCs.

The efficiency of Ig-mediated antigen internalization and subsequent presentation is because membrane Ig molecules specifically bind the antigen at low concentrations, and antigens endocytosed with Ig are delivered to the intracellular protein processing pathway that is especially efficient at generating class II MHC-peptide complexes. As a result, whenever antigen concentrations are limiting, specific B-cells are the preferential APCs. Third, as we shall discuss below, specific antigen recognition induces several surface molecules on the B-cells and helper T lymphocytes that bring the two cell types into direct contact. The B-cells in these T-B conjugates are exposed to signals delivered by T-cell surface molecules and to the highest concentrations of

T-cell help and are stimulated to proliferate and differentiate. The antibodies that are subsequently secreted are specific for conformational determinants of the antigen, because membrane Ig on B-cells is capable of binding conformational epitopes of native antigens. This feature determines the fine specificity of the helper T-cells in recognizing only linear epitopes of processed peptides. In fact, a single B lymphocyte may bind and endocytose a protein and present multiple different peptides complexed with class II MHC molecules to different helper T-cells, but the resultant antibody response remains specific for the native protein.

Although it is clear that B-cells need to function as APCs for MHC restricted T-cell-B-cell interactions to occur, it is likely that other APCs are required for initiating the activation of helper T-cells in primary antibody responses **(Figure 9.1)**. There are several reasons for this conclusion.

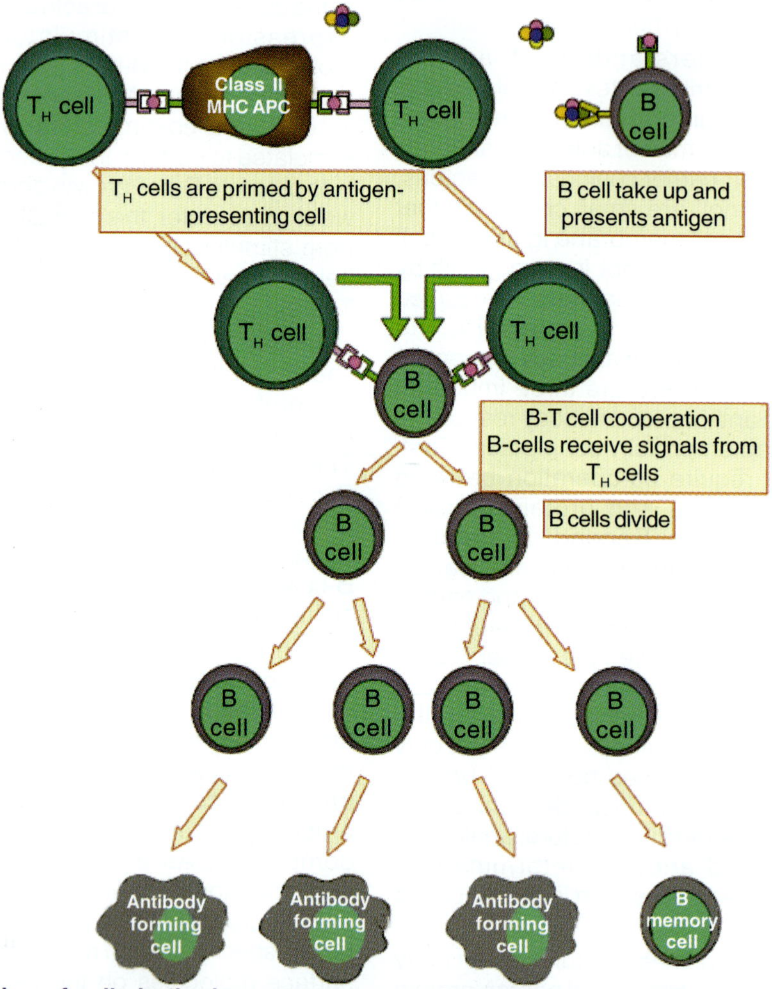

Fig. 9.1: Cooperation of cells in the immune response. Antigen-presenting cells (e.g. dendritic cells) present processed antigen to naive T cells, thereby priming them. B-cells also process the antigen and present it to the T cells. They then receive signals from the T cells that cause them to divide and differentiate. Some B-cells form antibody-forming cells while a few form B memory cells (Source: Nature Medicine 2001, Vol. 34, 56-78)

Naive B lymphocytes are inefficient at stimulating resting T-cells and may even induce T-cells tolerance, mainly because naive B-cells are deficient in co stimulators. In unimmunized individuals, there may be few B-cells specific for a particular antigen that they cannot effectively initiate a T-cell response. Furthermore, it is known that for generating optimal primary antibody responses to protein antigens the antigens have to be administered with adjuvants, and one function of adjuvants is to enhance the antigen-presenting functions of macrophages. Therefore, when an individual is exposed to a protein antigen for the first time, APCs such as macrophages and dendritic cells may process and present the antigen to naive helper T-cells. These activated T-cells then interact with B-cells that also present the antigen, and primary response ensues. In secondary responses, on the other hand, antigen-specific memory B-cells may be fully capable of functioning as APCs for the helper T-cells that have previously been stimulated to become effector cells. This is supported by the observation that secondary antibody responses in vitro require only activated B and helper T-cells and antigen.

Helper T-cell Mediated Activation of B Lymphocytes

The physical contact between B-cells specific for the native antigen and helper T lymphocytes specific for processed peptides is mediated by multiple ligand-receptor pairs, some of which deliver signals to the B-cells that are required for the full development of the humoral immune response. The two critical ligand-receptors pairs, in addition to antigen and antigen receptors, are B7 molecules: CD28 and CD40:CD40 ligand. As we mentioned previously, antigen recognition by B-cells enhances the expression of costimulators, first B7-2 and then B7-1. These consitmulators are recognized by CD28 on helper T-cells, which are, at the same time, interacting with peptide-class II MHC complexes on the B-cells. The helper T-cells thus receive the two sets of stimuli they need for their activation. Upon activation, helper T-cells express a 34-39 kD surface molecule called CD40 ligand, which specifically binds to a constitutively expressed B-cell receptor called CD40. CD40 is a member of a family of cell surface proteins that includes tumor necrosis factor (TNF) receptors and a protein called Fas. The interaction of CD40 ligand with CD40 triggers intracellular biochemical signals in B-cells which leads to their process of activation **(Figure 9.2)**.

Some studies suggest that the B7:CD28 and CD40 ligand: CD40 pairs may interact in the reverse sequence. T-cells are first activated by antigen presented by dendritic cells or macrophages, and this activation induces expression of CD40 ligand. When these helper T-cells see antigen presented by specific B-cells, CD40 ligand interacts with CD40 on the B-cells. This not only stimulates B-cells proliferation and differentiation but also leads to enhance expression of B7 molecules, thus causing more T cell activation. In either case, the interaction between helper T-cells and B-cells is bi-directional. Because the expression of both B7 and CD40 ligand is regulated, i.e., it is dependent on antigen mediated stimulation, only lymphocytes specifically stimulated by antigen interact bi-directionally with one another, thus maintaining the specificity of the immune response.

The critical role of this interaction in antibody production is illustrated by the findings that knockout mice lacking the gene for any member of the two ligand: receptor pairs, i.e., B7 (both B7-1 and B7-2), CD28, CD40 or CD40 ligand, exhibit profound defects in isotype switching, affinity maturation, and memory B-cell generation in response to protein antigens. Mutations in CD40 ligand are also responsible for an inherited immunodeficiency of humans, called the X-linked hyper IgM syndrome, in which patients are unable to produce normal amounts of most IgG, IgA and IgE antibodies against proteins.

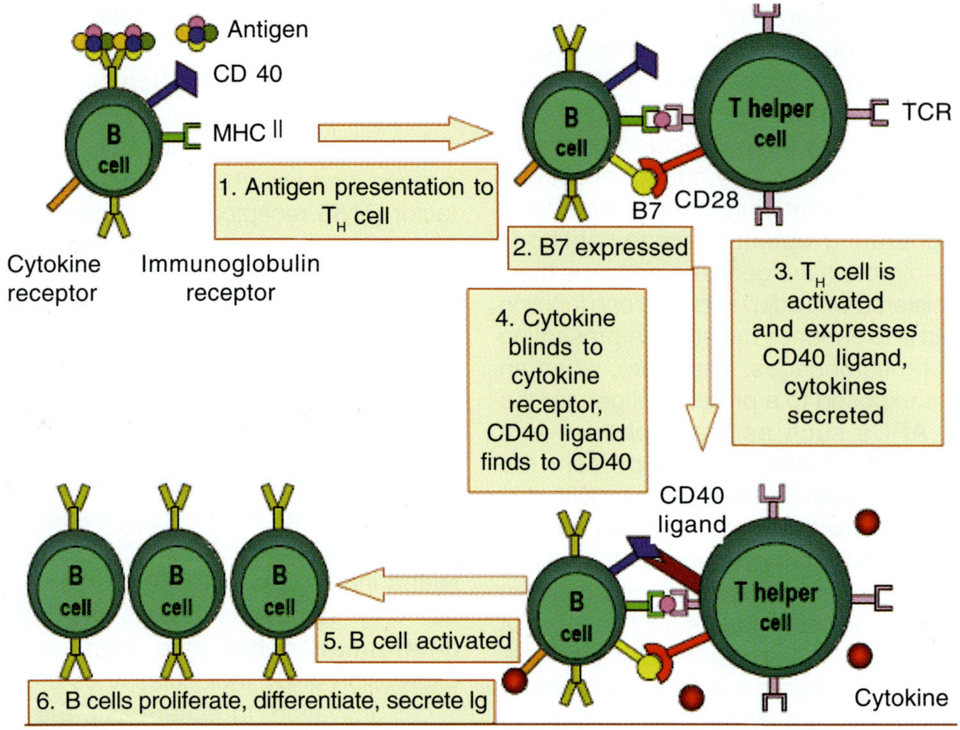

Fig. 9.2: Molecules involved in the interactions of B and T_H cells. Antigen is processed by B cell. Costimulators are expressed. The processed antigen peptide is presented in association with class II MHC. The T cell recognizes the peptide along with the MHC and the co-stimulators. The T cell expresses CD40 ligand. The latter binds to CD40 antigen on the B cell and the B-cells divide and differentiate. Antibodies are produced by the B cell
(Source: Nature Medicine 2001 Vol 34, 56-78)

Role of CD40 in Humoral Immune Responses

The requirement for physical contact between helper T and B lymphocytes in the generation of antibody responses was first suspected when it was found that the helper function of T lymphocytes could not be replaced by their secreted products (cytokines). Subsequent experiments showed that if helper T-cells are first activated with antigen, chemically fixed to render them incapable of producing cytokines, and then co-cultured with B-cells, they are still able to induce proliferation of the B-cells. The same responses are seen if the B-cells are cultured with purified plasma membranes of activated helper T lymphocytes. In the absence of cytokines, fixed T-cells or membranes induce only modest B cell proliferation. The full proliferation of B-cells and their differentiation into antibody-producing cells do require cytokines, as we shall discuss later.

Such results suggested that activated helper T lymphocytes express a membrane molecule(s) that binds to a receptor on B lymphocytes, and this interaction provides the stimulus that initiates B cell responses. Antibodies that blocked T-dependent B cell activation were used to identify the relevant surface molecules, which turned out to be CD40 on the B-cells and its ligand-receptor pair. Fibroblasts expressing CD40 ligand (by gene transfection) stimulate B-cells much like contact with helper T lymphocytes, and antibodies to CD40 can directly activate B-cells, presumably by functioning like CD40 ligand. The obligatory role of these molecules is demonstrated by gene knockout and inherited mutations, as mentioned above.

Members of the TNF receptor/Fas/CD40 family determine the fates of many cell populations in the immune system by regulating the choice between cell death and proliferation. Thus, these proteins serve a variety of roles in immune responses. CD40 ligand is a membrane protein that is structurally homologous to TNF and Fas ligand. CD40 ligand is rapidly induced on T-cells upon their activation. Its binding to CD40 results in oligomerization of CD40 molecules, and this apparently induces the association of cytoplasmic proteins (called TNF receptor-associated factors, or TRAFs) to the cytoplasmic C-terminal domains of CD40.

The TRAFs are in turn activated and, via kinases and biochemical intermediates that are not yet well defined, lead to the activation and nuclear translocation of transcription factors, including NFkB. The links between these transcription factors and changes in Ig gene expression, i.e., isotope switching, or induction of germinal center reactions, are not yet understood. T-cell- mediated macrophage activation may also involve the interaction of CD40 ligand on T-cells with CD40 on macrophages. Thus, this pathway of contact-mediated cellular responses is a general mechanism for the activation of target effector cells by helper T lymphocytes and is not unique to antibody production.

Interestingly, a DNA virus called Epstein Barr virus (EBV) infects human B-cells and induces their proliferation. This may lead to immortalization of the cells and the development of lymphomas. The cytoplasmic domain of a transforming protein of EBV associates with the same TRAF molecules as the cytoplasmic domain of CD40, and this apparently triggers B cell proliferation. Thus, the viral protein is functionally homologous to the physiologic B cell-signaling molecule, and EBV has apparently co-opted a normal pathway of B lymphocyte activation for its own purpose, which is to promote survival of cells the virus has infected.

B Lymphocyte Growth and Differentiation (Helper Factors)

Cytokines are soluble proteins secreted by T lymphocytes and by other cell types in response to activating stimuli. Cytokines mediate many of the effectors functions of the cells that produce them and are the principle mechanisms by which various immune and inflammatory cell populations communicate with one another. Although cytokines are produced as a result of the stimulation of specific T-cells by antigens, the cytokines themselves are not antigen-specific and do not bind to antigens. The roles of these secreted proteins in humoral immunity have been most clearly established by showing that various aspects of antibody responses can be inhibited by cytokine antagonists, or are deficient in mice in which particular cytokine genes are knocked out by homologous recombination.

Cytokines serve two principal functions in antibodies production by selectively promoting switching to different heavy chain isotypes, and they provide amplification mechanisms by augmenting B cell proliferation and differentiation. Different cytokines play distinct, but often overlapping, roles in antibody production, and their actions may be synergistic or antagonistic. Antigen recognition by B-cells enhances the expression of receptors for cytokines, and B-cells in direct contact with helper T lymphocytes are presumably exposed to high concentrations of these secreted proteins. As a result, antigen-specific B-cells respond to cytokines more than do "bystander" B-cells that are not specific for the initiating antigen but happen to be close to the antigen-stimulated lymphocytes.

Based on a variety of *in vitro* and *in vivo* studies, it is now possible to identify the cytokines that act at each stage of B cell activation.

1. *Proliferation:* Many different cytokines have been shown to stimulate the proliferation of B-cells *in vitro*. Three helper T cell-derived cytokines, interleukin IL-2, IL-4, and IL-5 all

contribute to B cell proliferation and may act synergistically. IL-6, which is produced by macrophages, T-cells, and many other cell types, is growth factor for already differentiated, antibody-secreting B-cells. Three other cytokines produced by macrophages, IL-1, IL-10 and TNF, also promote some B cell proliferation *in vitro*. The redundancy in the actions of these cytokines accounts for the observation that knockout of any one cytokine gene, or an antagonist that blocks the function of any one, has virtually no effect on B cell growth in response to protein antigens.

2. *Antibody secretion:* Antibody synthesis and secretion in response to protein antigens, like B cell proliferation, are also enhanced by cytokines. In the mouse, IL-4 and IL-5 are potent inducers of antibody secretion by B-cells. Human B-cells cultured with polyclonal activators secrete high levels of antibody if IL-2, IL-6 or IL-10 is added. It is not clear whether these differences in the cytokine responses of human and mouse B-cells are due to true species variations or merely reflect differences in experimental conditions.
3. *Isotype switching:* The most selective, and only obligatory, functions of different cytokines in humoral immune responses are in regulating the pattern of heavy chain isotype switching. We have mentioned previously that heavy chain isotype switching is typically seen with protein antigens and requires helper T-cells. Different T cell-derived cytokines selectively induce switching to particular Ig isotypes. For instance, IL-4 is the principal switch factor for IgE in all species examined. IgE production depends on IL-4, since IgE responses to antigen-specific or polyclonal stimulation *in vitro*, and to infection by helminthic parasites *in vivo*, are abrogated by antibodies that neutralize IL-4 and IL-4-deficient mice created by gene knockout. These findings have many practical implications, since IgE antibodies are involved in host defense against parasitic infestations and in immediate hypersensitivity (allergic) reactions.

The production of IgG2a in mice is dependent on interferon-γ (IFN-γ), which is also secreted by T-cells. Therefore, addition of IL-4 or IFN-γ induces switching to different isotypes in cultures of mature IgM and IgD-expressing B-cells stimulated with antigens or polyclonal activators. Interestingly, IFN-γ inhibits IL-4 induced B cell switching of IgE, and, conversely, IL-4 reduces IgG2a production. These are among the clearest examples of the antagonistic effects of different cytokines. Transforming growth factor-B, which is produced by many cell types, acts in concert with T cell-derived IL-5 to stimulate IgA production in mucosal lymphoid tissues. These two cytokines may, therefore, be especially important in mucosal immunity.

Cytokines induce switching to different heavy chain classes by triggering the process of switch recombination. In naive B-cells, which produce IgM, engagement of CD40 and exposure to a particular cytokine stimulates transcription through switch (S) regions located 5' of particular heavy chain constant (C) region genes. For instance, IL-4 induces transcription through the Se-Ce locus, and in mice IFN-γ through the Sγ2a-$C_{\gamma 2a}$ locus. This leads first to the production of sterile or "germline" transcripts. Subsequently, the rearranged VDJ complex in that B cell recombines with the downstream C ration that has become transcriptionally active, leading to the production of a new heavy chain with the same V region as the original IgM.

Germinal Center Reactions: Affinity Maturation and the Generation of Memory B-cells

The generation of high-affinity antibodies and memory B-cells in response to protein antigens occurs in germinal centers. Morphologic studies of antibody production *in vivo* show that the initial B cell response to protein antigens occurs mainly at the edges of T cell-rich zones, e.g., in the periarteriolar sheaths of the spleen. Within 4 to 7 days after antigen administration, some of the activated B-cells migrate into an adjacent lymphoid follicle and begin to proliferate rapidly, forming the lightly staining central region of the follicle, called the germinal center. The doubling time of germinal center B-cells is estimated to be 6 to 12 hours, so that within 5 days a single lymphocyte may give rise to almost 5000 progeny. The IgV genes of these rapidly dividing B-cells undergo somatic hypermutation, because of which V gene mutations accumulate sequentially in the progeny of the B-cells.

As these processes are going on in lymphoid tissues, antibodies that have been secreted into the circulation bind to residual antigen molecules and may activate the complement cascade. Antigen-antibody complexes with attached complement proteins are avidly bound to the surfaces of follicular dendritic cells in the germinal centers, because these cells express high-affinity receptors for complement proteins and for the Fc regions of IgG molecules. (Follicular dendritic cells are found only in germinal centers, do not express class II MHC molecules, and are different from the dendritic cells that present peptide antigens to CD4+ T lymphocytes). Somatically mutated B-cells whose membrane Ig molecules are able to recognize the displayed antigen are selected to survive. It is postulated that the survival signal may be delivered by antigen binding to membrane Ig and by CD40 ligand, expressed on follicular dendritic cells, binding to CD40 on the B lymphocytes. If somatic mutations have generated B cell antigen receptors that no longer recognize the antigen, these cells die by a process of apoptotic programmed cell death, because activated B-lymphocytes need to recognize antigen and other stimuli to be protected from programmed death. As the antibody response develops, the amount of antigen available for display on follicular dendritic cells decreases regressively. As a result, in order to be positively selected, the B-cells need to express Ig receptors with progressively higher affinity for the antigen. This is the basis for affinity maturation of the antibody response. Not surprisingly, many B-cells with V region mutations lose the ability to recognize antigen and cannot be selected, so that the germinal centers are sites of tremendous apoptosis. Macrophages present in the germinal centers rapidly phagocytose and clear these dead lymphocytes. During these selection processes, B-cells migrate from the basal dark zone of the germinal center, where the greatest proliferation occurs, to the basal light zone, which is the site of antigen-driven selection, and then to the apical zone, where additional isotype switching may occur. The cells then exit the germinal center and develop into high-rate antibody secretors in extra-follicular sites. Germinal centers gradually decrease in size and number and may involute by 1 to 2 weeks after immunization. At this time, affinity maturation also ceases unless the antigen is persistent or is re-administered.

Some of the B-cells do not develop into antibody secretors. Instead, they acquire the ability to survive for long periods, apparently without antigenic stimulation, and to circulate freely between the blood and lymphoid tissues, including germinal centers. These are memory cells, capable of mounting rapid responses to subsequent introduction of antigen. It is possible that memory cells are actually continually generated and maintained by low-level stimulation provided by antigen, which may be displayed on follicular dendritic cells for months or years. We do not know why some of the progeny of an antigen-stimulated B cell clone differentiate into antibody-secreting cells with brief life spans while others become functionally quiescent, long-lived memory cells.

The biochemical mechanisms of germinal center reactions are not well understood. These reactions require helper T-cells, because they are seen almost exclusively after immunization with protein antigens. A few CD4 T lymphocytes are found within germinal centers and have probably migrated after their activation in extra-follicular regions. It is not known if these T-cells provide specific contact-mediated signals or cytokines that stimulate somatic hyper mutation and memory B cell generation. Interactions between CD40 and CD40 ligand required for germinal center reactions do not develop in humans or mice with mutations or knockout of either CD40 or its ligand. As mentioned above, CD40 ligand on follicular dendritic cells may promote the survival of high-affinity B lymphocytes. The adhesion between follicular dendritic cells and activated B lymphocytes may be facilitated by the integrin VLA-4 (CD29CD49d), expressed on the lymphocytes, and its ligand, vascular cell adhesion molecule-1, on follicular dendritic cells. The same ligand-receptor pair promotes the migration of memory B-cells into germinal centers, where depots of antigen are displayed.

Sequence of Events in Antibody Response to Protein Antigens In Vivo

Now that we have described the cellular and molecular interactions that occur in different phases of helper T cell-dependent B lymphocyte activation. It is useful to summarize the sequence of events that occur in humoral immune responses *in vivo.* This process is best described in the spleen but is probably similar in lymph nodes and other lymphoid tissues.

Within 1 or 2 days after administration of a protein antigen to a naive individual, the antigen is processed and presented by dendritic cells and macrophages to specific CD+ T lymphocytes in the T cell-rich zones of the spleen and lymph nodes. Clusters of activated T-cells that express CD40 ligand and produce various cytokines are detectable in these regions. Specific B lymphocytes also encounter the antigen, are activated by helper T lymphocytes. As a result of cell-cell contact mediated by CD40 and CD40 ligand, as well as exposure to T cell cytokines, the antigen specific B-cells begin to proliferate, differentiate into antibody-secreting cells, and undergo heavy chain class switching.

Thus, by 4 to 7 days after antigen exposure, antibody-producing B-cells are found in close proximity to activated T lymphocytes. Antibody secretion and heavy chain class switching constitute the extra-follicular pathway of B cell differentiation. Some of the activated B-cells migrate into lymphoid follicles, form germinal centers, and undergo the sequential changes, described above, that culminate in affinity maturation and memory cell generation. These comprise the follicular pathway of B lymphocyte differentiation. The separation of these pathways is not absolute, because some isotype switching does occur in germinal centers; however, there is no evidence for extra-follicular somatic hyper-mutation of Ig V genes and affinity maturation. Antibody-secreting cells are found mainly in extra-follicular sites, such as the red pulp of the spleen and the medulla of lymph nodes. These cells also migrate to the bone marrow, and at 2 to 3 weeks after immunization the marrow may be a major site of antibody production. Secreted antibodies enter the circulation, but most antibody-producing cells do not circulate actively and have finite life spans (probably a few weeks).

Circulating antibodies bind antigens to initiate the effectors phase of humoral immune responses. Memory B-cells that exit germinal centers circulate in the blood and have a propensity to migrate through germinal centers. Memory cells typically bear high-affinity (mutated) antigen receptors and Ig molecules of switched isotypes more commonly than do naive B-lymphocytes. These processes are greatly accelerated in secondary antibody responses, because of the presence of memory cells in germinal centers and the rapid formation of immune complexes that can be concentrated by follicular dendritic cells.

Factors That Determine the Nature of Humoral Immune Responses to Protein Antigens

Different types of antigens and forms of antigen exposure stimulate antibody responses with distinct characteristics. The principal factors that determine the nature of antibody responses are the following:

1. *Types of cytokines produced:* An important general principle that has emerged from the study of cytokines is that the nature and magnitude of immune responses are influenced by the relative amounts of different cytokines produced at sites of lymphocyte stimulation. This is because, as described above, various cytokines have selective effects on B-cells, especially on heavy chain class switching, and because combinations of different cytokines may be synergistic or antagonistic. It is now clear that in different immune responses, helper T lymphocytes differentiate into effectors that produce different cytokines. The two most distinct, or polarized, populations of helper T-cells are called T_H1 and T_H2 subsets. The principal effectors cytokine of T_H1 cells is IFN-γ. IFN-γ promotes switching of B-cells to isotypes, such as IgG2a in mice that fix complement and promote phagocytosis by macrophages. IFN-γ also activates the microbicidal functions of macrophages. Therefore, T_H1 cells stimulate phagocyte dependent host reactions and are important for the elimination of intracellular microbes (cell-mediated immunity). T_H2 cells, in contrast, produce IL-4 and IL-5, IL-4 induces switching to IgE and to other isotypes, such as IgG4 in humans or its homolog IgGI in mice, that do not fix complement or bind to phagocyte Fc receptors. IL-5 activates eosinophils. Therefore, the T_H2 subset is important for phagocyte-independent, IgE and eosinophil-mediated defense, e.g., against helminths.
2. *Site of antigen exposure:* Antigens that enter the blood or lymph, and subsequently the peripheral lymphoid organs, such as the spleen and lymph nodes, induce the production of antibodies of multiple isotypes. Orally administered and inhaled antigens tend to stimulate high levels of IgA production, because B-cells in mucosal lymphoid tissues readily switch to IgA. This adaptation is important because IgA is the only antibody isotype that is actively secreted through epithelial cells into the lumen.
3. *Nature of the antigenic stimulus:* Large doses of antigens, especially if they are administered systemically without adjuvants, often inhibit antibody production by inducing tolerance, or unresponsiveness, in helper T or B lymphocytes.
4. Many of the features of secondary responses to protein antigens, and the differences from primary responses are due to the increased numbers of differentiated effectors CD4+ T-cells that are stimulated by the first exposure to antigen. Thus, heavy chain class switching, which is typical of secondary responses, is due to helper T-cells and their cytokines. Affinity maturation, which increases with repeated antigenic stimulation, is also a result of helper T cell-induced B cell activation. These features are usually seen in responses to protein antigens, because only proteins stimulate specific helper T-cells. The more rapid and larger secodnary response is because of the expansion of antigen-specific lymphocyte clones induced by prior antigenic stimulation.

ANTIBODY RESPONSES TO THYMUS INDEPENDENT ANTIGENS (Table 9.2)

The requirement for helper T-cells explains why thymus-dependent protein antigens do not induce antibody responses in T cell-deficient animals, such as congenitally athymic (nude) or neonatally thymectomized mice. In contrast, many non-protein antigens stimulate antibody production in athymic mice, and these antigens are termed thymus-independent (TI).

The most important TI antigens are polysaccharides, glycolipids, and nucleic acids, all of which induce specific antibody production in T cell-deficient animals. These antigens cannot be processed and presented in association with MHC molecules, and, therefore, they cannot be recognized by helper T-cells. Most TI antigens are polymeric, being composed of multiple identical antigenic epitopes; examples include dextrans and pneumococcal polysaccharide. Such multivalent

Table 9.2: Properties of thymus-dependent and thymus-independent antigens

Properties	*Thymus-dependent*	*Thymus-independent*
Chemical nature	Proteins	Polymeric antigens, especially polysaccharides; also glycolipids, nucleic acids
Antibody response in		
Athymic mice	No	
T cell-depleted cultures	No	Yes
Features of antibody response		May be reduced
Isotype switching	Yes	No (usually)
Affinity maturation	Yes	No
Secondary response (memory B cells)	Yes	No or low
Ability to induce delayed-type Hypersensitivity	Yes	No

antigens may induce maximal cross-linking of membrane Ig on specific B-cells, leading to activation without a requirement for cognate T cell help. B cell activation by TI antigens is one situation in which membrane Ig-mediated signal transduction may be critical for subsequent responses of the cells. It is not clear if B cell responses to TI antigens are dependent on any second signals. Experiments with mice suggest that antibody responses to polysaccharides do require the presence of small numbers of macrophages and/or helper T-cells. These cells may secrete cytokines that function as second signals for B cell responses to TI antigens, but neither the nature of these cytokines nor the mechanism(s) leading to their production are completely understood.

Responses to most TI antigens consists largely of IgM antibodies of low affinity and do not show significant heavy chain class switching, affinity maturation, or memory. However, some TI antigens do induce Ig isotypes other than IgM, probably because these antigens stimulate cytokine production. For instance, in humans the dominant antibody class induced by pneumococcal capsular polysaccharide is IgG2. In addition, despite their inability to generate good memory, many polysaccharide vaccines, such as pneumococcal vaccine, induce quite long-lived protective immunity. A likely reason for this is that polysaccharides are not degraded efficiently, persist for long periods in lymphoid tissues, and continue to stimulate newly maturing B-cells.

The practical significance of TI antigens is that many bacterial cell wall polysaccharides belong to this category, and humoral immunity is the major mechanism of host defense against such bacterial infections. For this reason, individuals with congenital or acquired deficiencies of humoral immunity are especially susceptible to life-threatening infections with encapsulated bacteria, such as *pneumococcus, meningococcus*, and *haemophilus*. Other examples of responses to TI antigens are natural antibodies, which are present in the circulation of normal individuals and are apparently produced without overt antigen exposure. Most natural antibodies are low-affinity anti-carbohydrate antibodies, postulated to be induced by bacteria that colonize the gastrointestinal tract.

Antibody responses to TI antigens may occur at particular anatomic sites in lymphoid tissues. Macrophages located in the marginal zones of lymphoid follicles in the spleen are particularly efficient at trapping polysaccharides when these are injected intravenosuly. Such antigens may either persist for prolonged periods on the surfaces of marginal zone macrophages, where they are recognized by specific B-cells, or they may be transferred from the marginal zone to the adjacent follicle. Marginal zones are present only in the spleen.

This is probably why spleenectomized individuals do not develop strong antibody responses to polysaccharides and are susceptible to infection by encapsulated bacteria like the pneumococcus.

Based on experiments with mice, TI antigens have been classified into two groups. Polysaccharides and the other TI antigens mentioned above are called "TI-2" antigen in mice is lipopolysaccharide (LPS), which stimulates B-cells by itself, without a requirement for any other cells. LPS, also called endotoxin, is a major component of the cell walls of many gram-negative bacteria.

At low concentrations, LPS stimulates specific antibody production in rodents. At high concentrations, it is a polyclonal B cell activator, stimulating the growth and differentiation of virtually all B-cells without binding to the membrane Ig. It is postulated that a component of the LPS molecule binds to B-cells and directly activates the cells, i.e., the antigen provides both the first and the second signals needed for B lymphocyte activation. However, neither the nature of the B cell receptor for LPS nor the biochemical mechanisms of LPS-induced B cell stimulation is clearly established. Also, LPS is a polyclonal B cell activator in mice but not in humans and most other species. In all species, LPS is one of most potent activators of macrophages known.

REGULATION OF HUMORAL IMMUNE RESPONSES BY COMPLEMENT, ANTIBODIES AND ACCESSORY CELLS

The production of antibodies is regulated by signals in addition to those provided by antigen and T-cells. These signals can both enhance and suppress humoral immune responses.

Role of Complement Proteins

The complement system consists of a set of proteins that are activated either by binding to antigen-complexes antibody molecules (the "classical pathway") or by binding directly to some polysaccharides and to microbial surfaces, in the absence of antibodies (the "alternative pathway"). Historically, much of the interest in complement has focused on its role as an effector mechanism of humoral immunity. Recent work has shown that complement also plays a role in the induction and amplification of antibody responses. Mice deficient in various complement components show profound defects in antibody responses to protein antigens. Conversely, attaching activated complement proteins to protein antigens increases the immunogenicity of these antigens more than 1000-fold.

The complement system augments antibody production by two mechanisms:

1. B lymphocytes express a receptor for a complement protein, C3d, called the type 2 complement receptor (CR2, or CD21) which transduces signals that enhance B cell proliferation and differentiation. C3d is generated by the proteolysis of the key component of complement, C3, and becomes covalently attached to antigens that trigger complement activation via the classical or alternative pathway. Binding of C3d to the B cell complement receptor recruits another B cell surface protein, CD19, into the complex. If the antigen receptor is also engaged by simultaneous binding of antigen, the response of the B cell is greatly enhanced. Knockout of the C3, CD21, or CD19 gene in mice results in defects in antibody production.
2. Complement proteins attached to antigens promote the binding of the antigens to follicular dendritic cells in germinal centers.

Follicular dendritic cells express a surface receptor for another C3 breakdown product, C3b; this receptor is called the type 1 complement receptor (CR1, or CD35). Complexes of antigens, antibodies, and C3b bind to the CR1 receptor on follicular dendritic cells, providing display of the antigens in germinal centers for the selection of high-affinity B-cells.

Since the complement system is usually activated after the binding of secreted antibodies to antigens, the question arises, how can complement be required for the induction of humoral immune responses? The likely answer is that in antibody responses to protein antigens, complement is essential for amplification. Thus, once a small amount of antibody is produced, it binds to the antigen, activates complement by the classical pathway, generates C3b and C3d, which bind covalently to the antigen, and the response is amplified by the two mechanisms mentioned above. Since IgM antibodies are produced first in humoral immune responses and are more potent activators of the complement system than all other Ig isotypes, they may provide the major amplification mechanism. In the case of T-independent antigens, many polysaccharides directly activate complement prior to specific antibody production, and the same sequence of events ensues. The complement system is an important component of innate immunity.

Antibody Feedback: The Inhibitory Function of Fc Receptors on B-cells

The simultaneous engagement of B cell Ig and Fcγ receptors by antigen-antibody complexes inhibits B cell activation. This is the explanation for a phenomenon called antibody feedback, which refers to the down regulation of antibody production by secreted IgG antibodies. Some antigen-complexes IgG isotypes bind to a B cell receptor for the Fc portion of these IgGs, called the Fcγ receptor II B (FcγRIIB, or CD323). The cytoplasmic domain of FcγRIIB binds to a protein tyrosine phosphatase that is found in many cell types. If the FcγRIIB is brought into close proximity to the B cell antigen receptor, the associated phosphatase may remove tyrosine residues from signaling molecules that have become attached to the B cell receptor complex and been tyrosine phosphorylated. This inhibits Ig mediated signal transduction and terminates the B-cells response.

Fc receptor-mediated antibody feedback is a physiologic control mechanism in humoral immune responses, since it is triggered by secreted antibody and blocks further antibody production. It is not clear under which circumstances secreted antibodies provide complement-mediated amplification or Fc receptor-mediated inhibition. A likely scenario is that early in humoral immune responses, IgM antibodies (which activate complement but do not bind to the Fc receptor) are involved in amplification, whereas increasing production of IgG leads to feedback inhibition.

Role of Accessory Cells

One of the first experiments suggesting the requirement for accessory cells in the responses of lymphocytes to antigens demonstrated that if spleen cells from unimmunized mice were depleted of adherenT-cells, they would not secrete antibody when stimulated by a model T cell-dependent antigen, sheep red blood cells. Responsiveness was restored by the addition of non-lymphoid cells such as macrophages, or, as shown later, by dendritic cells.

Macrophages and other accessory cells can perform various functions in the induction of humoral immunity.

1. Macrophages and dendritic cells are accessory for presenting antigens to naive helper T lymphocytes, thereby inducing proliferation of the T-cells and their differentiation into effector cells producing various cytokines. As discussed above, this is probably most important in primary antibody responses, because in secondary responses B lymphocytes are available for antigen presentation

to already differentiated effectors and memory T-cells. There is no evidence that B lymphocytes themselves need to recognize protein antigens presented by accessory cells. Two situations where B lymphocytes do recognize antigens displayed by other cells are in germinal center reactions, when follicular dendritic cells present antigens, and in responses to polysaccharides, which bind to marginal zone macrophages.

2. Macrophages secrete cytokines, which may augment the proliferation of both B and T lymphocytes. IL-1 and TNF may directly stimulate B-cells proliferation, IL-6 is a growth and differentiation factor for B-cells, and IL-12, stimulates the differentiation of CD+ T-cells into T_H1 effectors.

At this time you should know the following:

1. General characteristics of the specific immune response.
2. Differences between primary and secondary antibody responses.
3. Molecular events involved in class switching and membrane immunoglobulin expression.

Further Reading

1. A tassi MZ et al. Molecular Immunology. Marcel Decker, Inc. New York, 1984.
2. Harboe NMG and Ingild A. Scand J Immunol 1983;17:345-51.
3. Boenisch T. Appl. Immunohistochem 1999;7(4): 300-6.
4. Hornick CL and Karush F. Immunochemistry 1979;9:325-40.
5. Steward MW and Steensgaard J. Antibody Affinity: Thermodynamic Aspects and Biological Significance. Boca Raton: CRC Press, 1983.
6. Herschowitz HID Immunophysiology: Cell function and cellular interactions in antibody formation. In Bellanti JA. Immunology III. Philadelphia: Saunders, 1985.
7. Boenisch T. Appl Immunohistochem 2001; 9(2):176-9.
8. Boenisch T. Appl Immunohistochem 2005; 13(3):283-6.
9. A lexander J and Dayal Y. Appl Immunohistochem 1997; 5(4):252-3.
10. Smith RA. J Histotech 1990;13(4):255-69.
11. Martin CA and Badrán AF. Appl Immunohistochem 1998;6(2):84-8.
12. Boenisch T. Appl Immunohistochem 2002; 10(4):363-7.
13. Sternberger LA. Immunocytochemistry (2nd ed). New York: Wiley, 1979.
14. Underwood PA and Bean PA. J Immunol Meth 1985; 80:89-97.
15. Kirkwood TBL *et al.* Biometrics 1977;3:38-48.
16. Tydeman MS and Kirkwood TBL. J Biol Standard 1984;12:195-206.
17. Jackson CM. IVD Technology 1997;3:38-48.
18. van Erp R *et al.* J Biotech 1991;20:249-62.
19. Kim YC and Nishida TJ. Biol Chem 1979;254:9621-26, 64.

10

CHAPTER

Cells Involved in the Immune System

(Dr. Debapriya Bandyopadhyay and Dr. B K Gupta debudoc2000@gmail.com)

OBJECTIVES

1. To discuss a brief overview of the origin and development of immune cells and cell-mediated and humoral immunity.
2. To know different types and sub-population of lymphocytes, their characteristics and mechanism.
3. To describe antigen presenting cells and their types and functions.
4. To know a brief overview of granulocytes, their types and characteristics.
5. To know the abnormalities of immune cells.

INTRODUCTION

Immunity (derived from *immunitas*: Latin for exemption from civic duties and prosecution) means protection from disease and especially infectious disease. Cells and molecules involved in such protection constitute the immune system and the reaction against an introduced foreign agent is known as the immune response. Not all immune responses protect from disease; some foreign agents, such as the allergens found in house dust mite, cat dander or rye grass pollen, cause disease as a consequence of inducing an immune response. Likewise some individuals mount immune responses to their own tissues as if they were foreign agents due to autoimmunity. Thus, the immune response can cause the autoimmune diseases common to man such as multiple sclerosis, diabetes, rheumatoid arthritis or myasthenia gravis. Most individuals do not suffer from autoimmune disease because they have developed tolerance towards their own (self) antigens/tissues.

The cells involved in maintaining the immune system can be broadly classified into granulocytes, phagocytes and antigen presenting cells where granulocytes play a prominent role in primary immune responses arising due to infection or intrusion by a foreign particle, the antigen presenting cells are responsible for internalizing the invading pathogens by phagocytosis and presenting them in a processed form to lymphocytes. These lymphocytes circulate in the body and can migrate in the tissue space leading to subsequent T cell-B cell co-operation in order to activate and enhance the cellular and humoral immunity.

The immune system stockpiles a huge arsenal of cells, not only lymphocytes but also cell-devouring phagocytes and their relatives. Some immune cells take on all intruders, while others are trained on highly specific targets. To work effectively, most immune cells need the cooperation of their comrades. Sometimes immune cells communicate by direct physical contact and sometimes by releasing chemical messengers. The immune system stores just a few of each kind of the different T-cells needed to recognize millions of possible enemies. When an antigen appears, those few matching cells multiply into a full-scale army. After their job is done, they fade away, leaving sentries behind to watch for future attacks.

The Origin and Development of Immune Cells

All immune cells begin as stem cells in the bone marrow. They respond to different cytokines and other signals to grow into specific immune cell types, such as T-cells, B-cells, or phagocytes (**Figure 10.1**). Due to the unique property of multipotency of hematopoietic stem cells, researchers are currently investigating if a person's own stem cells can be used to restore normal cell count in autoimmune diseases and immune deficiency diseases. White blood cells play a major role by engulfing and destroying microorganism, presenting antigen on the surface and secreting cytokines. These lymphocytes circulate in the body and can migrate in the tissue space thus involving the immune system to great extent. Lymphocytes can be broadly differentiated into B-cells, T-cells and natural killer cells. Natural killer cells are large lymphocytes and do not display typical markers as B and T-cells have.

Naïve B and T cell are small, nonphagocytic in nature and cannot be distinguished morpho-

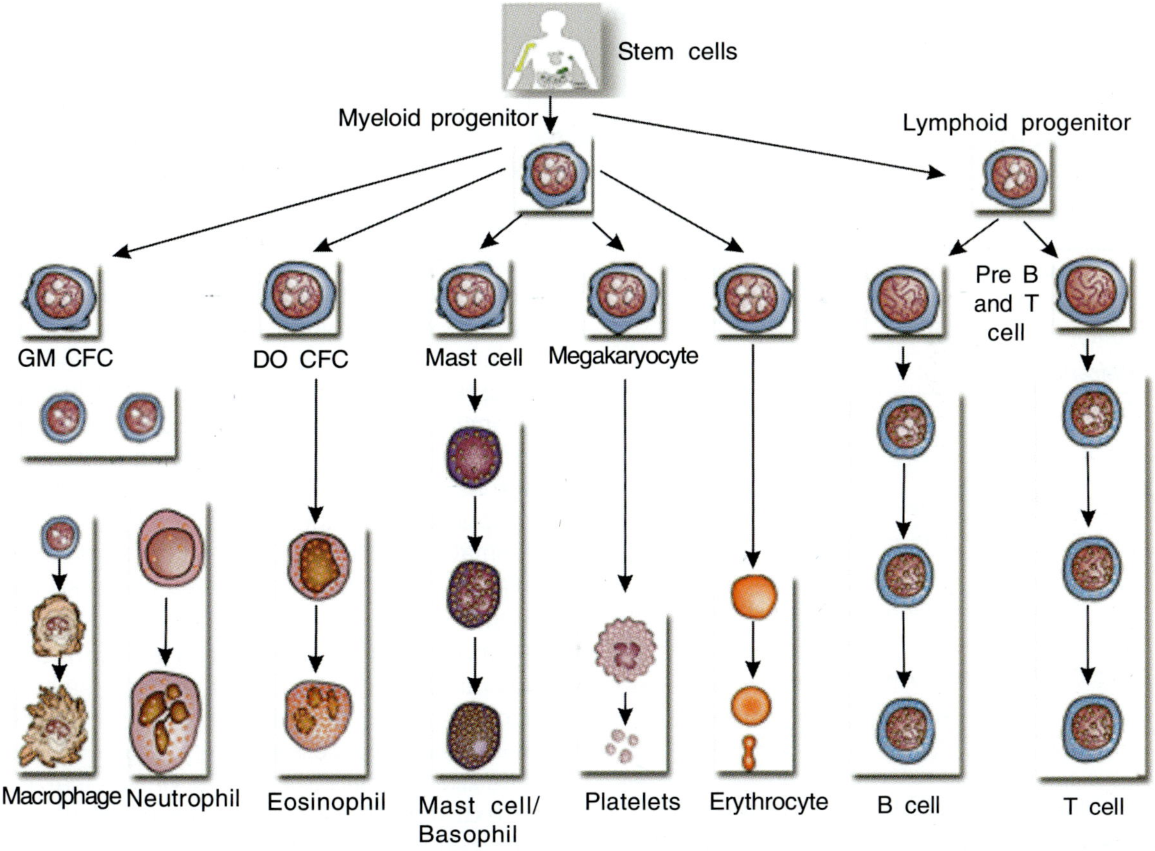

Fig. 10.1: Overview of hematopoiesis, stem cells in the bone marrow differentiate through two pathways, giving rise to lymphoid progenitor and myeloid progenitor cells from which, specialized cells such as lymphocytes originate by differentiation

logically. They have short life span. As they progress through life cycle the size increases from 6μm to 15μm. They are now called lymphoblast; they have ability to differentiate into effector cells or into memory cells. For example plasma cells, the effector cells of B cell differentiation can secrete antibodies against the antigen in large amount. Similarly effector cells of T cell differentiation include cytokine secreting T helper cell and memory cells which look like lymphocytes but can be distinguished from naïve cell by the presence of special cell membrane molecule. The presence of these cells gives life long immunity against many pathogens. Different lineages or maturational stages of lymphocytes can be distinguished by their expression of membrane molecules (surface markers) that can be recognized by particular monoclonal antibodies. All of the monoclonal antibodies that react with a particular membrane molecule are grouped together as a cluster of differentiation (CD).

This CD is distributed amongst different immune cells as shown in **Table 10.1**.

Table 10.1: Human leukocyte surface antigen—the cluster of differentiation (CD)

Cluster of differentiation	*Distribution*
CD 1	Cortical thymocytes, Langerhans type of dendritic cells
CD 2,3,4,7,8,28	T lymphocytes
CD 2,7	Natural killer cells
CD 19,20	Pan B cell marker (but absent in plasma cells)
CD 21,22,23	Mature B-cells
CD 28	Plasma cells
CD 45	Pan leukocyte marker
CD 80,95	Activated B and T-cells

Cell-Mediated and Humoral Immunity

Parts of the immune system are changeable and can adapt to attack the invading antigen better. There are two fundamental adaptive mechanisms: cell-mediated immunity and humoral immunity. B-cells are produced in the stem cells of the bone marrow; they produce antibody and oversee humoral immunity. T-cells are nonantibody-producing lymphocytes, which are also produced in the bone marrow but sensitized in the thymus and constitute the basis of cell-mediated immunity.

Cell-mediated responses are effective against intracellular pathogens, which reside in one of two major intracellular compartments:

1. *Cytosol* – Continuous with the nucleus through the pores in the nuclear membrane. Site of all viruses and some bacteria.
2. *Vesicular system* – Comprises endoplasmic reticulum, Golgi apparatus, endosomes, lysosomes, and other intracellular vesicles—site of some bacteria and some parasites.

Cells harboring pathogens in the cytosol are recognized and killed by cytotoxic T-cells, also known as CD8+ T-cells. A suitable example is the intracellular pathogen, *Mycobacteria* that infects macrophages. It prevents the fusion of cytoplasmic vesicles with lysosomes thereby resisting consequent destruction by macrophage bacteriocidal activity. However, when the appropriate T cell recognizes an infected macrophage it releases macrophage-activating molecules that induce lysosomal fusion and the activation of macrophage bactericidal activities. Cells harboring pathogens in the vesicular system are recognized by a subpopulation of helper T-cells, the T_H1 T cell or inflammatory T cell which releases products called cytokines that enable the infected cell to kill the pathogen.

Pathogens may elicit both an antibody (humoral) and cell-mediated response, each of which contributes to eliminate pathogen from the host. For example, cells with intracellular viruses can be killed by cytotoxic T-cells; viruses that are free extracellularly can be neutralized and opsonized by antibodies. A humoral or cell-mediated response may be insufficient to eliminate the pathogen by itself. In order to obtain a better immune response, a collective reaction of humoral and cell mediated immunity is required.

For example, *Mycobacterium leprae*, an intracellular bacterium that can cause leprosy. There can be two different responses to this infection:

1. In some, the major response is Immunoglobulin (Ig) production and *M. leprae* grows abundantly in macrophages leading to gross tissue destruction and development of lepromatous leprosy which is usually fatal.
2. In others, little Ig is produced, but there are few live intracellular *M. leprae* because a cell-mediated response has also occurred. Thus, disease progression is slow with a good outcome.

Lymphocytes

The lymphoid cells of the immune system are characterized by their capacity to recognize and respond to foreign pathogen in an exquisitely specific fashion. Part of this specificity is manifested by their ability to distinguish self from non-self, an essential prerequisite when directing a potentially lethal attack against an invading agent. Lymphocytes are broadly divided into two types termed "B-cells" and "T-cells". B-cells are responsible for antibody production. T-cells provide specific cellular immunity: this can involve direct killing of (particularly) virus-infected cells via cytotoxic T-cells (TC). For the majority of foreign pathogens, or antigens, B-cells need to interact with T_H cells in order to become antibody-producing plasma cells and to generate B memory cells for long-term immunity.

B Lymphocytes

B lymphocyte derived its letter designation from its site of maturation, in the bursa of fabricius in birds. Bone marrow is its major site of maturation in a number of mammalian species, including humans and mice. Mature B-cells are distinguished from other lymphocytes by the presence of membrane-bound immunoglobulin (antibody) molecules, which serve as receptors for antigen. B-cells are the generators of humoral immunity, so called because it consists of soluble proteins found in the "Humors" (Blood). Every B-cell has an Immunoglobulin (Ig) molecule on its surface that recognizes a unique three-dimensional epitope. In the bone marrow, millions of different B-cells are created every day, and then proceed to circulate throughout the bloodstream. Since each has a different immunoglobulin, each will bind to a different substrate. It is most often the case that a B-cell will find nothing to bind to in its short lifespan, and eventually be replaced by a new B-cell. In the event that a B-cell's immunoglobulin does find a substrate, that B-cell will clonally expand, resulting in many B-cells which recognize the same target. Over time, the clones' immunoglobulin genes will mutate to improve the affinity for the target even more. Based on the structure and function, the B-cells are divided into plasma cells and memory cells.

1. Plasma Cells

Plasma cells (also called plasma B-cells or plasmocytes) are cells of the immune system that secrete large amounts of antibodies. When a B cell encounters its triggering antigen, it gives rise to many large cells known as plasma cells. Every plasma cell is essentially a factory for producing an antibody. Each of the plasma cells descended from a given B cell manufactures millions of identical antibody molecules and pours them into the bloodstream (as shown in **Figure 10.2**). Plasma cells differentiate from B-cells upon stimulation by CD4+ lymphocytes.

When an offending pathogen is consumed by the B cell, B cell acts as an antigen presenting cell (APC). That pathogen gets taken up by the B cell by phagocytosis, and broken down within phagosomes after fusion with lysosomes releasing proteolytic enzymes onto the pathogen. Once the enzymes break down the pathogen, pieces of the pathogen (which are now known as antigenic peptides) are loaded onto MHC II molecules, and presented on its extracellular surface. Once on the extracellular surface, the CD4+ T-helper

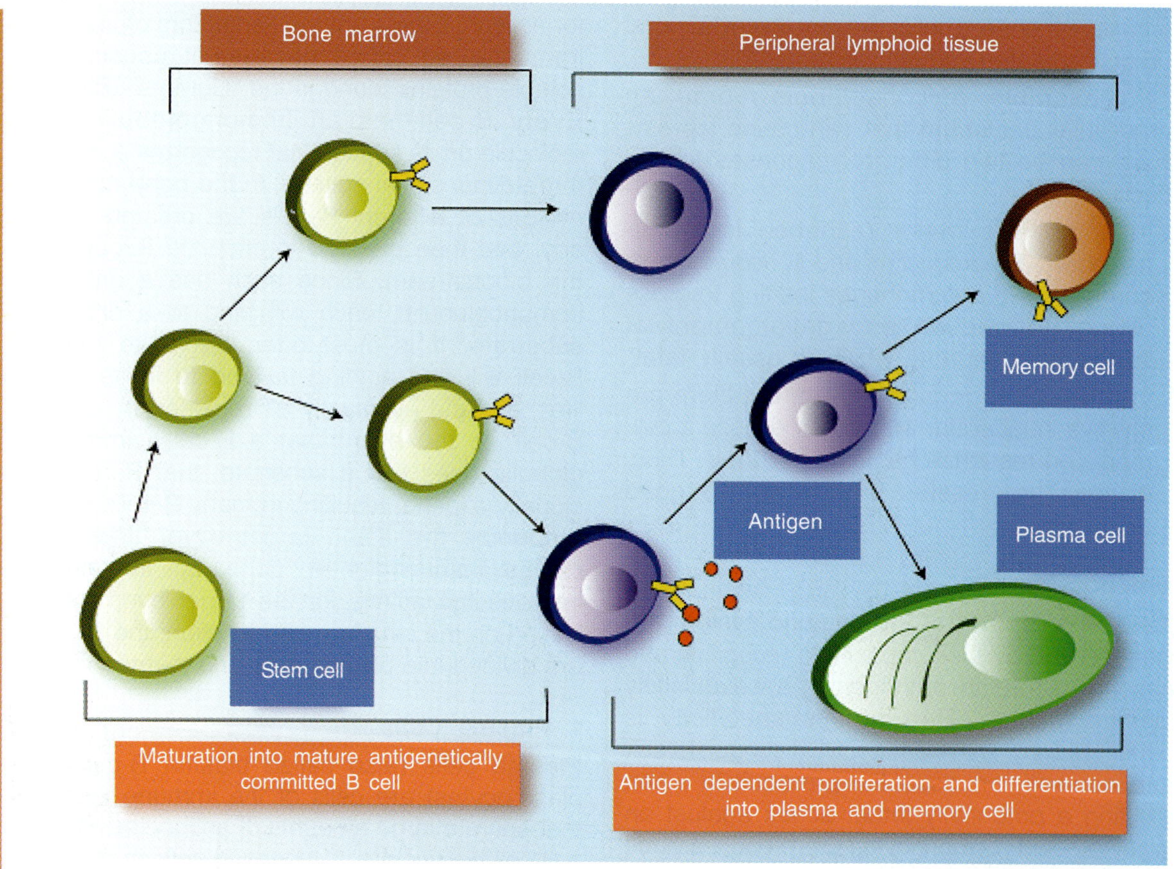

Fig. 10.2: Maturation of B-cell, on encountering an antigen, which binds to the Ig molecule on its surface, the B-cell divides and gives rise to many B-cells which recognize the same target

lymphocyte will bind to the MHC II/antigen molecule and cause activation of the B cell, which includes differentiation into a plasma cell, and subsequent generation of antibody against the phagocytized pathogen. These immunoglobulins will pass throughout the blood and attach to the foreign object (described in **Figure 10.3**).

2. Memory Cells

Memory cells are the main components of secondary immune system that have an affinity for a particular antigen as such molecular memory is programmed in these cells to enable the immunity for a particular antigen/pathogen. Like other B-cells, memory B-cells originate from lymphocytes that develop and are activated in the bone marrow. Memory cells by contrast are much smaller than plasma cells and don't immediately secrete anything. Instead, they persist in the body for a long time and may never be activated. However, in the event that the same foreign organism returns, they will develop into plasma cells much more rapidly than the original B-cells and proceed to secrete their immunoglobulin. They become antigen-specific when stimulated by interleukin-4 (IL-4).

Each B cell is programmed to make one specific antibody. For example, one B cell will make an antibody that blocks a virus that causes the common cold, while another produces an antibody that attacks a bacterium that causes pneumonia.

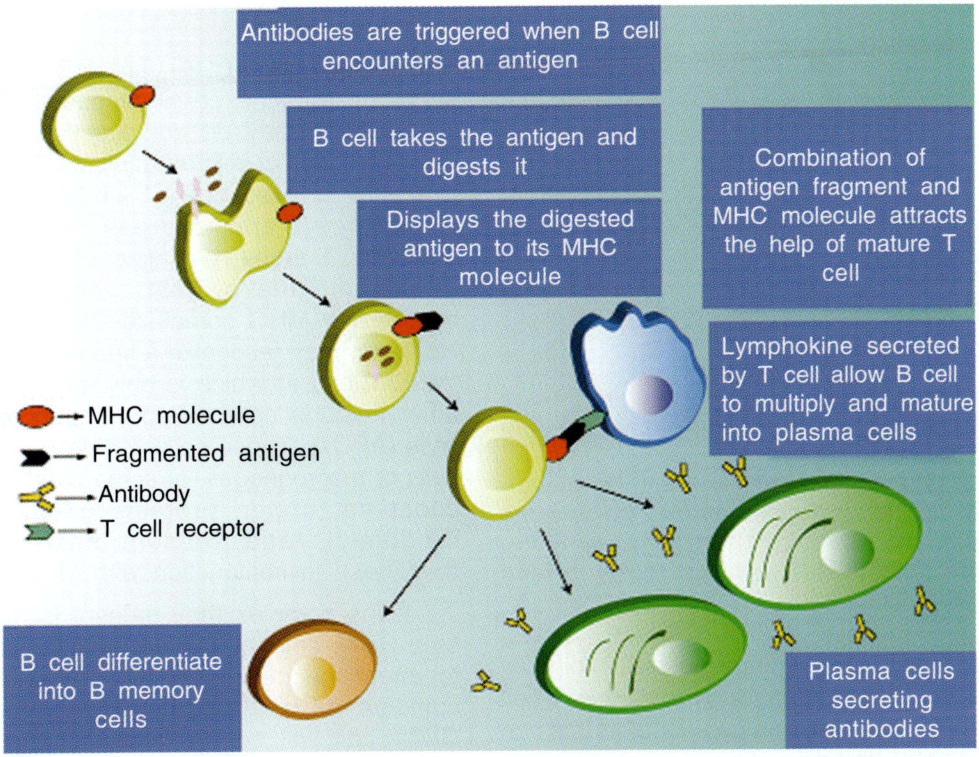

Fig. 10.3: B cell-T cell interaction. This diagram shows the role of B cell as an APC, and how it results in the activation of both T and B cell effector populations through chemical signals

An antigen matches an antibody much as a key matches a lock. Some match exactly; others fit more like a skeleton key. But, whenever antigen and antibody interlock, the antibody marks the antigen for destruction. Antibodies belong to a family of large molecules known as immunoglobulins. Different types play different roles in the immune defense strategy.

- Immunoglobulin G, or IgG, the most abundant immunoglobulin in the serum has subclasses and works efficiently to coat microbes, speeding their uptake by other cells in the immune system.
- IgM, a pentamer, and the first immunoglobulin to be produced in a primary response to the antigen, is very effective towards antigens.
- IgA, which may exist in polymeric forms, concentrates in body fluids like tears, saliva, the secretions of the respiratory tract and digestive tract – guarding the entrances to the body.
- IgE, whose natural job is probably to protect against parasitic infections, is responsible for the allergic reactions.
- IgD remains attached to B-cells and plays a key role in initiating early B-cell response.

T Lymphocytes

T-cells are responsible for destroying infected or cancerous cells, and for coordinating all acquired immune responses. For this reason, T-cell mediated immunity is generally called cellular immunity. Two sub-types of T-cells are responsible for cell mediated immunity:

1. Cytotoxic T-cell (CD8+); and
2. Helper T-cell (CD4+) (as shown in **Figure 10.4**).

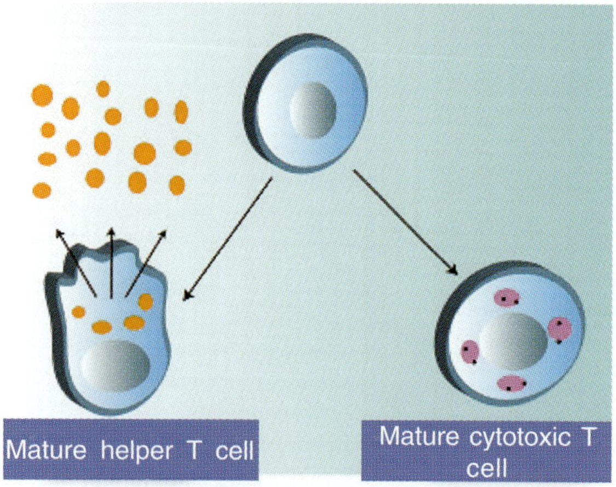

Fig 10.4: Differentiation of T-cell into its effector populations. Helper T-cell regulates the immune response by releasing myriad chemicals, whereas cytotoxic T-cells directly attack abnormal cells

Each T-cell has a unique surface molecule much like an immunoglobulin, called a T-cell receptor (TCR). Unlike immunoglobulins that can recognize any molecule, the TCR is restricted to recognize only short amino acid chains, displayed on the surface of cells, in conjunction with a molecule, called the major histocompatibility complex (MHC). Almost all the cells in the body are constantly producing MHC molecules and attaching processed antigenic peptides to them, for expression on their surface. T-cells probe the surface of all cells for MHC complexes. On finding the complex which their receptor recognizes they grow and divide into mature CD8+ T-cells and memory cells in an event similar to clonal expansion of B-cells.

Based on their function and surface markers, T-cells can be further classified into:

1. Helper T-Cell (CD4+).
2. Cytotoxic T-Cell (CD8+); and
3. T suppressor (TS) cells.

Like memory cells for B lymphocytes, memory cells exist for T-cells also.

1. Helper T-Cell (CD4+)

The helper T-cells (CD4+) are probably the most important immune cells, despite the fact that by definition they do not directly destroy any diseased cells or microorganisms. Rather, they produce a plethora of chemical factors (Cytokines), and express many surface elements, thereby regulating all other aspects of the immune system. They too act by recognizing MHC complexes with their TCRs. However, they recognize a special type of MHC (MHC Class II) which is only found on certain other immune cells called, antigen presenting cells (APCs). These cells, whether they are B-cells or macrophages, or some other leukocyte, consume foreign proteins (specifically or randomly), and present small portions (peptides), in conjunction with MHC Class II.

If the complex they present is recognized by a CD4+ cell, the cell will produce chemicals to affect the cell, which presented the MHC complex, as well as other immune cells. The CD4+ cell will go on to divide and mature, producing more cytokines that activate other effector cells and memory cells (as shown in **Figure 10.5**). Helper T-cells coordinate immune responses by communicating with other cells. Some stimulate nearby B-cells to produce antibody, others call in microbe-gobbling cells called phagocytes, and still others activate other types of T-cells. No acquired immune response could take place without the signal chemicals that a CD4+ cell produces, and its absence, as seen in cases of HIV infection, results in a collapse of the active immune system.

2. Cytotoxic T-Cell (CD8+)

Cytotoxic T lymphocytes or CTLs, also called killer T-cells, perform a different function. These cells directly attack other cells carrying certain foreign or abnormal molecules on their surfaces. Mature CD8+ cells move throughout the body, searching for cells that possess complexes, to

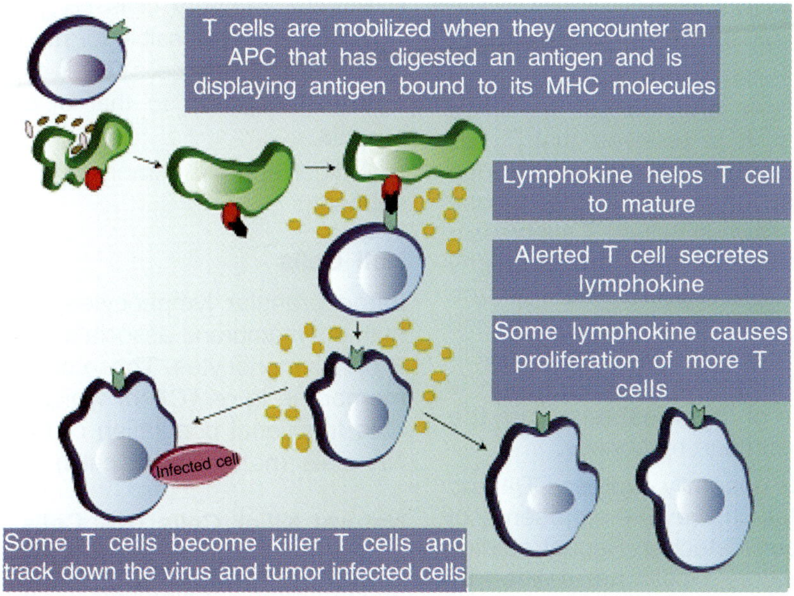

Fig. 10.5: Following antigen presentation, the activated T-cells secrete chemical mediators and exist cell mediated immune response

which the T cell receptor (TCR) will bind and proceed to destroy those cells. Memory CD8+ cells function like memory B-cells, they persist and will multiply and mature if they are re-exposed to the same MHC complex. CTLs are especially useful for attacking viruses because viruses often hide from other parts of the immune system while they grow inside infected cells. CTLs recognize small fragments of these viruses peeking out from the cell membrane and launch an attack to kill the cell. In contrast to T_H cells, most CTLs secrete few cytokines, but instead, CTLs have the ability to recognize and eliminate altered self-cells.

T cells express two types of glycoproteins CD4 and CD8, cells with CD4 are restricted to recognize antigen bound to class II MHC molecule, where cells with CD8 marker, will bound to antigen combined with class I MHC molecule. Presence of CD4 and CD8 guides the two major populations of the T lymphocytes. This ratio is approximately 2:1 in normal human peripheral blood. Any immune related disease in the organism may cause alteration in this ratio.

The classification of CD4 class II binding cells as TH cells and CD8 class I binding cell as TC cell is not well differentiated. Some CD4 can act as killer cells. Some TC cells show secretion of some kind of cytokine also as of T_H cells. T_H cell gets activated by binding itself with MHC II molecule of the antigen presenting cell combined with an antigen. Then, it proliferates to give clone of effector cells; these cells also secrete various cytokines, which play an important role in activation of B, T-cells and other cells. T_H1 response secrete a plethora of cytokine that causes inflammation and activates T-cells and macrophages while T_H2 response activates mainly B-cells that causes production of antibodies. TC cells are activated when they interact with MHC I molecule complexed with antigen on virus infected cells or tumor cells in the presence of appropriate cytokine. This causes proliferation of TC cells into cytotoxic T lymphocyte (CTL) or killer cell.

3. T Suppressor (TS) Cells

Another type of T cell is gaining its recognition as T suppresser cells. Some T-cells help to suppress the humoral and the cell mediated immune responses. It is believed that T cell mediated suppression in some systems is due to the activities of T_H and TC cells, whose activities are suppressive in nature. T suppressor or T regulatory cells (as they are popularly known) mainly down regulate the immune responses after skirmishing foreign intruders and also prevent immune responses against self-antigens/tissues. Hence their main function is the maintenance of homeostasis and the prevention of autoimmune responses.

Suppressor cells generally express CD4 and CD25 on their surface however the presence of CD8+ has also been detected. Recent studies suggest that regulatory T-cells are defined by expression of the fork-head family transcription factor Fox P3 (fork-head box p3). Expression of Fox P3 is required for regulatory T cell development and appears to control a genetic program specifying this cell fate. Typically, high levels of cytotoxic T-lymphocyte associated molecule-4 (CTLA-4) and glucocorticoid-induced TNF receptor (GITR) are expressed on regulatory T-cells; however the functional significance of this expression is yet to be explored.

4. T Memory Cells

Similar to B memory cells, memory T-cells are specific in identifying foreign agents, which were encountered in a previous incidence of infection/vaccination. Subsequent exposure to the same agent may generate an immediate and heightened immune response. Three distinct subpopulations of these cells are present which are:

- Central memory cells (T_{CM}) – Which have self renewal capacity like stem cells due to hyper phosphorylation of STAT5 transcription factor. These cells express L-selectin and CCR7 receptors and secrete IL2 but do not secrete INF-γ and IL4.
- Effector memory cells (T_{EM}) and (T_{EMRA}) – Which are responsible for mediating functions similar to CD8+ cells. Their expression profile is just opposite to that of central memory cells.

Antigen specific memory cells are found in both subsets.

Null Cells

Large granular lymphocytes that lack surface markers/membrane associated proteins of either B or T lymphocytes. These cells fail to express membrane Ig or TCR or typical CD molecules. One functional population of these cells is the NK cells (natural killer cells).

Natural Killer Cells (NK Cells)

Natural killer cells (**Figure 10.6**) are also known as large granular lymphocytes (LGL). Of all the cells involved in immunity natural killer cells (NK cells) are the most aggressive. They act as the first line defense system against mutant and virus infected cells. They are lymphocytes with no immunological memory and are part of innate immune system. NK cells make up about 5 to 16% of the total lymphocyte population. Their specific function is to destroy infected and cancerous cells. Their mode of operation is shown in **Figure 10.7**.

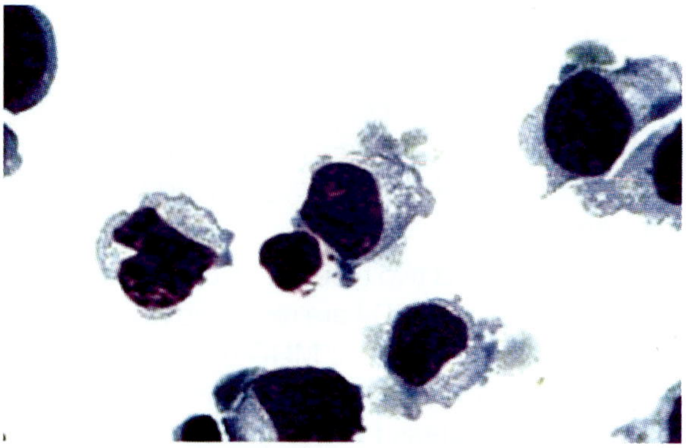

Fig. 10.6: Natural killer cell (Source: http://cae2k.com/photos-de-studio-0/natural-killer-cell.html)

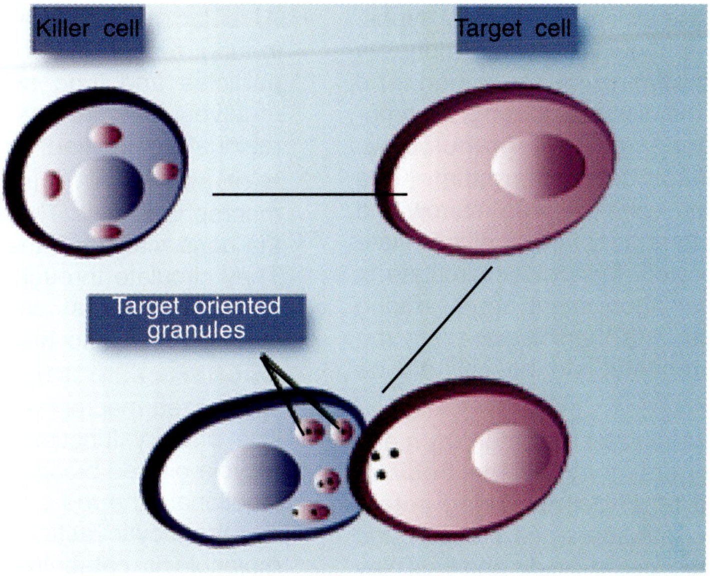

Fig. 10.7: Modus operandi of NK cells, on seeing an abnormal display of surface antigens on the target cell; NK cells destroy the cell by the release of specialized granules containing hydrolytic enzymes

NK cells kill the infected cell by two mechanisms:

1. It looks for the abnormality in the cell like decrease in the display of class I MHC molecule or unusual presence of surface antigen on some tumor cell or cells infected with some virus.
2. Another way is that it recognizes the cell by seeing some antibodies on the infected cell that are produced by the immune system against the displayed antigen on the surface of the cell. It attaches itself to the Fc region of the antibodies and destroys the targeted cell. This process is known as Antibody Dependent Cell Mediated Cytotoxicity (ADCC).

In addition to their role in the control of infections, NK cells help in the regulation of other aspects of the immune system that contributes overall health. Immunotherapy to increase NK cell population is becoming available and will become more widely used as knowledge of the immune system increases. Certain cell type of NK cells like NK1-T cell has some of the characteristics of both T-cells and NK cells. Like T-cells, NK1-T-cells have T cell receptors (TCRs). Unlike most T-cells, the TCRs of NK1-T-cells interact with MHC-like molecules like CD1 rather with class I or class II MHC molecules. Variable levels of CD16 and other receptors typical to NK cells are there with NK1-T-cells. A population of triggered NK1-T-cells can rapidly secrete large amounts of the cytokines required to support antibody production by B-cells as well as inflammation and the development and expansion of cytotoxic T-cells.

Phagocytes

Phagocytes (means-cell eaters) are large white cells that can engulf and digest microorganisms and other antigenic particles. Some phagocytes also have the ability to present antigen to lymphocytes. Important phagocytes are monocytes and macrophages. Monocytes circulate in the blood and then migrate into tissues where they develop into macrophages (means—big eaters). Macrophages are seeded throughout body tissues in a variety of types. The mononuclear phagocytic system consists of monocytes circulating in the blood and macrophages in the tissues. During hematopoiesis in the bone marrow, granulocyte-monocyte progenitor cells differentiate into promonocytes, which leave the bone marrow and enter the blood, where they further differentiate into mature monocytes. Monocytes circulate in the bloodstream for about eight hours, during which they enlarge; and then migrate into the tissues and differentiate into specific tissue macrophages.

Macrophages are versatile cells that play many roles. As scavengers, they rid the body of wornout cells and other debris. Being potent antigen presenters, macrophages process and present antigenic peptides to T-cells and thus play a crucial role in initiating the immune response. As secretory cells, monocytes and macrophages are vital to the regulation of immune responses and the development of inflammation; they churn out an amazing array of powerful chemical substances (monokines) including enzymes, complement proteins, and regulatory factors such as interleukin-1. At the same time, they carry receptors for lymphokines that allow them to be "activated" into single-minded pursuit of microbes and tumor cells.

Macrophages are not the only cells to present antigen to lymphocytes. Other antigen-presenting cells include B-cells, dendritic cells and irregularly shaped white blood cells found in the spleen and other lymphoid organs. Dendritic cells typically have long threadlike tentacles that enmesh lymphocytes and antigens. Langerhans cells are dendritic cells that travel in the skin, picking up antigen and transporting it to nearby lymph nodes. Many other types of body cells, when properly stimulated, can also be recruited to present antigens to lymphocytes. Macrophages have amoeboid movement within the tissues. Macrophages, according to location (tissues), have different function to perform and are named according to tissue location:

1. **Alveolar macrophages:** Macrophages found in lung, responsible for clearance of inhaled particles and lung surfactant. Often have multivesicular bodies that may represent residual undigested lung surfactant.
2. **Histiocytes:** A histiocyte is a tissue macrophage cell. These cells migrate from the bone marrow to the blood as monocytes. They circulate through the body and stop in various organs where they undergo differentiation into histiocytes.
3. **Kupffer cells:** Kupffer cells which are specialized macrophages located in the liver. The primary function of Kupffer cells is to recycle old red blood cells that are no longer functional. The red blood cell is broken down by phagocytic action and the hemoglobin molecule is catabolized.
4. **Mesangial cells:** Mesangial cells are specialized cells around blood vessels in the kidneys, at the mesangium that takes care of the kidney from suspicious particles.
5. **Microglial cells:** Microglia is a type of glial cell that act as the immune cells of the central nervous system (CNS). Being, the smallest of the glial cells, they can act as phagocytes, cleaning up CNS debris. Most serve as representatives of the immune system in the brain and spinal cord.
6. **Osteoclasts:** An osteoclast is a type of bone cell that removes bone tissue by removing the bone's mineralized matrix. This process is known as bone resorption.

One important main role of macrophage is the removal of necrotic debris and dust in the lungs. The removal of dust and necrotic tissue is to a greater extent handled by fixed macrophages, which will stay at strategic locations such as the lungs, liver, neural tissue, bone, spleen and connective tissue, ingesting foreign materials such as dust and pathogens, calling upon wandering macrophages if needed. When a macrophage ingests a pathogen, the pathogen becomes trapped in a food vacuole, which then fuses with a lysosome. Within the lysosome, enzymes and toxic peroxides digest the invader. However, some bacteria, such as *Mycobacterium tuberculosis*, become resistant to these methods of digestion. Macrophages can digest more than 100 bacteria before they finally die due to their own digestive compounds.

Macrophages are involved in cell-mediated immunity in conjunction with NK cells and cytotoxic T-cells. After digesting a pathogen, a macrophage will present the *antigen* of the pathogen to a corresponding *helper T cell*. The presentation is done by integrating it into the cell membrane and displaying it attached to a *MHC* class II molecule, indicating to other white blood cells that the macrophage is not a pathogen, despite having antigens on its surface. Eventually the antigen presentation results in the production of *antibodies* that attach to the antigens of pathogens (opsonization), making them easier for macrophages to adhere to with their cell membrane and phagocytize.

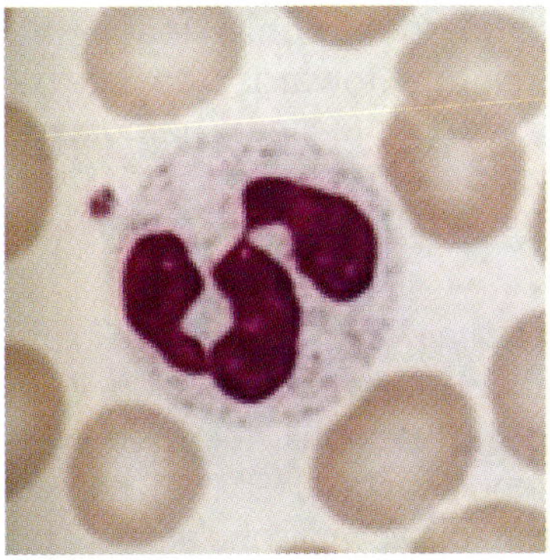

Neutrophil[β]

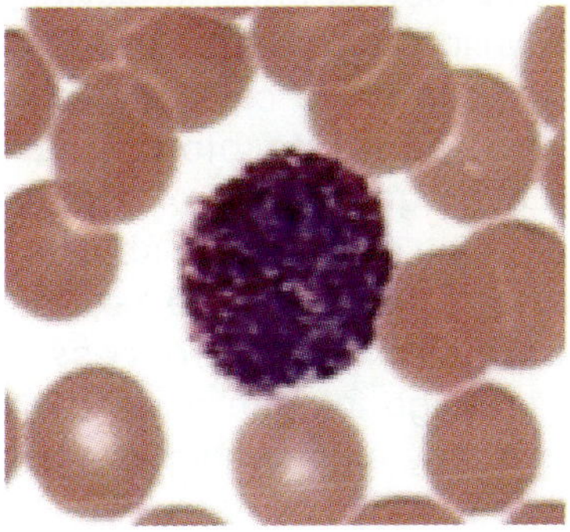

Basophil[α]

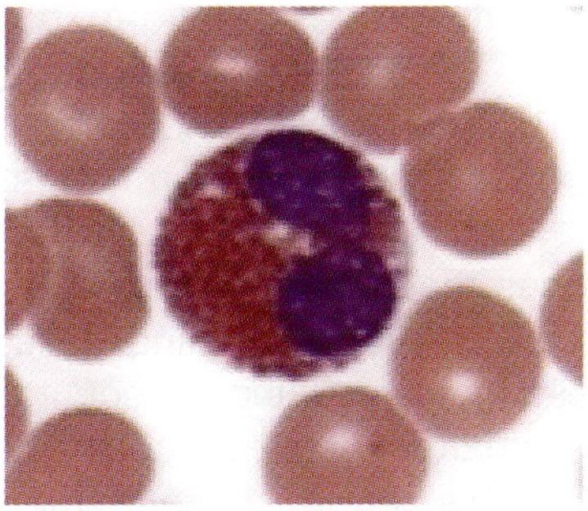

Eosinophil[β]

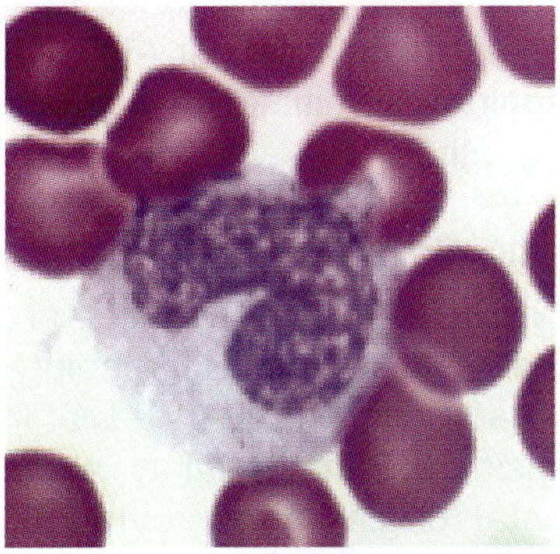

Monocyte[α]

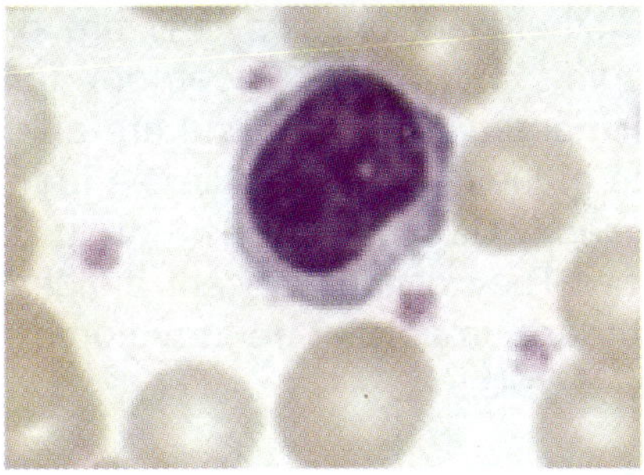

Lymphocytes[α]

Fig. 10.8: Cells of the immune system

α (Reproduced from Practical Hematology, 8th edition, John V Dacie, S M Lewis, Churchill Livingstone 1999) β (Reproduced from Text and Practical Hematology for MBBS, Dr. Tejinder Singh, Arya Publications 2010)

Dendritic Cells

There are two cell types with similar names but different functions. Cells of the dendritic cell (DC) lineage are bone marrow derived. In the skin they are known as Langerhans Cells (LC).

These cells efficiently process antigen but cannot present it to T-cells. LC have been shown to pick up antigen in skin and carry it via afferent lymphatic vessels to lymph nodes. Dendritic cells in lymph are known as "veiled" cells. In lymph nodes the cells, now known as tissue dendritic cells or inter-digitating cells, may efficiently present antigen if they encounter the right T cell. Immature dendritic cells are also called veiled cells, in which case they possess large cytoplasmic 'veils' rather than dendrites. In fact, these are the best APC, far fewer DC are required to initiate an immune response than any other APC.

Follicular Dendritic Cells (FDC)

These are found in lymphoid follicles. They are called dendritic because of their morphology rather than any lineage relationship with DC. In fact, there is considerable uncertainty about their developmental origin (some evidence suggests that they are long-lived bone marrow derived cells, other data projects they are of epithelial origin). FDC have receptors for immunoglobulin and complement and are able to trap antigen at their cell surface, in the form of antigen/antibody/C3d complexes, for long periods of time. They cannot present antigen to T-cells but are important in developing responses by B-cells.

Granulocytes

Granulocytes are a category of *white blood cells* characterized by the presence of *granules* in their cytoplasm. They are also called polymorphonuclear leukocytes (PMN or PML) because of the varying shapes of the *nucleus*, which is usually lobed into three segments. In common parlance, the term polymorphonuclear leukocyte often refers specifically to *neutrophil granulocytes*, the most abundant of the granulocytes. Granulocytes or PMN are released from the bone marrow by the regulatory *complement* proteins. Granulocytes are broadly classified as:

1. Neutrophil.
2. Eosinophil.
3. Basophil.

Both neutrophils and eosinophils are phagocytic, while basophils are not. Neutrophils, comprises 50%–70% of the white blood cells population, where as eosinophils and basophils comprises just (1%-3%) and (<1%) respectively.

Neutrophils

Neutrophilic granulocytes, generally referred to as neutrophils, are the most abundant type of white blood cells and form an integral part of the immune system. Their name arrives from staining characteristics on hematoxylin and eosin (H and E) histological preparations. Basophilic cellular components stain dark blue in contrast to bright red of eosinophilic components and neutral pink of neutrophilic components. These phagocytes are normally found in the blood stream. However, during the acute phase of inflammation, particularly as a result of bacterial infection, neutrophils leave the vasculature and migrate towards the site of inflammation in a process called chemotaxis. They are the predominant cells in pus, accounting for its whitish/ pale yellowish appearance.

Neutrophils react within an hour of tissue injury and are the hallmark of acute inflammation. With the eosinophil and the basophil, they form the class of polymorphonuclear cells (PMNs), named for the nucleus' characteristic multilobulated shape (as compared to lymphocytes and monocytes, the other types of white cells). Neutrophils are the most abundant white blood cells and they account for 70% of all white blood cells (leukocytes). The average half-life of a non-activated neutrophil in the circulation is about 4-10 hours. Upon activation, they marginate (position themselves adjacent to the blood vessel endothelium) and undergo integrin dependent adhesion after which they migrate into tissues, where they survive for 1-2 days.

Neutrophils are much more numerous than the longer-lived monocyte/macrophages. The first phagocyte a pathogen (disease-causing microorganism) is likely to encounter is a neutrophil. Some experts feel that the short span of neutrophils is an evolutionary adaptation to minimize propagation of those pathogens that parasitize phagocytes. The more time such parasites spend outside a host cell, the more likely they will be destroyed by some component of the body's defenses. However, because neutrophil antimicrobial products can also damage host tissues, other school of thought believes that their short life is an adaptation to limit damage to the host during inflammation process.

Neutrophils undergo a process called chemotaxis that allows them to migrate towards the sites of infection/inflammation. Cell surface receptors are able to detect chemical gradients of molecules such as interleukin-8 (IL-8), interferon gamma (IFN-γ), and C5a which these cells use to direct the path of their migration. Neutrophils are phagocytes, capable of ingesting microorganisms or particles. They can internalize and kill many microbes, each phagocytic event resulting in the formation of a phagosome into which reactive oxygen species and hydrolytic enzymes are secreted. The consumption of oxygen during the generation of reactive oxygen species has been termed the "respiratory burst", although it actually has nothing to do with respiration or energy production.

The respiratory burst involves the activation of the enzyme NADPH oxidase, which produces large quantities of superoxide, a reactive oxygen species. Superoxide dismutates, spontaneously or through catalysis via the enzyme catalase, to hydrogen peroxide, which is then converted to hypochlorous acid (HOCl, also known as chlorine bleach) by the green heme enzyme myelo-peroxidase. It is thought that the bactericidal properties of HOCl are enough to kill bacteria phagocytized by the neutrophil, but this has not been proven conclusively. The type of granules and the protein they secrete is given in the **Table 10.2.**

Eosinophils

Eosinophilic cells like neutrophils are motile but their phagocytic role is less pronounced. Nonetheless, they play a key role in defense against parasitic organisms and are known to control mechanisms associated with asthma and allergy. Eosinophils develop and mature in bone marrow. They differentiate from myeloid precursor cells in response to the granulocyte macrophage colony-stimulating factor (GM-CSF). When stained, the staining is concentrated in small granules within the cellular cytoplasm, which contain many chemical mediators, such as histamine and proteins such as eosinophil peroxidase, RNase, DNases, lipase, and plasminogen. These mediators are released by a process called degranulation following activation of the eosinophil, and are toxic to both parasite and host tissues.

Eosinophils make up to nearly about 1-5% of white blood cells, and are about 10-12 micrometers in size. They are found in the medulla and the junction between the cortex and medulla of the thymus, and in the lower gastrointestinal tract, ovary, uterus, spleen, and lymph nodes, but not in the lung, skin, esophagus, or some other internal organs under normal conditions. The presence of eosinophils in these latter organs is associated with disease. Eosinophils persist in the circulation for 6-12 hours, and can survive in tissue for an additional 2-3 days in the absence of stimulation. After maturation, eosinophils circulate in blood and migrate to inflammatory sites in tissues, or to sites of helminth infection in response to chemokines. At these infectious sites, eosinophils are activated by Type 2 cytokines released from a specific subset of helper T-cells. Eosinophils have some important functions related to the performance of:

Table 10.2: Granulocytes and mast cells showing comparative analysis

Granulocyte	*Nuclear morphology*	*Size*	*Granules*	*Protein*	*Function*
			Secondary granules	Lactoferin and cathelicidin	
Neutrophil	Horse-shoe shape	12-15μ	Azurophilic granules	Myeloperoxidase, bactericidal/permeability increasing protein (BPI) defensins and the serine proteases neutrophil elastase and cathepsin G	Active phagocytosis
			Tertiary granules	Cathepsin, gelatinase	
Basophil	Bi-lobed nucleus	8-12μ	Large cytoplasmic	Proteolytic enzyme example elastase	Allergic reactions
Eosinophil	Dumble shaped nucleus	10-12μ	Small granules	Peroxidase	Combating infection by parasite
Mast cell	Bi-lobed		Numerous granule rich in heparin and histamine	Nil	Allergic and anaphylaxis reaction

- Cytokines such as IL-1, IL-2, IL-4, IL-5, IL-6, IL-8, IL-13 and TNF alpha.
- Enzymes, such as elastase.
- Reactive oxygen species such as superoxide.
- Cationic granule proteins and their release by degranulation.

In addition eosinophils play a role in fighting viral infections, which is evident from the abundance of RNAses they contain within their granules and in fibrin removal during inflammation. Eosinophils are considered the main effector cells in allergic responses and asthma pathogenesis and are associated with disease severity. They also fight helminth colonization and their level may be slightly elevated in the presence of certain parasites. Eosinophils are also involved in many other biological processes, including post-pubertal mammary gland development, oestrus cycling, allograft rejection and neoplasia. They have also recently been implicated in antigen presentation to T-cells.

Basophils

Basophils are the least common of the granulocytes, representing about 0.01% to 0.3% of circulating leukocytes (white blood cells). They contain large cytoplasmic granules which obscure the cell nucleus under the microscope. However, when unstained, the nucleus is visible and it usually has 2 lobes. The mast cell, a cell in tissues, has many similar characteristics.

For example, both cell types store histamine, a chemical that is secreted by the cells when stimulated in certain ways (histamine causes some of the symptoms of an allergic reaction).

Like all circulating granulocytes, basophils can be recruited out of the blood into a tissue when needed. When activated, basophils degranulate to release histamine, proteoglycans (e.g., heparin and chondroitin), and proteolytic enzymes (e.g., elastase and lysophospholipase). They also secrete lipid mediators like leukotrienes, and several cytokines. Histamine and proteoglycans are pre-stored in the cell's granules while the other secreted substances are newly generated. Each of these substances contributes to inflammation. There are other substances that can activate basophils to secrete, which suggests that these cells have other roles in inflammation.

Mast Cells

A mast cell (or mastocyte) is a resident of several types of tissues and contains many granules rich in histamine and heparin. Although best known for their role in allergy and anaphylaxis, mast cells play an important proactive protective role as well, being intimately involved in wound healing and defense against pathogens. Mast cells have large granules that led to the mistaken belief that they existed to nourish the surrounding tissue, and were named as "mastzellen", meaning "feeding cells". Nowadays, they are considered part of the immune system. Mast cells are very similar to basophil granulocytes in blood; the similarities between mast cells and basophils have led many to speculate that mast cells are basophils that have "homed in" on tissues. However, current evidence suggests that they are generated by different precursor cells in the bone marrow.

Two types of mast cells, one from connective tissue and the other from mucosal cell, are recognized. The activities of the latter are dependent on T-cells. Mast cells are present in most tissues in the vicinity of blood vessels, and are especially prominent near the boundaries between the outside world and the internal milieu, such as the skin, mucosa of the lungs and digestive tract, as well as in the mouth, conjunctiva and nose.

Abnormalities of Immune Cells

Abnormalities found in immune cells are generally inherited defects which are found in either specific or non-specific immune mechanisms. Individuals suffering from such abnormalities are susceptible to a variety of infections and the type of infection depends on the nature of the abnormality. They can be classified as B cell, T cell or phagocytic abnormalities depending on their site of occurrence. These abnormalities are responsible for some specific diseases as shown in **Table 10.3**.

Phagocytic Abnormalities

Defects in phagocyte function can be classified as either intrinsic, i.e., related to the inherent properties or extrinsic. Intrinsic disorders related to different stages of differentiation and function of phagocyte have been identified, in addition to those associated with abnormal chemo-attraction to the site of microbial assault and intracellular killing of the microbe. Extrinsic defects result from deficiency of antibody/complement or suppression of phagocytic activity by glucocorticoids/autoantibodies.

Abnormalities of B Lymphocytes

These defects, mainly arise due to the abnormal development of the B cell system. Some abnormalities may also arise due to blockage in certain steps of B cell maturation. An example is Bruton's disease, in which B cell precursors do not develop resulting in severe deficiency of B-cells and very few antibodies in circulation. The lack of antibodies means that patients suffer from recurrent infections. Other B cell abnormalities may arise due to the defective regulation by T-cells. In common

Table 10.3: Abnormalities of the immune cells, which are responsible for certain diseases/malfunction

Abnormality	*Disease/Mechanism*
Stem cell differentiation	Neutropenia—very few neutrophils
Lack of adhesion to endothelium	Leukocyte adhesion deficiency—Lack of expression of CD18 molecule
Defective phagocytosis	Chediak Higashi syndrome—Lack of fusion of phagosome with lysosome
Defective intracellular killing	Chronic granulomatous disease—Defective genes encoding for NADPH oxidase involved in oxygen mediated killing
Defective IFN-γ or IL-12 receptors	Failure to activate NADPH oxidase.

variable Immunodeficiency B-cells may not respond to signals from other cells. These abnormalities can lead to a condition of transient hypogammaglobulemia, where levels of certain immunoglobulins are downregulated due to poor T cell help.

Abnormalities of T Lymphocytes

These abnormalities are rare, and are mainly due to defects during development. The most clearly defined disorder of T-cells is DiGeorge's syndrome which is caused due to a defect in the thymic embryogenesis. No genetic disposition is clear and not all DiGeorge's babies have thymic aplasia. Cases have been reported on stem cell defects where the patient has an abnormality in the chain used by many cytokine receptors; hence he/she cannot respond to or produce IFN-γ. T cell abnormalities may also arise due to lack of coordination of movement as seen in ataxia telangiectasia or due to reduced T cell functions which progressively worsen as in the case of Wiskott Aldrich syndrome. Individuals having a defect in MHC Class II transactivator (CIITA) and transport associated protein (TAP) have deficiencies in CD4 and CD8 cells respectively.

Conclusion

The immune system is a versatile defense system which protects organisms from invading pathogenic microbes. It has the ability to generate myriad varieties of cells and molecules capable of recognizing and eliminating an enormous number of foreign intruders which may or may not be pathogenic. Cells of the immune system are classified into three classes namely- lymphocytes, granulocytes and antigen presenting cells. All immune cells originate in the bone marrow from stem cells. They respond to different signals, undergo selection pressures, mature and grow into specific cell types such as T-cells, B-cells, granulocytes and phagocytes. Immune cells act with a synchronization and synergy depending on the situation, which is influenced by various intrinsic and extrinsic factors. The effector response generated by these cells to neutralize the antigen depends on the type of the cell, as well as the nature of the antigen. Some cells are also dedicated towards generation of a memory response, marked by an immediate and heightened immune reaction on subsequent exposures to foreign invaders. The lymphocyte is the only cell to possess the immunological attributes of specificity, diversity, memory and self/non T self recognition.

The immunoglobulins bound to the membrane of B lymphocytes are effective in neutralizing numerous antigens. On target recognition, these cells expand clonally. With time, affinity maturation of the immunoglobulin through gene rearrangement makes them effective mediators of humoral immunity. T lymphocytes mediate the cellular arm of immunity. They recognize antigenic peptides in conjunction with MHC. CD8+ (TC) cells are MHC-1 restricted, whereas CD4+ (TH) cells are MHC-2 restricted. The T_H1 activates T-cells and phagocytes whereas T_H2 response activate mainly antibody mediated responses by co-operating with B-cells.

The large and granular natural killer cells are also lymphocytes but do not express the set of surface markers characteristic of B and T-cells. They detect and attack mainly virus infected self cells. Irregularities in the 'surface antigen profile' of infected cells mark them for destruction by NK cells. The gigantic phagocytes engulf micro-organisms and also clear the cellular debris. They effectively process and present antigens to lymphocytes. Granulocytes namely neutrophils, basophils, eosinophils and mast cells vary widely in their morphology, abundance and staining pattern. They play prominent roles in a gamut of immune responses ranging from anaphylaxis to inflammation. Hematopoiesis is closely regulated to assure steady state levels of different types of cells. Cell division and differentiation of each of the lineages is balanced by programmed cell death. The origin of immune cells from multipotent self renewing stem cells holds promise in cell based therapy for autoimmune and immunodeficiency disorders and a potential cure for leukemia.

At this time you should know the following:

1. A brief overview of the origin and development of immune cells and cell-mediated and humoral immunity.
2. The types and sub-population of lymphocytes, their characteristics and mechanism.
3. Antigen presenting cells and their types and functions.
4. Granulocytes, their types and characteristics
5. Abnormalities of immune cells.

Further Reading

1. http://pathmicro.med.sc.edu/bowers/immune%20cells.htm
2. http://bcs.whfreeman.com/thelifewire/content/chp18/1802001.html
3. http://www.microbiologybytes.com/iandi/2a.html
4. http://www.merckmanuals.com/home/sec16/ch183/ch183b.html

11

CHAPTER

Major Histocompatibility Complex (MHC) and T-Cell Receptors

(Dr. Parul Goel and Dr. Mohd. Suhail parul006@gmail.com**)**

OBJECTIVES

To understand the structure and function of cell surface molecules involved in immune cell interactions:

- Major histocompatibility complex molecules.
- The T cell receptor (TCR).
- The CD3 complex; and
- Accessory and costimulatory molecules.

INTRODUCTION

Each mammal possesses a tightly linked cluster of genes called the major histocompatibility complex (MHC) that play a role in intercellular recognition, discrimination between self and non-self, organ transplantation, and autoimmunity. The human MHC complex is called human leukocyte antigen (HLA) complex and is 4-megabase (Mb) region on chromosome 6.

MAJOR HISTOCOMPATIBILITY COMPLEX

A. History

1. In transplantation studies, MHC gene products were identified as responsible for graft rejection.
2. It was determined that antigen-specific T-cells recognize portions of protein antigens that are bound to MHC gene products.
   a. Helper T-cells recognize peptide bound to class II MHC gene products.
   b. Cytotoxic T-cells recognize peptide bound to class I MHC gene products.
3. The complete three-dimensional structure for both class I and class II MHC molecules was determined by X-ray crystallography.

B. Structure of MHC Molecules

1. Class I MHC

Class I MHC molecule is a glycoprotein and contains two separate polypeptide chains:

1. MHC-encoded alpha (or heavy) chain; 43 kDa.
2. Non-MHC-encoded beta chain (β_2 microglobulin) 12 kDa.

There are four separate regions:

1. Peptide-binding region is a groove formed from the alpha 1 and alpha 2 regions which interact to form a "floor" of an 8-stranded, beta-pleated sheet with two opposite "walls" consisting of parallel strands of a α-helix (alpha 1 and alpha 2 each contribute 4 strands of beta-pleated sheet and one alpha-helix). A peptide 8-10 amino acid long sits in the groove. The greatest variability in amino acids occurs in the alpha 1 and alpha 2 sequences that form the groove that interacts with

amino acids of the peptide fragment. Thus, the polymorphism among class I MHC gene products creates variation in the chemical surface of the peptide-binding groove. For any given MHC molecule, binding of a peptide usually requires the peptide to have one or more specific amino acids at a fixed position, frequently the terminal or penultimate amino acid of the peptide. Binding of the specific amino acid in the groove of the MHC molecule occurs in what is termed anchor site(s). The other amino acids can be variable so that each MHC molecule can bind many different peptides. Other polymorphic residues of the MHC molecule are those in contact with the T cell receptor (TCR), which interacts with both peptide and the MHC molecule itself.

2. Immunoglobulin-like region is composed of an alpha 3 segment that is highly conserved and is homologous to Ig constant domains and non-covalently bound to beta 2 microglobulin (100 amino acids), an invariant molecule, also homologous to Ig constant domains. These two interact with alpha 1 and alpha 2 to maintain their proper conformation.

   The importance of the highly conserved region of alpha 3 is that CD 8, a molecule expressed on cytotoxic T-cells that recognizes class I MHC molecules, binds to this region.

3. Transmembrane region is a stretch of ~25 hydrophobic amino acids.
4. Cytoplasmic region is the carboxy terminal 30 amino acids. It contains phosphorylation sites and provides binding sites for cytoskeletal elements.

2. Class II MHC

MHC class II molecule contains two non-covalently associated polypeptide chains

1. Alpha chain; 34 kDa
2. Beta chain; 28 kDa

There are four separate regions:

1. Peptide-binding region is formed by interaction of the alpha1 and beta1 segments. There is a groove having a "floor" of 8 beta-pleated strands and two "walls" with alpha-helices; alpha1 and beta1 make equal contributions to this structure. As in the case for class I MHC, the greatest polymorphic variability is in the amino acids facing the groove. Thus, as for class I MHC, the genetic polymorphism determines the chemical structure of the groove and influences the specificity and affinity of peptide binding and T cell recognition. Peptides associated with class II MHC are 13-25 amino acids long; the longer peptides project from the ends of the groove. As with class I MHC, anchor sites for one or more amino acids also exist in the groove of the class II MHC molecule, but these occur at more variable locations.
2. Immunoglobulin-like region formed by alpha 2 and beta 2 is folded into Immunoglobulin (Ig)-like domains. These are largely non-polymorphic. The correlation of CD4 expression on helper T-cells with a specific TCR for class II MHC molecules is due to binding of the CD4 molecules to the Ig-like non-polymorphic beta 2 domain of the class II MHC molecules.

3. & 4. Transmembrane and cytoplasmic regions have proposed functions similar to their counterparts in class I MHC.

C. Similarities and Differences Between Class I and Class II MHC Molecules

Despite differences in the two-chain composition of class I and class II MHC molecules, they are quite similar structurally and both are made up of glycoproteins **(Table 11.1)**.

Table 11.1: The MHC I and MHC II

Properties	***Class I***	***Class II***
Distribution	Most of the somatic cells (Nucleated Cells), More on lymphocytes and less on hepatocyte, Fibroblasts, muscle cell and neurons	Limited to APC, macrophage, dendritic cells, thymic epithelial cells, B cells
Location	2-Mb and on telomeric end	1-Mb and on centromeric end
Constituents	α1, α2, α3 on chromosome 6 and β2 on chromosome 15	α1, α2, β1 and β2 on chromosome 6
Peptide binding domain	α1 / α2, intrachain dimer	α1/β1, interchain dimer
Nature of peptide binding cleft	Closed at both ends	Open at both ends
General size of bound peptides	8–10 amino acids	13–18 amino acids
Peptide motifs involved in binding to MHC molecule	Anchor residues at both ends of peptide; generally hydrophobic carboxyl terminal anchor	Anchor residues distributed along the length of the peptide
Nature of bound peptide	Extended structure in which both ends interact with MHC cleft but middle arches up away from MHC molecule	Extended structure that is held at a constant elevation above the floor of MHC cleft
Expression	Expressed in intracellular infection (Listeria, Plasmodium), Tumor antigen, minor histocompatibility antigen and certain auto antigens	Expressed in immune response in general
Functions	HLA-A and HLA-B: Present antigen to CD8 + T cell HLA-C: Target of NK cell recognition HLA-G: Express on trophoblasts, maintaining maternal foeto tolerance	Bind to antigenic peptide and present antigen to CD4 + Helper T-cell Class II DO molecule: Expressed in thymus and mature B-cell
Commonly associated with	Ankylosing spondylitis, Reiter's syndrome, T-cell psoriatic spondylitis, Behcet's disease, myasthenia gravis, congenital adrenal hyperplasia	Celiac disease, Goodpasteur's syndrome, pemphigus vulgaris, Sjögren's syndrome, SLE, Rheumatoid arthritis, DM type I.

D. Important Aspects of MHC

1. Since MHC molecules are membrane-associated and not soluble, T-cells must make cell to cell contact with cells expressing MHC molecules.
2. In general, peptide fragments of proteins in the cytosol associate with class I MHC; those of vesicular proteins associate with class II MHC. Each is recognized by functionally distinct T cell populations. CD8+ T-cells recognize class I MHC-peptide while CD4+ T-cells recognize class II MHC-peptide.
3. There are many different MHC gene products for class I and class II in the human population (polymorphism), only some of which are found in an individual. The maximum number of class I MHC gene products expressed in an individual is six; that for class II MHC products can exceed six but is also limited. Whether or not a peptide fragment can associate with a given MHC product determines whether there will be an immune response. This is one level of control of immune responses.
4. Mature T-cells respond to foreign antigens, but not self protein. The repertoire of antigen recognition is based on selection processes involving MHC molecules that occur mainly in the thymus. This is another level of control of immune responses.
5. Only a single binding site exists on a class I or class II MHC molecule; all peptides it is capable of binding must bind to the same site.
6. The MHC polymorphism is determined only in the germ line. There is no somatic DNA recombination that occurs for antibodies and for the TCR, so the MHC genes lack recombinational mechanisms for generating diversity. As a result, the affinity and selectivity of MHC molecules for foreign proteins are considerably lower than those of antibodies and T cell antigens.
7. Because each MHC molecule can bind many different peptides, the binding is said to be degenerate. Compared with the restricted binding of a hormone to a receptor, for example, where a difference in even one amino acid may impair binding.
8. Cytokines, especially interferon gamma (IFN-gamma), increase the level of expression of class I and class II MHC molecules.
9. Alleles for MHC genes are co-dominant, i.e. each gene product is expressed on the cell surface (Contrast this with allelic exclusion).
10. Why the high polymorphism of MHC molecules? Although an individual may not possess MHC molecules capable of binding certain antigenic peptides, say for example against a virulent organism, the likelihood is great that other MHC in the species can do so. Overall this affords an evolutionary protection for the continuation of that species.
11. MHC class I expression is reduced during malignancy and viral infection (Cytomegalo virus, Hepatitis B, Adenovirus) which is recognized by NK cells resulting in the destruction of affected host cells.

3. MHC III

Several structurally and functionally diverse proteins are encoded within the third region of the MHC. It is 1 Mb in size and situated between II and I MHC gene. These class III molecules include several complement components (C2, C4a, C4b and Factor B), two enzymes (21 hydroxylases α and β), inflammatory cytokines (tumor necrosis factors α and β) and two heat shock proteins.

The class III molecules are not membrane proteins and are not related structurally to class I and II. They play some role in immune functions including components of the complement system and inflammation but have no role in antigen presentation.

T-CELL RECEPTOR (TCR)

The three-dimensional structure of the TCR has been determined by X-ray crystallography. It is a heterodimer of two polypeptide chains, alpha (40-50 kDa) and beta (35-47 kDa), covalently linked by a disulfide bond. Both alpha and beta chains are similar to immunoglobulin, each consisting of a variable (V) and constant (C) region. The variable region also has a joining (J) segment, and for the beta chains only, a diversity (D) segment as well. Both chains contribute to the receptor formed by the V regions. There are hypervariable regions in the V regions; these contribute to the diversity of the TCR. The cytoplasmic tail for each chain is short and not involved in signal transduction. The TCR is present on both helper and cytotoxic T-cells. A given T cell expresses TCR of only a single specificity. The TCR recognizes portions of both the MHC molecule and the peptide bound in the groove.

There is also a small population of T-cells that expresses a TCR comprised completely different chains, the γ chain and the δ chain. These T-cells are termed γδ T-cells to distinguish them from the more prevalent alpha-beta T-cells. Most gamma delta T-cells do not express CD4, characteristic of helper T-cells, or CD8, characteristic of cytotoxic T-cells. They appear earlier in development than αβ T-cells and have a TCR that does not recognize MHC-peptide. The functions of γδ T-cells are still being elucidated.

The diversity of TCRs is estimated to be as high as 10^{16}. This is due to the many possibilities for combining V, D and J regions, N-region diversification, joining-site variation and multiple D regions. This number is considerably higher than the number of T-cells leaving the thymus, as is true for the number of possible immunoglobulin specificities relative to the number of B-cells produced **(Table 11.2)**.

CD3 Complex

CD3 complex is a group of five proteins that are physically associated with the TCR. It consists of α γ chain, δ chain, 2 ε chains, and 2 ζ chains.

The γ, δ and ε chains are produced by three closely linked genes and are highly homologous. The ζ chain is the product of a single gene and is

Table 11.2: Comparison of the major properties of immunoglobulin (Ig) and T-cell receptor (TCR) genes and proteins

	GENES	
Properties	Ig	TCR
Many VDJs, Few C's	Yes	Yes
VDJ rearrangement	Yes	Yes
V pairs form antigen-recognition site	Yes	Yes
Somatic hypermutation	Yes	No
	PROTEINS	
Transmembrane forms	Yes	Yes
Secreted forms	Yes	No
Isotypes with distinct functions	Yes	No
Valency	2	1

involved in signaling. All four are invariant and do not contribute to the specificity of binding of the TCR. Do not confuse the $\gamma\delta$ chains of the T cell receptor on $\gamma\delta$ T-cells with the γ chain and δ chain of the CD3 complex; they are distinctly different molecules.

The functions of the CD3 complex are:

1. To ensure the cell surface expression of the TCR. The synthesis of the TCR and the CD3 complex, their assembly, and surface expression are tightly coordinated.
2. To transduce activating signals to the interior of the T cell when the associated TCR binds peptide-MHC. The CD3 complex thus performs a signaling function similar to that of the Ig-alpha and Ig-beta molecules associated with the immunoglobulin receptor on B-cells.

CELL SURFACE MOLECULES INVOLVED IN CELL-CELL INTERACTIONS

Engagement of a TCR and the peptide-MHC complex it recognizes is not sufficient to activate a T cell. Other cell surface molecules between the two interacting cells also engage. These form two groups termed accessory molecules and costimulatory molecules **(Table 11.3)**.

1. Accessory molecules

When the TCR of a T cell recognizes the peptide-MHC molecule on another cell, the accessory molecules attach non-covalently to ligands on that cell.

2. Costimulatory molecules

Engagement of the TCR with peptide-MHC delivers one signal to the T cell that alone is insufficient to activate a T cell. Costimulatory molecules when bound to their ligand deliver a second signal required for the T cell to become activated. The most critical costimulatory molecule on the T cell is CD28, which binds to either B7-1 (CD80) or B7-2 (CD86). All three molecules are non-polymorphic and invariant.

At this time you should know the following:

1. The basics of cell surface involvement in immune interaction.
2. Major histocompatibility complex molecules and their mechanism of action.
3. Basic of the T cell receptor (TCR) and their mechanism of action.
4. Basic of the CD3 complex and their mechanism of action; and
5. Accessory and costimulatory molecules and their mechanism of action.

Further Reading

1. Roitt's Essential Immunology: Delves, Martin, Burton and Roitt.
2. Cellular and Molecular Immunology: Abbas, Lichtman, Pillai.
3. Janeway's Immunobiology: Murphy, Travers, Walport.

Table 11.3: Important ligand-receptor interaction

T cell molecule	*Ligand on second cell*
CD4 on helper T cells	Class II MHC molecules
CD8 on cytotoxic T cells	Class I MHC molecules
LFA-2	LFA-3
LFA-1	ICAM-1, ICAM-2

LFA = Leukocyte Function-associated Antigen

ICAM = Intercellular Adhesion Molecule

12

CHAPTER

Response to Antigen

(Dr. Rashid Ali and Dr. B K Gupta *raliamu@yahoo.com*)

OBJECTIVES

1. Different types of antigen recognized by T and B-cells.
2. Various pathways operating for antigen processing and presentation.
3. Role of class I and class II MHC molecules.
4. Class I and class II restricted antigens and peptide binding sites.
5. Role of thymus in determining T-cell repertoire.
6. Significance of costimulators and accessory molecules.

INTRODUCTION

B and T-cells recognize different substances as antigen in different forms after processing by two different pathways. The B-cell recognizes antigen by surface-bound Ig as a receptor and its specificity is the same as Ig that plasma cell is able to secrete after cell activation. A variety of cell molecules are recognized by B-cells having altogether different immunogenicity. However, the majority of antigens for T-cells are proteins. These are changed to immunogenic peptides by processing and require association with MHC class I and class II molecules. Helper T-cells recognize only those peptides associated with class II MHC molecules, and cytolytic T-cells (CTLs) recognize only those peptides that are associated with class I MHC molecules.

BIOCHEMISTRY OF PROCESSING AND PRESENTATION

The Role of Class II MHC Molecules

The interaction of T-cell and class II MHC molecules became evident when antibodies against class II MHC profoundly inhibited T-cell activation. The restriction in T-cell activation are also imposed by the different alleles of the Class II region of the MHC gene complex (**Figure 12.1**). The antibodies to class II MHC bind to these molecules on the APC surface and stop the cell from recognizing the immunogen and adhering to the APC, the result is a lack of T-cell stimulation. The requirement of T-cells to recognize protein antigen molecules by APC that contained class II MHC molecules has been definitely established. The cells do not respond in the absence of APC and their receptors do not interact or bind to the protein directly.

The APC recognizes the antigen only subsequent to its interaction with class II MHC bearing macrophage. The recognition of antigen on the APCs results in a close cellular contact for several hours. By about 24 hours after contact, the T-cells proliferate and abandon the surface of the macrophage. The three experimental system in which MHC restriction was discovered, involves (**Figure 12.2**):

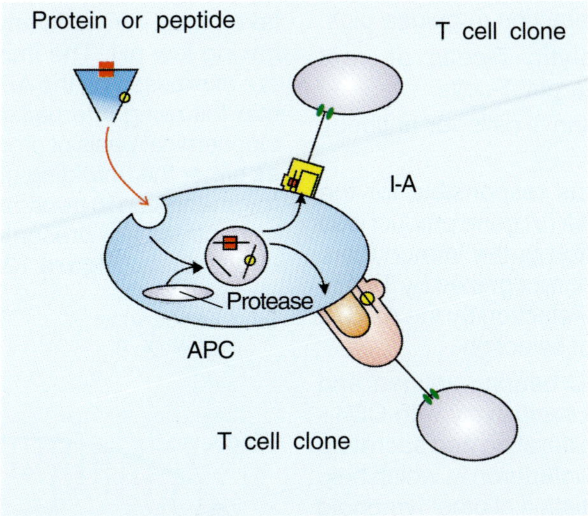

Fig. 12.1: Steps in antigen presentation. Soluble antigen enters the presenting cell by phagocytosis, pinocytosis, or receptor-mediated endocytosis. It is partially degraded to peptide fragments by acid-dependent endosomal proteases. If antigenic peptides are formed, they will associate with MHC class II molecules (I-A or I-E in the mouse) to form an antigenic complex on the cell surface. Binding of T-cell receptors to the complex triggers the T-cell to divide, resulting in clonal expansion of antigen specific T-cells

(Source: Fundamental Immunology, second edition, 1989 (Ed. W. Paul), Raven Press, New York, Page 189)

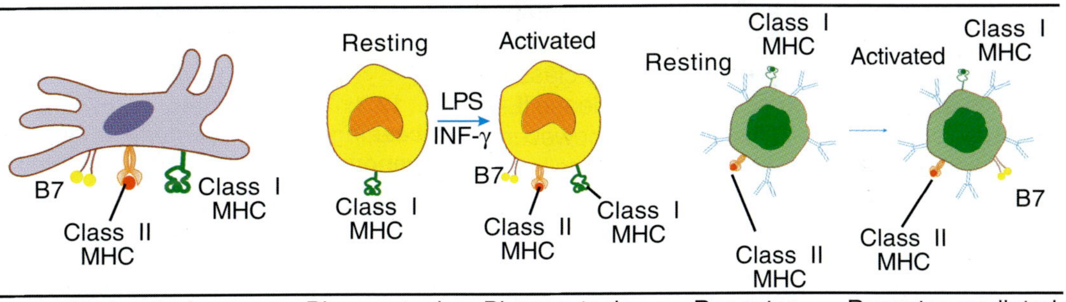

	Dendritic cell	*Macrophage* (Resting)	*Macrophage* (Activated)	*B Lymphocyte* (Resting)	*B Lymphocyte* (Activated)
Antigen uptake	Endocytosis phagocytosis (by Langerhans cells)	Phagocytosis	Phagocytosis	Receptor mediated endocytosis	Receptor-mediated endocytosis
Class II MHC expression	Constitutive B7 (+++)	Inducible (–)	Inducible (++)	Constitutive (++)	Constitutive (+++)
Co-stimulatory activity	Constitutive B7 (+++)	Inducible B7 (–)	Inducible B7 (++)	Inducible B7 (–)	Inducible B7 (++)
T-cell activation	Naive T cells Effector T cells Memory T cells	(–)	Effector T cells Memory T cells	Effector T cells Memory T cells	Naive T cells Effector T cells Memory T cells

Fig. 12.2: Differences in the properties of professional antigen-presenting cells affect their ability to present antigen and induce T-cell activation

1. Macrophage-T-cell interaction in guinea pigs.
2. Recognition of cytolytic T-cells of viral antigens in infected target T-cells.
3. The interaction of B and T-cells for antibody formation.

Thus one cellular locus responsible for the effects of immune response (Ir) gene product was the APC by its presentation to the immunogen. The antigenic determinant recognized by T-cells depends on a process of selection by the APC. It is referred as 'determinant selection'.

The interaction of APC bearing antigen and class II MHC molecule is exclusively with CD4+ cells, they respond by proliferating and secreting lymphokines like IL-2 and interferon λ, which help in the growth and differentiation of other lymphoid cells—thus the name helper or inducer T-cells given to them.

In contrast, the CD8 bearing cell recognizes antigen in the context of class I MHC molecules and responds by producing a lytic lesion on the target cells (cytolytic T-cell). The correlation between helper and cytolytic function with recognition of class II and class I molecules, respectively, is not always true as some CD4 cells produce lysis of the target cells bearing class I MHC molecules while some CD8 cells release IL-2 and can act as helpers. The correlation, however, is consistant between the presence in T-cells of CD4 or CD8 molecules and the interaction of their receptors with either class II MHC or class I MHC molecules, respectively.

A globular protein antigen induces an antibody in which the antibodies recognize conformational determinants of the antigen. These determinants are expressed in the folded protein, which involve areas normally separated in the unfolded molecule. This indicates that B-cell clones are selected by an antigen that is not biochemically altered by the host metabolic processes. In striking contrast. The T-cell responses—delayed sensitivity or proliferation to antigen presented by APC—are elicited by denatured proteins or partially fragmented antigens.

Most protein antigens require their internalization and a biochemical processing event that take place intracellularly, in vesicles of the APC having low pH. The immunogenic determinants are expressed on the APC surface within 30 to 60 min following internalization of the protein. The biochemical basis of processing has been defined as either the unfolding of the protein antigen or its fragmentation to peptides. The denatured protein or peptides are presented to APCs without their endocytosis (**Figure 12.3**).

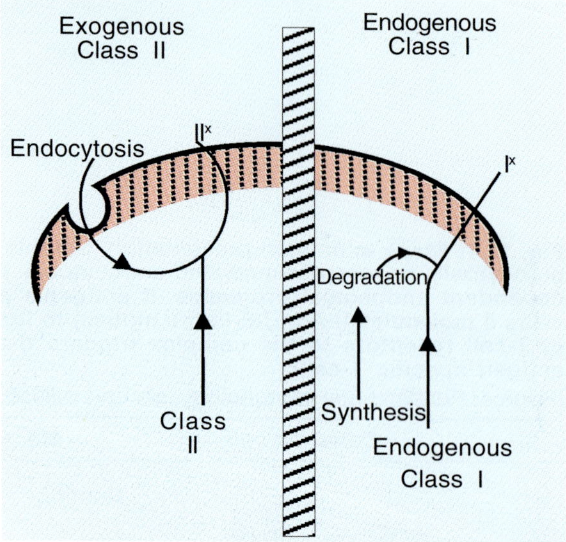

Fig. 12.3: Two possible pathways of antigen processing and presentation. On the left the exogenous or class II MHC-restricted pathway, on the right the endogenous or class I MHC-restricted pathway. Exogenous antigens that enter a cell by endocytosis, either receptor mediated or fluid phase, may be degraded in endocytic vesicles which eventually fuse with vesicles containing available class II molecules but not available class I molecules. The degradation of proteins made endogenously on free or membrane-bound ribosomes results in the peptides binding to class I molecules (Source: Fundamental Immunology, second edition, 1989 (Ed. W. Paul), Raven Press, New York, Page 556)

Some T-cell clones recognize the denatured protein while others recognize peptide fragment. Exposure of peptide fragments to the live macrophage resulted in their presentation for processing. Peptide fragments of about 10 to 12

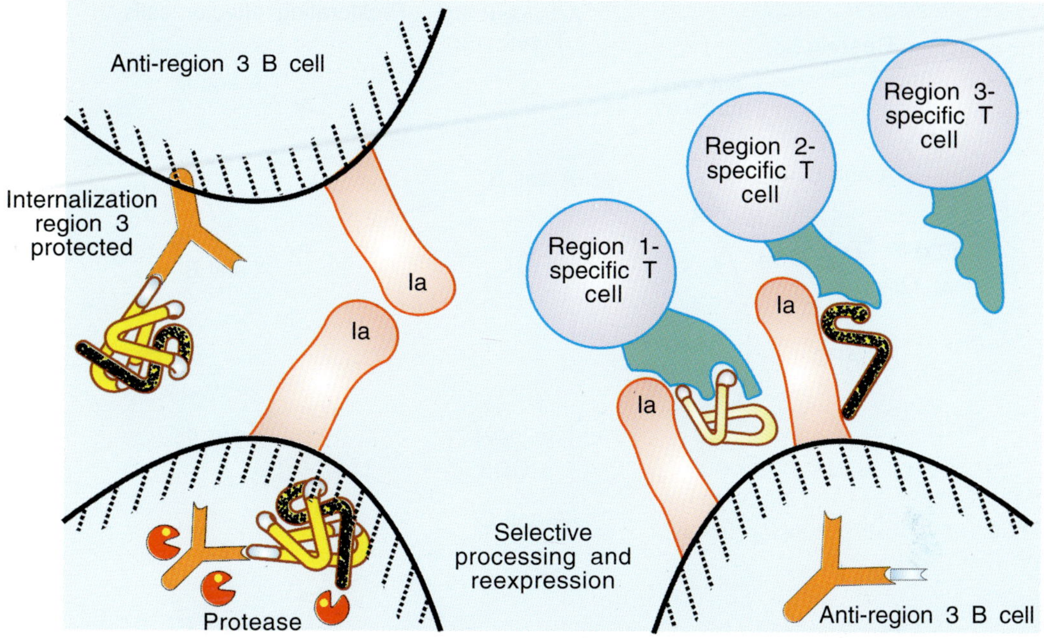

Fig. 12.4: Salient features of biochemical response to antigen
(Source: Fundamental Immunology, second edition, 1989 (Ed. W. Paul), Raven Press, New York, Page 200)

amino acids are presented to the T-cell. The salient features of biochemical processing are as follows (**Figure 12.4**):

1. The antigenic determinants from a protein recognized by T-cells vary depending on the halotype of the class II MHC molecules. For a given peptide from the protein, some strains are responders and others non-responders.
2. In a complex protein, there are more than one epitopes which are potentially immunogenic but the T-cell are usually directed to the immunodominant peptides.
3. The antigenic peptides may be located in areas of the protein antigen that are hidden or buried in the cell. Antibody response is directed which is usually located in the periphery of the protein.
4. A single peptide can stimulate more than one set of clone of T-cells which recognize it with subtle differences in specificity (**Figure 12.5**).

MHC molecules interact with antigens to form bimolecular complexes recognized by T-cells, the protein binds immunogenic peptides. The association between class II MHC protein and immunogenic peptides is slow accompanied by very slow rate of dissociation. There is a close relationship between the degree of binding of a peptide to class II MHC molecules and its recognition and presentation by APCs. A correlation between this binding and peptides *in vivo* imunogenicity has been noticed. The role of class II MHC molecules is to bind and transport peptide for processing.

A single class II MHC molecule contains one combining site that accommodates a single peptide. The binding site accommodate peptides of different structure and is quite diverse. Physicochemical studies have given strong structural evidence for a combining site on class I MHC protein. The combining site is represented by a groove situated on the outermost region of the molecule, made up of a platform of β-pleated sheets surrounded by two α-helices. Both the α_1 and α_2 domains of class I MHC contribute to the platform and the helices. The area of the α-helices

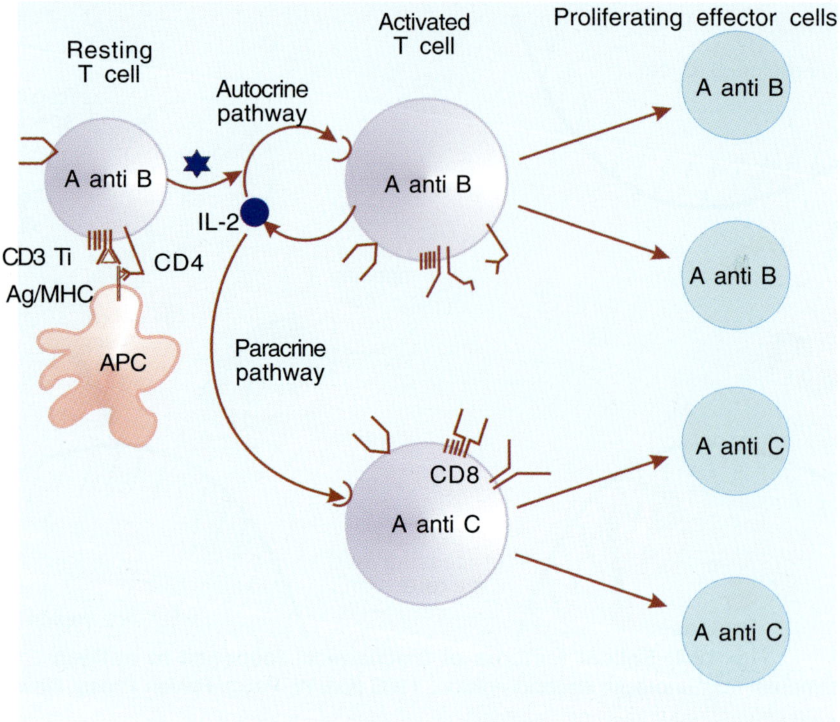

Fig. 12.5: Model of autocrine and paracrine pathways of T cell proliferation (Source: Fundamental Immunology, second edition, 1989 (Ed. W. Paul), Raven Press, New York, P-376)

and platform contains most of the amino acids responsible for allelic polymorphism or for mutations that affect presentation.

The peptides that bind to class II MHC have amino acid residues that contact the MHC molecules intermixed with other residues that are primarily recognized by the T-cell receptor. It has been observed that the MHC contact and T-cell contact residues were three amino acids apart. The peptides bind to MHC and adopt novel conformation imposed by the MHC combining site. Perhaps the slow association rate of binding may reflect the time required to develop novel conformation.

The T-cell receptor will therefore recognize those amino acid side chains of the peptide facing out from the groove that comprises the putative combing site. The novel peptide configuration together with the class II MHC residues of α helix of combining site would constitute the structure to which the T-cell receptor binds.

Pure polysaccharides do not stimulate T-cell immunity as they do not bind class II MHC molecules because of their large hydrophilicity. Polysaccharides affect antigen presentation probably by interfering with the coupling of peptides with class II MHC molecules. Certain microbes having large polysaccharide contents have poor presentation of their own antigen.

Antigenic Competition

Peptide binding to a single site on class II MHC indicates competition for presentation not only among foreign peptides but also between foreign and autologous peptides. Antigenic competition was shown to take place at the level of APC among peptides by the same class II MHC molecules and the molecule does not make any discrimination between foreign and self structures. Such discrimination, however, is made by the T-cell system.

Some of the MHC molecules have peptides already bound to them from processing of self proteins. That self peptides are being presented as important in the context of autoimmunity as well as self-tolerance in the thymus. A higher mass (i.e. aggregating, precipitation in alum, incorporation in lipids) of immunogen in the APC overrides the physiological competition between foreign and autologous proteins.

Cellular Studies

During protein processing, a great majority end up in lysosomes and undergo extensive degradation to amino acids or small peptides. Some partially catabolised becomes available to the immune system. These fragments are released from time to time from the macrophage and also detected on the plasma membrane. These fragments, however, are not in the final form that associate with class II MHC and are not presented.

Trypsin treatment of macrophage, which removes surface-bound peptide, does not alter the presentation of the class II MHC-peptide complex and therefore does not impair antigen presentation. Thus, immunogenic peptide is protected from proteolysis.

The immunogenic peptides are generated in an acid compartment compatible with endosomes. Class II MHC molecules serve as a transport system that binds to the peptide generated in endosomes and transport them to the membrane, thus protect it from further proteolysis. Antigen presentation is not an exclusive property of APCs from lymphoid tissues. Cells can be made to express MHC molecules by treatment with interferon γ or by transfecting them with the genes encoding for α and β chains of class II MHC. Endothelial cells, fibroblast and a variety of epithelial cells have the capacity to present antigen.

Co-Stimulators and Accessory Molecules

Stimulation of T-cells, a complex phenomenon, is by a number of accessory molecules expressed by both T-cell and APC. These molecules are:

1. Those that promote the physical contact of APCs and CD4 lymphocytes.
2. Those that promote the growth/activation of the T-cell.

Cell adhesion molecules promote contact between the APCs and CD4 T lymphocytes, one such molecule is LFA-1. The stimulator molecules are required for the initiation of growth and activation of T-cells. They may act by inducing early release of lymphokines that promote T-cell growth factor and/or expression of surface receptors for growth factors. The best known example of stimulator is IL-1, has multiple effects of stimulation of IL-2 release and increase in the number of IL-2 receptors. IL-1 has complex effects on mixtures of T-cells and APCs like:

1. Promoting the antigen-presenting functions of APCs.
2. Promoting the cell to cell adhesion.

There is more than one co-stimulator and that the presence of one or the other influence how T-cells are activated.

Tolerance to the proteins can be passed if the immune system is activated at the time of antigen administration. Lymphocyte activation after its recognition of antigen requires a triggering signal. Macrophages are excellent producers of IL-1. Its expression is not constitutive and the expression is induced by microbial products including LPS. Its expression is also induced by membrane activation of macrophages. During antigen presentation IL-1 is produced by:

1. The intimate cell contact involving the recognition of MHC class II-restricted antigen by the T-cell.
2. Secretions by cells following their recognition of class II MHC proteins, of TNF-α and lymphotoxin.

The second co-stimulatory molecule is by contact with lymphokines like interferon γ and is not related to the expression of class II MHC molecules or IL-1.

Cell surface molecules show lateral movements like IgG receptors, readily move when anti-Ig cross-linked Ig molecules. By the movement of the receptors, they form cap (capping). After capping, Ig receptors are endocytosed and then regenerated on the surface about 15 to 20 hours later. Therefore, capping formation may be responsible for the endocytosis and processing of antigen molecules by B-cells. Antigen molecules are endocytosed, processed and the fragments are expressed on the surface of B-cells as a complex with class II MHC Ia molecules. These complexes are then recognized by helper T-cells in T and B interaction. Therefore, capping may be one of the essential processes for B-cell activation.

Processing of MHC Class II-Restricted Antigens

The T-cell recognition of antigen depends on APCs unlike B-cells (**Figure 12.6**). The functions of APCs are as follows:

1. To take up the antigen by phagocytosis, pinocytosis or in some cases receptor mediated endocytosis.
2. To partially degrade foreign antigens into discrete antigenic fragments that can be recognized by T-cells.
3. To display these antigenic fragments on the cell surface in association with class II MHC molecules.

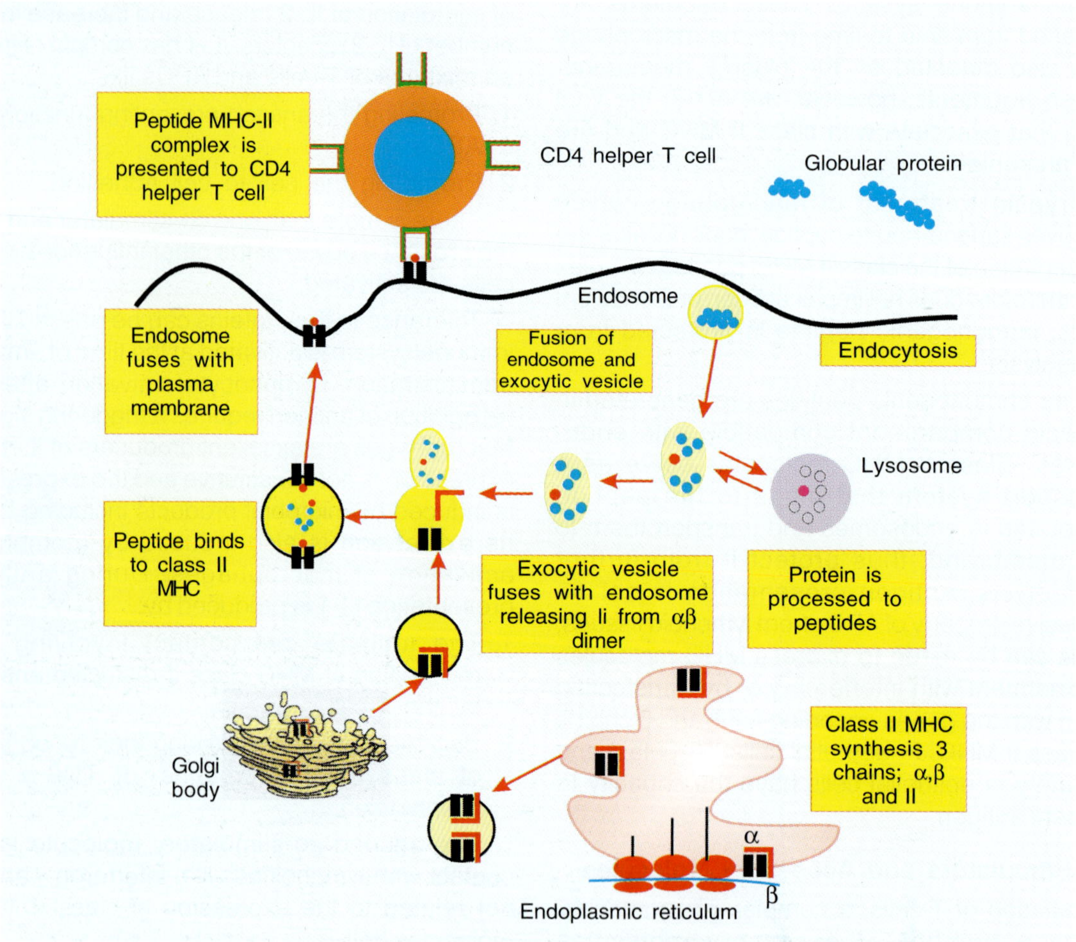

Fig. 12.6: Pathway of class II MHC-restricted presentation of an exogenous antigen

Focusing of antigen on APC surface provide an effective antigenic stimulus to T-cells. The stimulation *in vitro* is not only by native protein but also by denatured protein and fragments of native protein. The stimulatory peptide must contain all the information required for antigen presentation and T-cell stimulation. The antigenic peptide may not be long enough to have secondary structure. Therefore, the amino acid sequence of antigenic peptide may serve as the common molecular signal that is recognized by T-cells responding to either native or denatured antigen.

T-cell recognizes processed antigen as established by the use of inhibitors. The inhibitors of processing can block antigen presentation. Processed peptide plus class II MHC alone act as trigger of T-cells. The antigen processing may uncover functional sites that are buried in the native protein structure. The requirement for processing may simply be a steric requirement to uncover the two sites needed to form the trimolecular complex between antigen and MHC and between antigen and T-cell receptor. For protein unfolding may be sufficient without proteolysis. Unfolding rather than size reduction is the primary goal of antigen processing. Antigen presentation by MHC class II molecules or T-cell receptor recognition frequently requires exposure of residues, not normally exposed on the surface of the native protein.

Processing of MHC Class I-Restricted Antigens

In contrast to class II-restricted T-cells, it was widely assumed that class I-restricted T-cells, such as cytolytic T-cells (CLTs) specific for virus infected cells, respond mainly to unprocessed viral glycoproteins expressed on the surface of infected cells. Subsequent studies have demonstrated that antigen presentation in association with class I molecules requires processing into antigenic fragments. Surface expression of antigen is not required for antigenicity, implying that it is the processed antigen that stimulates a T-cell response (**Figure 12.7**).

The antigen processing pathway leading to class I presentation is apparently quite different from the endosomal pathway leading to class II presentation. Class I MHC pathway is not inhibited by class II MHC pathway inhibitors. However, different form of the same antigen can be processed exclusively by one pathway or the other. Some of the observations are clearly depicted below:

Processing	Inhibitors	Affect	Conclusion
MHC II	Chloroquine, NH_4Cl, leupeptin	Inhibited	Endosomal processing
MHC I	—do—	Insensitive	Non-endosomal processing

UV-inactivated influenza virus is processed by endosomal pathway whereas live virus does not. UV-inactivated virus plus cells are recognized by class II restricted CTLs. On the other hand live virus plus cells is recognized by class I-restricted CTLs.

Therefore, it can be concluded that endogenous synthesis of viral proteins led to the non-endosomal processing of defective or excess proteins and the resultant peptides were displayed on the cell surface with class I MHC molecules. The pathway would be inaccessible to exogenous proteins, accounting for their failure to be presented with class I MHC antigens. The two processing pathways begin with different substrates, proceed to different types of antigen presentation, restricted to either class I or class II antigens. In fact, the processing pathway would determine the class restriction.

The distinction between pathways may be cytoplasmic versus endosomal rather than endogenous versus exogenous synthesis. Thus, two distinct processing pathway apparently exist, each leading to a different MHC association, but entry to each pathways is not strictly limited

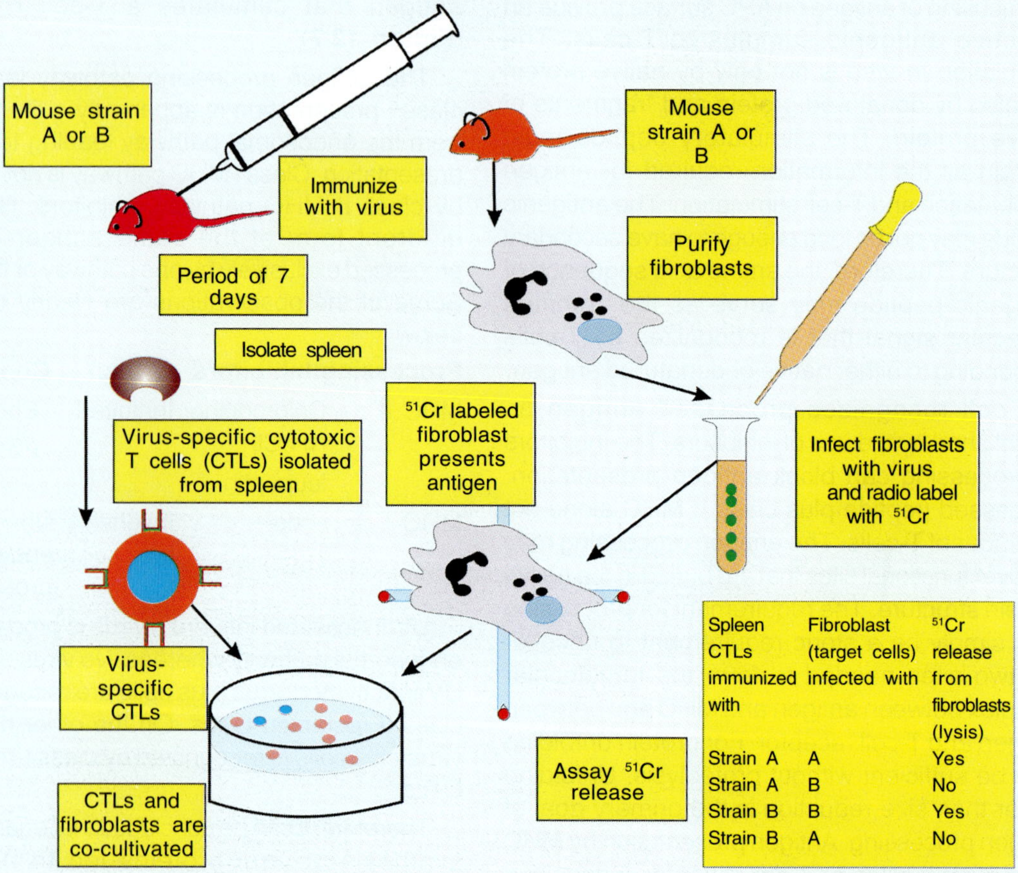

Spleen CTLs immunized with	Fibroblast (target cells) infected with	^{51}Cr release from fibroblasts (lysis)
Strain A	A	Yes
Strain A	B	No
Strain B	B	Yes
Strain B	A	No

Fig. 12.7: Virus-specific CTLs from a strain A or strain B mouse lyse only syngeneic target cells infected with aspecific virus. The CTLs do not lyse uninfected target cells and are not alloreactive. Further analysis has shown that the CTLs and target cells must come from animals that share class I MHC alleles in order for the target to present viral antigens to the CTLs

according to the endogenous or exogenous synthesis of the antigen.

Antigen Processing and T-Cells Repertoire

Antigen processing plays a critical role in determining which potential antigenic sites are recognized and therefore what part of the potential T-cell repertoire is expressed from immunization with a protein antigen. T-cell does not see the native antigen but only the products of antigen processing (**Figure 12.8**). The nature of these products would at least partly determine which epitopes could be recognized by T-cells. A number of evidences employing peptide versus native molecule established that processing plays a major role in T repertoire. The failure to respond to the native molecule was apparently not due to suppressor cells induced by native molecule. The peptide, not the native molecule, induces T-cell specific for this site, and these T-cells did not cross react with the native molecule.

A number of other studies provided evidence that a structure outside the minimal site can hinder presentation in association with a particular MHC

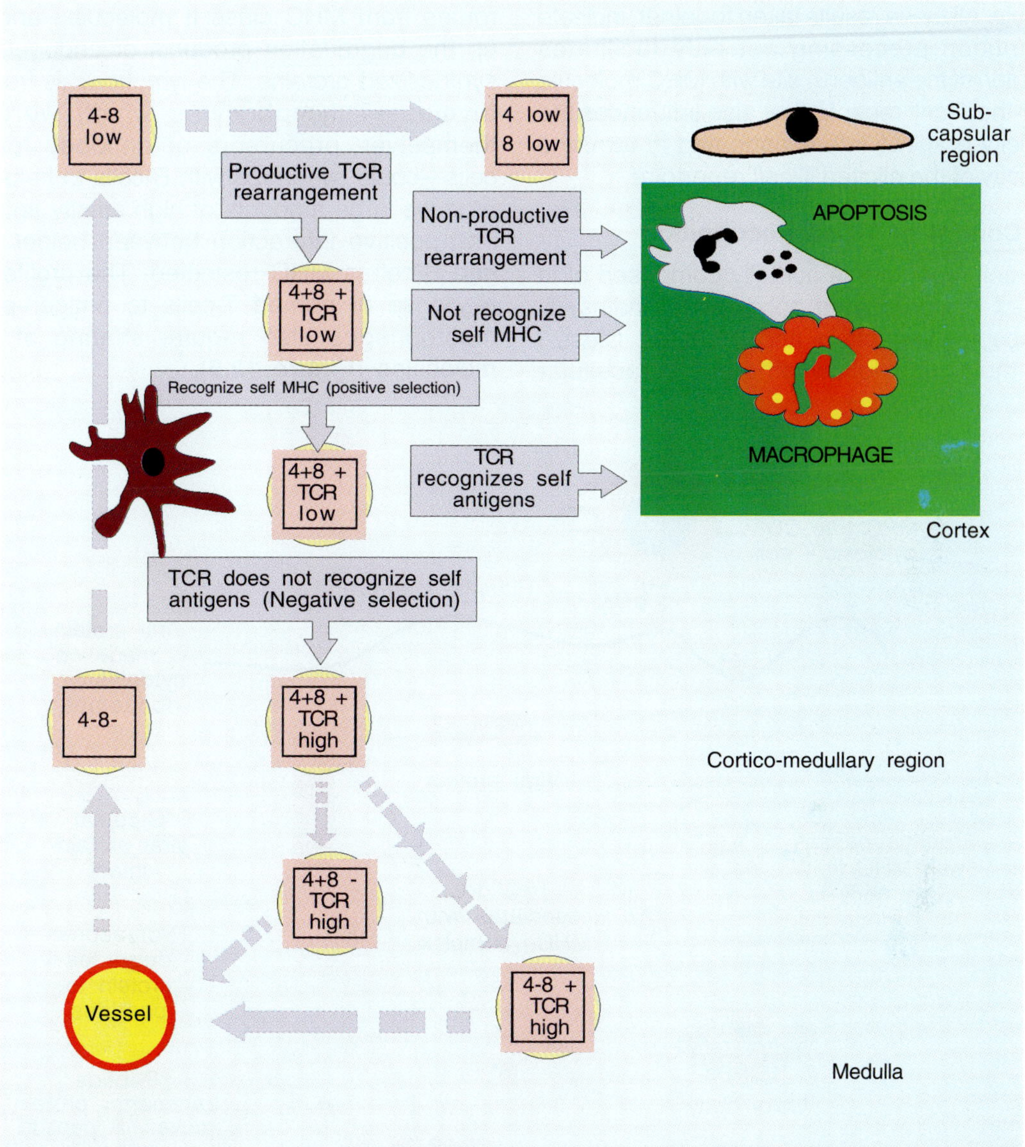

Fig. 12.8: Prethymic T-cells enter the thymus rudiment and proliferate as large lymphoblasts in the sub capsular region of the thymus. The lymphoblasts replicate resulting in a pool of cells that differentiate. Here the cells become CD8 and CD4 positive but expression is low. TCR genes are also rearranged in these cells and the products may also be expressed on the cell surface at low levels. As the cells mature, they move into the cortex where they adhere to cortical epithelial cells which are long and branched, providing a large surface area to interact with other cells. TCRs on the surfaces of thymocytes interact with the MHC molecules on the cortical epithelial cells leading to positive selection. The cells that are not selected are subject to apoptosis and are phagocytosed by macrophages. As the thymocytes migrate further into the cortex of the thymus, the expression of CD3, CD4, CD8 and TCR increase

molecule. All these results taken together, indicate that antigen processing not only facilitates interaction of the antigenic site with MHC molecule and/or the T-cell receptor but also influences the specificity of these interactions and in turn, the specificity of the elicited T-cell repertoire.

MHC Control of T-Cell Recognition

The T-cell repertoire is actually composed of in terms of its component polypeptide chains, T-cell receptor variable α and β chains. Class I MHC molecules follow different intracellular routes from MHC class II molecules and pick up the degradation products of endogenously synthesized proteins. The lymphocytes from the thymus—T lymphocytes which were not themselves precursors of antibody forming cells—could synergize with B-cells to help them produce large amounts of high affinity antibody. The positive interaction between helper T-cell and B-cell is MHC restricted. The proliferative response of primed T-cells to antigen-pulsed macrophages also require sharing of MHC molecules (**Figure 12.9**).

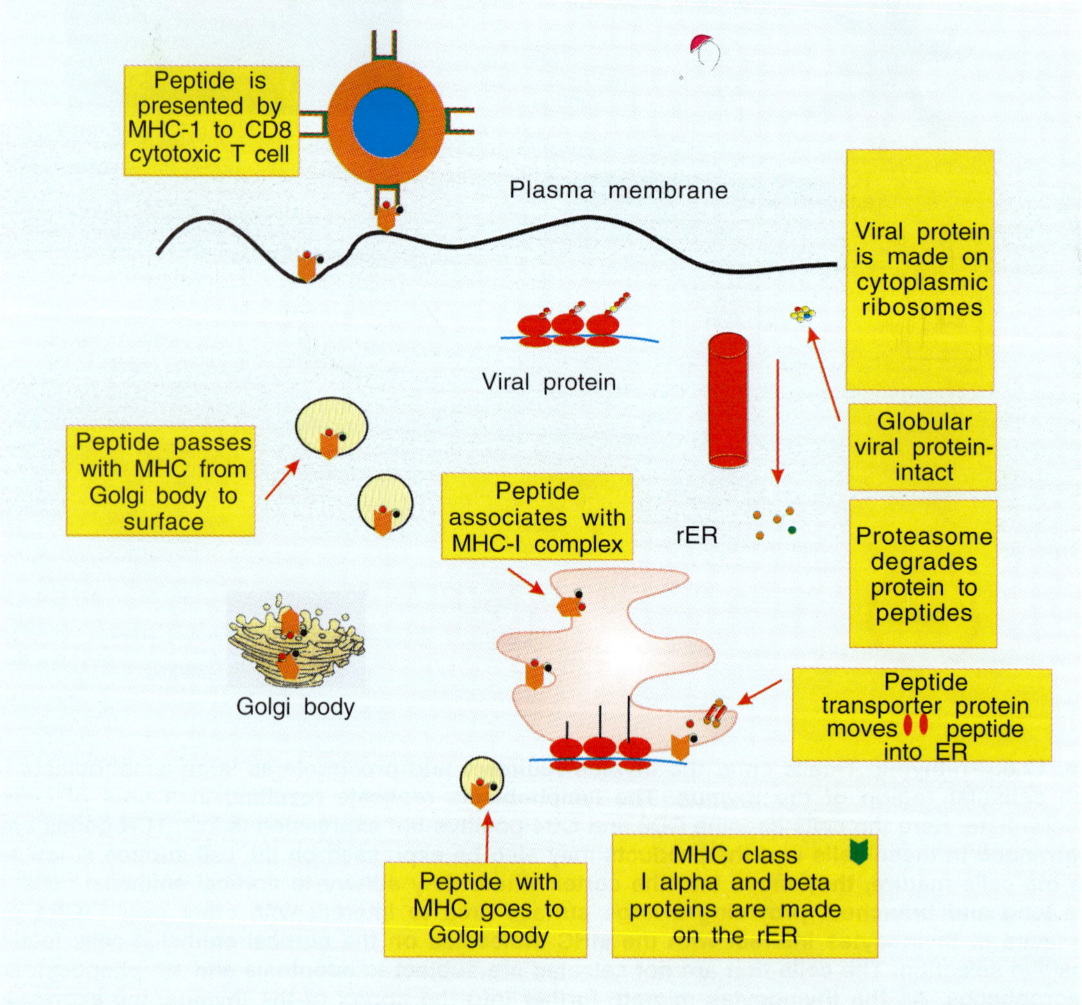

Fig. 12.9: Pathway of class I MHC restricted presentation of an endogenously synthesized antigen. An example of such an antigen would be a viral protein made in the cell as a result of infection

CTLs generated against virus-infected or chemically modified syngeneic cells were specific for a self class I antigen in addition to the foreign antigenic stimulus. A number of specific illustrative examples showed MHC class I-restricted CTL-mediated cytotoxicity. Normal cellular components or any minor histocompatability antigen could serve to generate class I-restricted CTLs in a genetically different host. The genetic control of the immune response was first demonstrated at the level of the immunogenicity of simple amino acid polymers, by immune response genes (Ir). The immune response or *I*region is made up of two sub-regions encoding class II glycoproteins (Ia molecules), I-A and I-E of the MHC. Ir genes encodes the T-cell receptor (TCR) for antigen thus controlling the ability of T-cells to respond to a specific antigen.

There have been two broad classes of explanation for MHC-linked control of T-cell recognition.

1. T-cell recognizes epitopes on the foreign antigen and on the self-MHC-encoded marker somewhat independently. Thus it has two receptors.
2. T-cell has one receptor that can bind the complex of foreign antigen plus self-MHC.

Various experimental studies argued against the independent recognition of class II MHC and antigen. It has been established that T-cell recognition involves a molecular complex of TCR, antigen and MHC. And the data is against the notion that foreign antigen and the MHC-restricting element could be recognized independently.

Two hypotheses namely altered-self model and determinant–selection model have been proposed for MHC control of immune response. Non-responsiveness can be explained as a failure to elicit T-cells specific for certain combinations of MHC products (class I or class II) and foreign antigens.

The non-responsiveness could be due to two possibilities:

1. The complex forms but there are no T-cells that recognize it; or
2. The complex does not form.

Certain combinations of MHC products and antigen cannot exist. Failure of a given antigen to elicit a response within a non-responder results from defective antigen presentation by the individual's MHC products. A given combination of MHC product and antigen is permissible and does indeed forms, recognition of this pair is limited by the T-cell repertoire.

MHC Class I Restricted Antigens

The class I MHC-associated antigen was likely to exist as a fragmented form of a viral gene product. The results of a number of studies suggested that the degradation of the endogenous gene product was likely to be a general requirement for class I-restricted T-cell recognition. It has been established that a processed form of the antigen and not the native molecule was the form relevant to class I-restricted T-cell recognition.

There is an absolute requirement for cellular processing of the T-cell antigen. This was first demonstrated for MHC class II restricted antigen. It became apparent that macrophages played a central role in taking up and retaining antigen during antibody formation. Processed and macrophage-associated antigen was in fact far more efficient in eliciting an immune response than the free form of the same antigen. The antigen processing was in fact dependent on antigen degradation. Intracellular degradation is a key pathway of antigen handling by accessory cells.

The results of various experimental studies strongly suggest that antigen degradation resulting in the production of peptide fragments was the necessary and sufficient step in accessory cell processing of soluble antigen. T-cell recognizes peptides in association with the class II MHC gene products, the Ia molecules. It has been clearly demonstrated that the only feature necessary for T-cell recognition were the appropriate Ia molecules and peptide fragments.

Ir Genes

Cell surface glycoproteins coated by the MHC bind peptide fragments produced by intracellular degradation and present them for T-cell recognition. This results in either an antibody response or unresponsiveness. The selective unresponsiveness is due to an apparent defect in antigen presentation. Not all peptides presented by the MHC molecules elicit a T-cell response due to limitations on the pool of T-cell receptors, the so called holes in the T-cell receptor repertoire.

Ir genes which encode MHC molecules, appeared to act through effects of T-cell help, could influence the specificity of antibodies produced to a given antigen. The explanation suggested was that the Ir genes first select which helper T-cells are activated and these in turn influence which B-cells, specific for particular epitopes, could be activated. For cognate help, the B-cell has to present the antigen in association with a MHC molecule to the helper T-cell. The Ir gene control of antibody specificity must operate at least partly at this step by selecting which helper T-cell can be activated by and help a given B-cell.

Selection of T-cell Repertoire by Thymus

It has been experimentally established that the thymus is the site in which most or all T-cells differentiate. It is now well accepted that both class I-restricted CTLs and class II-restricted helper T-cells are selected by the MHC antigens expressed in the thymus such that only thymus-restricted T-cells are allowed to emigrate. Each immune T-cell is restricted by only one MHC product. It thus appears that the critical cell type is a thymic epithelial cell and not an emigrant, bone marrow-derived cell (**Figure 12.10**).

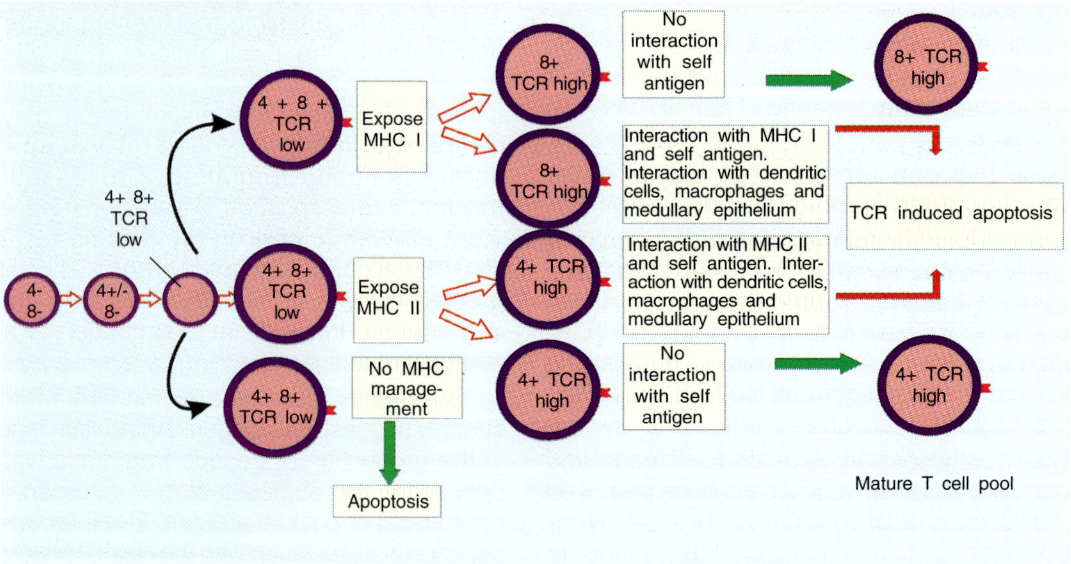

Fig. 12.10: CD4⁻ CD8⁻ precursor thymocytes become double positive, CD4⁺ CD8⁺ cells expressing low levels of the alpha and beta chains of the T cell receptor (TCR). Positive selection for interaction with self MHC-I or MHC-II molecules occurs in the cortical epithelium. The majority of the cells are unselected and undergo apoptosis. The cells that remain either interact with MHC-I and lose their CD4 antigen or interact with MHC-II and lose their CD8 antigen. Autoreactive cells are then removed as a result of their interaction with self antigen-peptides that are presented by cells in the corticomedullary junction and the medulla of the thymus

Endogenous and Exogenous Pathways

Endogenously synthesized proteins provide peptides for class I MHC presentation while exogenously added proteins that are endocytosed provide peptides that associate with class II molecules. Introduction of live infectious virus will induce class I-restricted CTLs; a killed version of the same virus in general does not. In general, class I-restricted CTLs recognize cell-associated antigens such as those on virus-infected cells or cells expressing foreign alloantigens.

Class II-restricted T-cells, on the other hand, recognize antigens that enter the system as soluble components. These antigens are derived from proteins taken up by antigen-presenting cells from the external medium. Therefore, when a soluble antigen is introduced into the immune system, class II restricted but not class I restricted T-cells, are activated.

Responsiveness to Class II-Associated Antigens

The class I and class II MHC glycoproteins function by binding peptides derived from intracellular processing and present them on the cell surface for T-cell recognition. T-cells of either class-specific use the same receptor. The distinction between class I and class II antigen presentation is probably achieved by differential processing mechanisms. The putative binding site can accommodate peptides of between 8 and 20 amino acid residues. Most of the known polymorphic residues are located on the top of the MHC protein around the putative peptide binding cleft and are inaccessible to the T-cell receptor. The ability of the MHC products to bind to given peptides would then determine the responsiveness to that particular MHC-combination. The inability to bind would result in non-responsiveness.

Experimental data suggests that specific Ia peptide binding is necessary for a peptide to be immunogenic. The immune response is controlled by the ability of MHC proteins to from a stable association with a given peptide derived from intracellular processing. Stable peptide-MHC complexes must form prior to T-cell recognition and inability to form such complexes would result in non-responsiveness. The amino acid residues located within the MHC binding cleft play a decisive role in MHC-peptide interactions. Holes in the T-cell repertoire sometimes contribute to MHC-linked non-responsiveness. MHC proteins can bind to many different but not to all, peptides. While this binding is necessary, it does not ultimately fully control the immune response, which rests at the level of T-cell repertoire generation and selection.

Peptide Binding of Class I MHC

The class I molecules would have peptide binding abilities, analogous to those attributed to the detergent solubilised form of Ia, notably a single binding site that forms a very stable association with peptide. This would be consistent with the strong sequence homology between both classes of MHC gene products which predicts closely related protein structures. Class I MHC most likely binds peptide antigens in a manner analogous to that defined for the Ia molecule.

The HLA antigen binding cleft was almost completely occupied by a mixture of peptide antigens. The presence of a prominent groove on the top of the HLA-A2 molecule, consisting of walls formed by two α helices, one from the α_1 domain of the HLA molecule and the other from the α_2 domain. The floor of the groove is formed by a series of β strands from both the α_1 and α_2 domains. The overall structure consists of a cleft that is presumed to be peptide binding sites. The HLA antigen binding cleft was found almost completely occupied by a mixture of peptide antigens.

Peptide Binding of Class II MHC Molecules

Since T-cells recognize a combination of antigen and MHC products, the question arise about the stability of complex and role of TCR. Peptides represent the actual form of antigen associated with class II MHC molecules. It has been successfully demonstrated that indeed a stable specific complex is formed between a short immunogenic peptide and its purified Ia restricting element. Experiments have demonstrated peptide-Ia binding which is relevant to T-cell recognition. Therefore, Ia had a single site capable of trapping peptide antigens in a stable, immunogenic form.

At this time you should know the following:

1. A clear role of MHC of class I and class II in immunogenicity or cytolytic activity through the help of lymphocytes.
2. Recognition of antigen or virus infected cells by respective MHC products followed by relevant processing by APCs.
3. The processing of T-cell-restricted MHC class I and class II antigens.
4. The difference between two pathways of processing namely endosomal and non-endosomal.
5. The role of co-stimulator and accessory molecules in immune response.
6. Generation of T-cell repertoire, their selection in thymus and role of Ir gene products in immune response.

Further Reading

- Ivan Roitt and others (Eds), Immunology, 1985, Gower Medical Publishing, New York.
- Unanue (1984) Antigen presenting function of the micropage. Annu. Rev. Immunol 2, 395.
- William Paul (Ed.), Fundamental Immunology, second edition, 1989, Raven Press, New York.
- M. Howard and W. Paul (1983), Recognition of B cell growth and differentiation by soluble factors. Annu. Rev. Immunol 1, 307.

13

CHAPTER

Cell Interaction in Specific Immune Response

(Dr. K N Krithika, Dr. M V R Reddy and Dr. Mythily Srinivasan
knkodumu@iupui.edu)

OBJECTIVES

1. To know the immune system as a "Sensory organ".
2. Co-stimulatory signals essential for T-cell activation.
3. Membrane proteins involved in the interaction between a CD4 T lymphocyte and an antigen-presenting cell (APC).
4. $CD4^+$ T_H interaction with $CD8^+$ T-cells.
5. T_H 17 subset of $CD4^+$ T-cells.
6. Natural killer T-lymphocytes (NKT cells).
7. T regulatory cells (T reg cells).

INTRODUCTION

The cell-cell interaction that we have described in this chapter:

- Provides an overview of the types of cell interactions and molecules required for specific immunity.
- Describes specific immunity and the cells involved.

The Immune System as a "Sensory Organ"

A key attribute of an effective immune system is to be able to detect the presence of trouble—this could be dead or damaged cells, tumor cells or infection with viruses, bacteria or eukaryotic parasites. The immune response is defined by three principles: discrimination between self and non self, specificity and memory. This chapter discusses the cell interactions in specific immune response.

Immunity has two arms represented by non-specific and specific immunities. The non-specific immunity which is also referred to as natural or native or as innate immunity is the defense system that comes in action prior to exposure to antigen, lacks discrimination among antigens and can be enhanced after exposure to antigen through effects of cytokines. The specific immunity also referred to as acquired or adaptive immunity on the other hand is induced by antigen, shows fine discrimination among antigens and is enhanced by antigen.

The hallmarks of the specific immune system are memory and specificity. It "remembers" each encounter with a microbe or foreign antigen, so that subsequent encounters stimulate increasingly effective defense mechanisms. The specific immune response amplifies the protective mechanisms of non-specific immunity, directs or focuses these mechanisms to the site of antigen entry, and thus makes them better able to eliminate foreign antigens.

Lymphocytes: The Orchestrators of Specific Immune Response

The lymphocytes are the most important cells of the immune system that participate in most of the immune reactions due to their ability to interact specifically with antigenic substances and to react to nonself antigenic determinants. Lymphocytes differentiate from stem cells in the fetal liver, bone marrow, and thymus into two main functional classes. They are found in the peripheral blood and in all lymphoid tissues.

B-Lymphocytes

B-cells are responsible for humoral immunity. B lymphocytes or B-cells are so named because the Bursa of fabricius, a lymphoid organ located at the caudal end of the gut in birds, plays a key role in their differentiation. A mammalian counterpart to the avian bursa has not yet been found. Some investigators believe that the bone marrow is the most likely organ for B Lymphocyte differentiation, while others propose that the peri-intestinal lymphoid tissues play this role.

Antigen recognition by B-cells: B lymphocytes carry immunoglobulins on their cell membrane, which enable them to recognize the appropriate antigen. If the B-cell comes into contact with the specific type of antigen to which it is targeted it divides rapidly to form a clone of identical cells. On recognition of the antigen they migrate to the secondary lymphoid tissues and proliferate to form daughter lymphocytes that develop into short-lived plasma cells. The plasma cells release specific antibodies into the circulation to fight the invading pathogen. The antibodies circulate as part of the gamma globulin fraction of the blood plasma. In the event of subsequent infection with the same pathogen, this circulating antibody acts quickly to destroy it. Some of the activated B-cells do not become plasma cells instead they turn into memory cells which continue to produce small amounts of the antibody long after the infection has been overcome. Upon re-encounter with the antigen the memory cells quickly divide to produce new clones of the appropriate type of plasma cell. B lymphocytes can also play the role of antigen-presenting cells, which is usually attributed to cells of monocytic / macrophagic lineage (see **Figure 13.1**).

T Lymphocytes

T lymphocytes or T-cells are so named because the thymus plays a key role in their differentiation. The functions of the T lymphocytes form the basis of cell-mediated immunity (CMI). T lymphocytes have a longer lifespan than B lymphocytes. Long-lasting lymphocytes are particularly important because of their involvement on immunological memory.

Antigen recognition by T-cells: T lymphocytes do not express immunoglobulins but detect the presence of foreign substances by way of surface proteins called T-cell receptors. T-cell

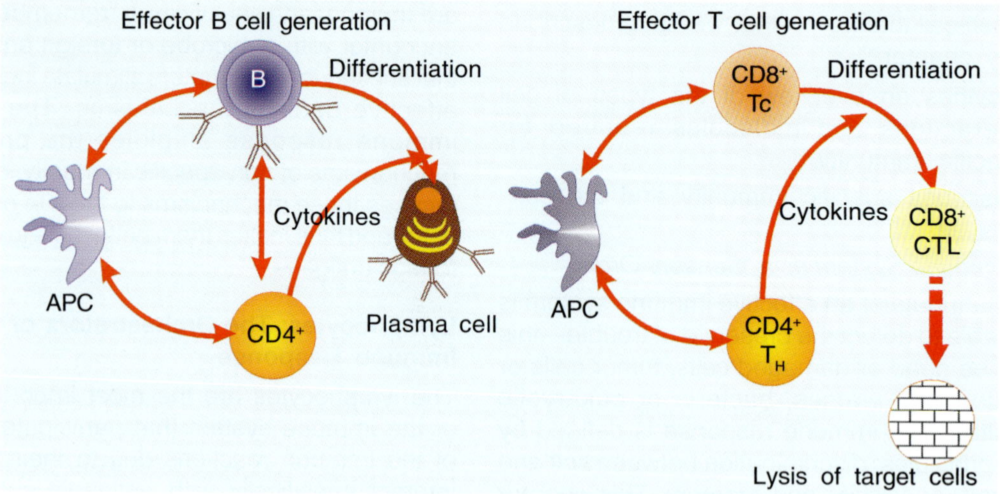

Fig. 13.1: Effector B and T cell generation

diversity is attained by a complex 5-stage genetic rearrangement that occurs at random in the developing T-cells in the thymus. Each lymphocyte (or possibly a small number of similar T-cells) is thus able to react with one antigen. T-cells are tested for their ability to recognize and bind to antigens in the thymus. It is thought that this occurs by positive and negative selection. The postulation is that positive selection eliminates T-cells that do not bind tightly enough to antigen type molecules produced in the thymus and negative selection eliminates T-cells that bind too tightly to self type molecules found in the thymus. It is suggested that T-cells that recognize antigens of the body's own cells are excluded by this process. It is known that approximately 95% of all developing T-cells die in the thymus. This produces mature T-cell repertoire that is potentially capable of recognizing 'self' from 'non-self' and only reacting against the 'non-self' molecules.

Unlike immunoglobulins, the T-cell receptor (TCR) proteins are never secreted, and hence T-cells lack the ability to act at long distance. Instead, they exert their protective effects either through direct contact with a target or by influencing the activity of other immune cells. Furthermore, T-cells can detect foreign substances only in specific contexts. Thus, T lymphocytes recognize a protein only if it is first broken down into small peptides, which are then displayed on the surface of a second host cell, called an antigen-presenting cell (APC). Although most host cells can present antigens, cell types specially adapted for this purpose include macrophages, B lymphocytes, and a family of bone-marrow-derived cells known as dendritic cells. The APC present peptides derived from the antigen within the groove of a cell surface molecule called the major histocompatibility (MHC) complex (or the human leukocyte antigen complex in humans). Two major classes of MHC molecules, MHC class I and MHC class II are known to exist and present peptides predominantly from the extra-cellular or intracellular pathogens respectively.

Several subpopulations of T lymphocytes with separate functions have been recognized. These mature functional T lymphocytes express a number of characteristic surface proteins in addition to T-cell receptors. The two main populations are the helper T lymphocytes, which are involved in the induction and regulation of immune responses, and the cytotoxic T lymphocytes, which are involved in the destruction of infected cells. The helper T-cells express CD4 protein on their surface while cytotoxic T-cells express CD8 proteins on their surface. Mature, functional T lymphocytes almost always express only one of these two proteins, and this correlates with important differences in cell function. The TCR on the surface of $CD4^+$ T helper cells recognize antigenic peptides presented by the APC in the groove of MHC class II molecule. A sub-population of T lymphocytes with suppressor functions called regulatory T-cells has been recognized recently.

Co-stimulatory Signals Essential for T-cell Activation

As stated above each T-cell carries a unique TCR that recognizes only one MHC-antigen complex. This interaction delivers an antigen-specific signal, essential but not sufficient, for T-cell activation. Co-stimulatory signals are delivered by the APCs with which activated T-cells establish strong adhesive interactions. In the absence of co-stimulatory signals, TCR occupancy, by itself, induces T-cell unresponsiveness or anergy. The delivery of co-stimulatory signals requires close interactions between helper and effector cells. Multiple sets of costimulatory molecules have been identified to date. Interaction between specific pairs of costimulatory molecules influences the immune response distinctly. The interactions between the molecules CD2/CD58 and LFA-1/ICAM-1 play a primary role in T lymphocyte: APC adhesion, allowing the proper delivery of co-stimulatory signals. Some of the most significant co-stimulatory signals result from cell-cell interactions mediated by membrane proteins, such as those involving the interactions between CD28 and B7 family members and between CD40L and CD40.

The Immune Response Develops Sequentially and Requires Cellular Co-operation

The introduction of antigen into an immunologically naive host starts multiple sequential events that lead to an immune response. These events can be broadly classified into three groups. The initial response is the non-specific innate immune response. Next is the central phase that involves cellular interactions between the lymphocytes, antigen presenting cells and/or specific soluble factors leading to functional differentiation of the lymphocytes. The final effector phase consists of differentiated B and T lymphocytes eliciting specific immune responses. The B-cells differentiating into plasma cells secrete antibodies while the differentiated effector T-cells induce cell mediated immune responses either by (CD8) mediating cytotoxic activity or by (CD4) promoting proliferation, maturation, and immunologic function of other cell types.

Membrane Proteins Involved in the Interaction Between a $CD4^+$ T Lymphocyte and an Antigen-Presenting Cell (APC)

T- and B-cell cooperation is needed to produce antibody

Although B-cells can recognize soluble antigens through their surface receptors, efficient humoral immune response requires additional help from $CD4^+$ T helper cells. Furthermore, certain antigens can trigger antibody synthesis only in the presence of T-cells; others do not need T-cells. These antigens are called thymus (T)-dependent and thymus (T)-independent antigens, respectively. Most protein antigens fall into the T-dependent category. Following the initial recognition of a specific soluble antigen by the B-cell, redistribution of antigen-BCR complex to one pole of the B-cell membrane occurs. There is also upregulation of co-stimulatory molecules such as CD86 and CD40. The antigen is then internalized, processed and presented in the context of the MHC molecule that is recognized by $CD4^+$ T-cells with specific TCR, initiating cytokine secretion. This leads to B-cell proliferation, differentiation into plasma cells and secretion of antibodies.

The delivery of T-cell help is divided into a recognition phase and an effector phase. During the recognition phase, the appropriate resting $CD4^+$ T_H cells recognize the complexes of processed antigen–class II MHC molecule displayed on the surface of B-cells. The T-helper (T_H) cell–B cell conjugate is further stabilized by the binding of CD54 to CD11a/CD18 and by the binding of CD4 to monomorphic domains of the class II MHC molecules. These interactions lead to the clustering of T-cell surface molecules (TCR, CD4, and CD11a/CD18) and subsequent induction of T_H cell effector functions. However, B-cell induction into the cell cycle occurs only after a constitutively expressed B-cell surface molecule known as *CD40* interacts with a transiently expressed T-cell surface glycoprotein called *gp39 (CD40-L)* on activated T_H cells. The entry of B-cells into the cell cycle initiates the second phase, known as the *effector phase*. As this phase proceeds, the dominant interaction becomes the recognition of nonpolymorphic domains of B-cell class II MHC molecules by T-cell CD4 molecules and increases the B-cell responsiveness to T_H cell cytokines. IL-4 helps to promote the transition from G_1 to S, while other cytokines, such as IL-5 and IL-6, participate as differentiation factors.

Cellular interactions in cell mediated immune responses

The T_H1 and T_H2 immune responses: As stated above T-cells do not recognize soluble nominal antigen; the protein antigen must be processed and presented as immunogenic peptides by APCs, usually macrophages. The T_H cells are activated when they "corecognize" foreign peptides and specific sites (non-polymorphic) on class II MHC molecules plus CD28 coreceptor on its surface interacting with the CD80/CD86 ligands on the APC. These interactions can lead to the development of functionally distinct $CD4^+$ T_H cell subsets. T-helper 1 (T_H1) cells and T-helper 2 (T_H2) cells are distinguished based on their ability to secrete distinct cytokines.

Activated T_H1 cells produce IL-2, IFN-γ, and TNF-β, use IL-2 as an autocrine growth factor, and mediate cytotoxicity and delayed-type hypersensitivity responses. In contrast, activated T_H2 cells produce IL-4, IL-5, IL-6, IL-10 and IL-13, use IL-4 for autocrine growth, and fail to induce delayed-type hypersensitivity responses. T_H2 cells primarily provide help to B-cells. Factors such as the density of the antigen–MHC ligands, the cytokines elicited by antigen, the type of APC, and the MHC haplotype influence the differentiation of naive $CD4^+$ T-cells into specific T_H subsets. The mechanism whereby one subset is activated over the other is unclear, but APCs presenting low densities of peptide-MHC ligands induce naive $CD4^+$ T-cells to differentiate into T_H2 cells, while presentation of high densities induces them to differentiate into T_H1 cells. T_H2 cells seem less susceptible to being turned off by inappropriate stimulation than are T_H1 cells; therefore, if antigen is low or too high, T_H2 cells have the advantage.

Polarized human T_H1 type and T_H2 type responses play different roles in mediating protection against infections. While T_H1 responses are effective in the defense against intracellular pathogens, the T_H2 responses protect against intestinal nematodes. Skewed polarization towards T_H1 or T_H2 is responsible for different types of immuno pathological reactions. Tissue injury and inflammation caused by T_H1 cells and activated macrophages are the hallmarks of delayed type hypersensitivity reactions (DTH). DTH reactions may occur as collateral damage during a protective T_H1 response to a microbe, or DTH may be entirely pathologic, as in the setting of certain autoimmune diseases. Many of the disorders caused by abnormal immune responses are called immune mediated inflammatory diseases. T_H1 dominated responses may be involved in the pathogenesis of organ specific autoimmune disorders, acute allograft rejections and some chronic inflammatory disorders of unknown etiology. In contrast, T_H2 type responses are responsible for reduced protection against some intracellular pathogens, transplantation, tolerance, atopic disorders and some systemic autoimmune diseases (see **Figure 13.2**).

$CD4^+$ T_H interaction with $CD8^+$ T-cells

The collaborative interaction between macrophages, $CD4^+$ T helper cells and $CD8^+$ cytotoxic T-cells is complex. When they exit the thymus, the cytotoxic T-cells are immature and are called the pre-Tc cells.

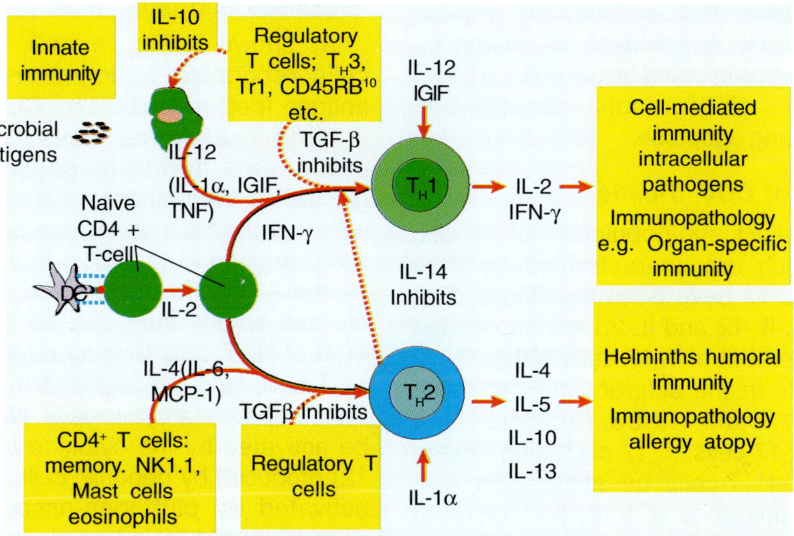

Fig. 13.2: Schematic representation of T_H1/T_H2 immune response

The differentiation of pre-T_C-cell to mature functional effector T_C cells requires two distinct signals. The first signal is interaction of TCR with a protein antigen fragment bound to MHC class I molecules on a target cell. The second signal consists of T_H-cell-derived cytokines such as IL-2 and IFN-γ. The contribution by these cytokines implies that both $CD4^+$ and $CD8^+$ T-cells must be stimulated by the same antigen but in association with class II and class I MHC molecules, respectively, to generate functional T_C cells. This differentiation process causes T_C cells to develop membrane-bound cytoplasmic granules called *perforins* and to develop the ability to transcribe and secrete cytokines such as IFN-γ and TNF-β and, to a lesser extent, IL-2.

$CD8^+$ CTLs kill virally infected cells (also known as target cells). The required activation signals are recognition of antigen, i.e., co-stimulatory signals from virus-specific $CD4^+$ T_H cells. This is another example of the requirement for cell-cell interaction to generate an immune response; in this case a cell mediated immune response. Here $CD4^+$ T_H cells recognize viral antigen displayed on APCs; activation of the $CD4^+$ T_H cell causes release of IL-2, which stimulates viral antigen-specific $CD8^+$ T-cells. TCR recognition of viral antigen, plus a second signal via IL-2 receptor (IL-2R) stimulates differentiation of the $CD8^+$ T-cell in to an effector CTL, capable of cell killing on encountering a virus infected target cell. CTLs kill target by exchanging granule contents and eventually inducing apoptosis.

Th 17 subset of $CD4^+$ T-cells

Recently, a distinct sub-population of T-cells, T_H17 cells which are characterized by their production of IL-17 have been described. Two other cytokines, IL-12 and IL-23 are associated with the development of T_H17 cells. While IL-12 plays a key role in the differentiation of naïve T-cells to T_H1 cells, IL-23 promotes the expansion of T_H17 cells. T_H17 cells differentiate from naïve $CD4^+$ T-cells by stimulation with antigen in the presence of IL-6, IL-1 or other proinflammatory cytokines. This new wave of studies has resulted in the recognition of the role of IL-23 and T_H17 cells in inflammatory conditions, such as arthritis and inflammatory bowel disease. There is also the speculation about a possible role in type 1 diabetes. It is postulated that IL-6 and other inflammatory cytokines may be produced early at sites of tissue damage, and these promote the subsequent destructive T_H17 response.

Natural Killer T-lymphocytes (NKT Cells)

Natural Killer T (NKT) cells are a small subset of unconventional T cells that has features of both T cells and NK cells. These cells recognize lipid antigens presented by the non-classical MHC class I molecule CD1d that binds self and foreign lipids and glycolipids. It is now generally accepted that the term "NKT cells" refers to CD1d-restricted T cells. NKT cells are a subset of T cells that co-express an αβ T cell receptor (TCR), but also express a variety of molecular markers that are typically associated with NK cells, such as NK1.1.Ligation of the NKT- T cell receptor (TCR) leads to a rapid production of protypical T_H1 and T_H2 cytokines such as IFN-gamma and IL-4, and in some cases, GM-CSF, IL-10, IL-13, TGF-beta and other cytokines and chemokines and thus influence diverse immune responses and pathogenic processes.

As shown in **Figure 13.3**, the TCR of NKT cells recognize endogenous self glycolipid antigen (def) presented by CD1d molecules on antigen presenting cells (APC). Antigen-presenting dendritic cells engulf certain glycolipids from human cells and degrade them with their lysosomes. These glycolipid epitopes are then bound to CD1d molecules produced by the APC and transported to the surface of the cell where they can be presented to the TCR of NKT cells to induce NKT cell activation. NKT cells also mediate perforin-dependent and FasL dependent cytotoxicity. NKT cells can also be activated by the cytokine Interleukin-12 (IL-12) produced by dendritic cells and also become activated by pathogen-associated molecular patterns (PAMPs) of microbes binding to the toll-like receptors (TLRs) of the dendritic cells which in turn produces copious amount of T_H1/ T_H2 cytokines. These cells play an important role in the development of autoimmune diseases and transplantation tolerance.

Pathogens may not directly activate NKT cells. The TCR of NKT cells recognize endogenous self glycolipid antigen (def) presented by CD1d molecules on antigen presenting cells (def) (APCs) as shown in **Figure 13.3**. Antigen-presenting dendritic cells engulf certain glycolipids from human cells and degrade them with their lysosomes. These glycolipid epitopes are then bound to CD1d molecules produced by the APC and transported to the surface of the cell where they can be presented to the TCR of NKT cells to induce NKT cell activation. NKT cells can also be activated by the cytokine Interleukin-12 (IL-12) produced by dendritic cells that have themselves become activated by pathogen-associated molecular patterns (PAMPs) of microbes binding to the toll-like receptors (TLRs) of the dendritic cells. Once activated, the NKT cells rapidly produce large quantities of T_H1 cell and T_H2 cell cytokines, including interferon-gamma (IFN-gamma), IL-4, IL-2, IL-10, TNF-alpha, IL-13, and chemokines. They also produce perforins and granzymes like those produced by CTLs and NK cells to induce apoptosis in infected cells and tumor cells. These cytokines, in turn, promote both innate and adaptive immunity and may also help to regulate the immune responses. Large amounts of IFN-gamma are especially produced by activated NKT cells. IFN-gamma activates NK cells and macrophages as a part of innate immunity; it also promotes the maturation of dendritic cells so that they induce a T_H1 cell response to induce adaptive immunity. If the NKT cell is repeatedly stimulated by the body's own glycolipids in the absence of microbes then this might stimulate the NK T-cell/dendritic cell interaction to produce signals that inhibit T_H1 cell response and possibly stimulate the production of regulatory T lymphocytes (T-reg cells). In this way it might suppress autoimmune responses and prevent tissue damage.

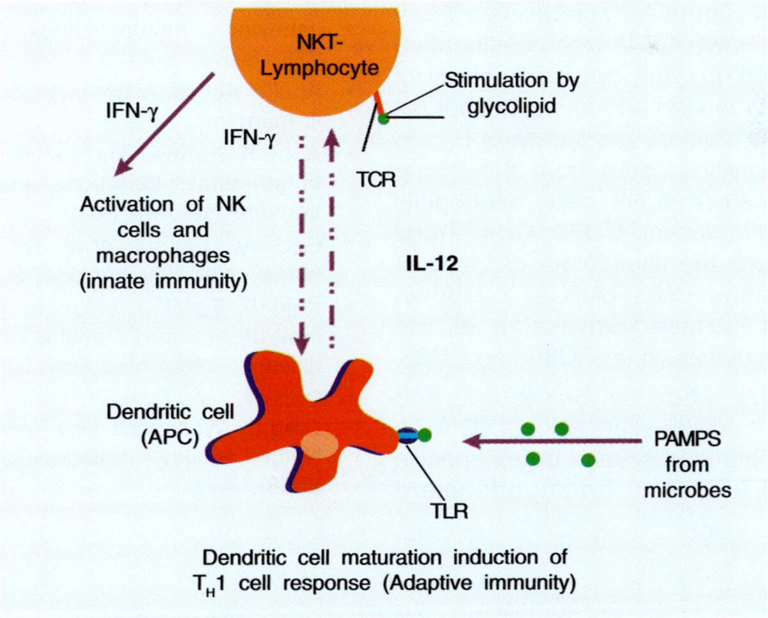

Fig. 13.3: Activation of an NKT lymphocyte and NKT cell induction of innate immunity and adaptive immunity
(Soruce: http://student.ccbcmd.edu/courses/bio141/lecguide/unit5/intro/NKTcell/nkt.html)

T regulatory cells (Treg cells)

For cells of adaptive immune system, the capacity to distinguish between self and foreign antigens is acquired during B and T lymphocyte development and maintained in the periphery. T-reg cells are a subpopulation of $CD4^+$ T-lymphocytes. In addition to T-cell receptors (TCRs) and CD4 molecules on their surface, they have a receptor for the cytokine interleukin-2 (IL-2) containing CD25. These suppressor T-cells have first been described in the early 1970s, but since the hypothetical soluble suppressor factor could not be identified on a molecular level and since appropriate cellular markers were lacking, the suppressor T cell concept vanished for considerable time. $CD25^+$ $CD4^+$ T-cells were named regulatory T-cells (Treg). It functions in cell-intrinsic peripheral tolerance mechanisms such as anergy induction and peripheral deletion play indispensable roles in the maintenance of natural self-tolerance, inverting autoimmune responses, as well as in controlling inflammatory reactions. $CD25^+$ $CD4^+$ Treg cells are pluripotent suppressors modulating many different immune reactions. They efficiently inhibit naïve $CD4^+$ T-cell proliferation and differentiation, prevent cytotoxic activity of $CD8^+$ T-cells both *in vitro* and *in vivo*, suppress the activation and antibody production of B-cells and limit the activity of cells from the innate immune system such as NK cells, neutrophils and monocytes. Moreover, $CD25^+$ $CD4^+$ Tregs can efficiently limit the stimulatory capacity of antigen presenting cells (APCs) by down regulating cell surface expression of co-stimulatory molecules such as CD80 and CD86.

The discovery made by Sakaguchi and coworkers, that the adoptive transfer of $CD25^+CD4^-$ depleted T-cells induced several organ specific autoimmune diseases in immunodeficient recipients has put the suppressor T-cell model back into the focus of many immunologists.

Their regulatory functions include:

1. Preventing autoimmunity: They help to prevent the immune system from attacking the body by producing a suppressor protein FOXP3 that helps to convert developing T-lymphocytes into T reg and suppresses autoreactive T lymphocytes.
2. Promote anamenestic response (immunologic memory) to resist repeat infections by the same microbe.

At this time you should know the following:

- Describe humoral and cell mediated immunity.
- Describe $CD4^+$ T_H interaction with B-cells.
- Describe $CD4^+$ T_H interaction with $CD8^+$ cells.
- Explain the process of generation of T and B-cells.
- Explain the role of T_H1, T_H2 cells and the profile of cytokines involved.
- Explain Nature Killer T-cells.
- Explain Regulatory T-cells.

Further Reading

- Janeway's Immunobiology, 7th edition, Volume 978, Issues 0-4129, 2008.
- Abul K Abbas, Andrew H Lichtman – 2006. Basic immunology.
- Abul K Abbas, Andrew H. Lichtman Basic Immunology: Functions and Disorders of the Immune System, 2010.
- Godfrey, D I, and *et al.,* NKT cells: What's in a name? Nat Rev Immunol 2004, 4(3): 231-7.
- Kidd P, T_H1/T_H2 balance: The hypothesis, its limitations, and implications for health and disease. Altern Med Rev. 2003 Aug;8(3):223-46.
- Dario A. A. Vignali1, Lauren W. Collison1 and Creg J Workman1 How regulatory T cells work Nature Reviews Immunology 8, 523-532 (July 2008).

14

CHAPTER

Immune Regulation

(Dr. Man Updesh Singh Sachdeva drmanupdeshpgi@yahoo.co.in)

OBJECTIVES

1. To define immune regulation.
2. To discuss "Central" and "Peripheral" mechanisms of immune regulation.
3. Role of negative and positive selection in thymus.
4. To know the role of Autoimmune Regulator (AIRE) gene and co-stimulatory molecules.
5. How immune mechanism deviates?
6. Mechanism of Activation Induced Cell Death (AICD).
7. To know the role of regulatory/suppressor cells.

INTRODUCTION

The immune system evolved to protect organisms from a virtually infinite variety of disease-causing agents but to avoid harmful responses to self. Because immune protective mechanisms include the elaboration of potent inflammatory molecules, antibodies and killer cell activation–which together cannot only destroy invading microorganisms, pathogenic auto reactive cells, and tumors, but also mortally injure normal cells. The immune system is inherently a "double-edged sword". Therefore, the antibody and cell-mediated immune responses must be closely regulated following antigenic stimulation; otherwise, our bodies would be overwhelmed by proliferating clones of lymphocytes and their products. Immune responses to foreign antigens are self-limiting and diminish as the antigens are eliminated, leading to a return of the immune system to a resting state.

Definition: Any process that modulates the frequency, rate or extent of the immune response, the immunological reaction of an organism to an immunogenic stimulus.

IMMUNE REGULATION BY CENTRAL SELECTION

The T-cell precursors migrate from the bone marrow to the corticomedullary zone of the thymus, where they begin to differentiate, rearrange their variable region genes, and proliferate. This complex program ends in the medullary region of the thymus, from which the mature T-cells exit. During this process of maturation, the T-cells (thymocytes) begin to express T-cell receptors (TCRs) for antigen. The majority of these receptors have two chains, α and β, and are called α/β receptors. The receptors recognize an immunogenic peptide held in the cleft of a major histocompatibility complex (MHC) molecule – the MHC antigen peptide complex. In the thymus, epithelial cells and other antigen-presenting cells display a wide variety of complexes composed of self peptides bound to MHC molecules. At the stage when thymocytes express the TCR and both the CD4 and CD8 co-receptors (the "double-positive" stage), thymocytes undergo apoptosis if they receive no TCR stimulation. This has been called as "death by neglect". This process eliminates thymocytes that have not productively rearranged the TCR genes or have no capacity to recognize antigen in the context of self-major histocompatibility complex (MHC). "Low-level" stimulation of the TCR antagonizes death by neglect. This protective event ensures MHC-specific antigen recognition by T-cells and is called "positive selection". While weak TCR signals can deliver an anti-apoptotic stimulus, strong TCR engagement of double positive thymocytes delivers a pro-apoptotic signal. This event, termed "negative selection" prevents the emergence of strongly autoreactive lymphocytes from the thymus. Therefore, whether the cell lives or dies depends on the binding affinity of its antigen receptors to peptides within the thymus. If the binding affinity is high, the cell dies; if there is no affinity, the cell dies. If the affinity is just right, the cell lives. Survival of the developing T-cell because of "just-right" affinity is called positive selection; the "wrong" affinity dooms the cell to death by apoptosis (negative selection). This deletion step is a major mechanism of central tolerance and the prevention of autoimmunity. Only 3 percent of the T-cell precursors that enter the thymus survive positive and negative selection. Curiously, the emigrants from the thymus were selected for survival because of their ability to bind to self peptides with low avidity, yet they constitute the population of T-cells that deal with foreign antigens. An explanation for this paradox is that a given T-cell receptor shows degeneracy and can cross-react with multiple peptides; this cross-reactivity maintains the flexibility required by the immune system to adapt to changing environment.

Ectopic Autoantigens in the Thymus

It is rather amazing that thymic epithelial cells produce and display ectopic autoantigens. A major leap forward in the understanding of this phenomenon was made with the identification of a gene, the product of which termed as AIRE (Autoimmune Regulator), is a large protein of 545 amino acids with several domains reminiscent of those found in transcriptional regulators. This locus was identified as the underlying susceptibility to the polyendocrine autoimmune disease known as APECED (autoimmune polyendocrinopathy-candidiasis-endodermal dystrophy), characterized by a set of three abnormal features–chronic muco-cutaneous candidiasis, hypoparathyroidism, and adrenal insufficiency. Autoimmune regulator (AIRE) promotes the ectopic transcriptional activity of a large number of chromosomal locations, thereby enhancing the expression by medullary epithelial cells (MECs) of genes that would normally only be expressed in specific tissues. This 'shadow' of the peripheral self in MECs is then presented to immature thymocytes, either directly by the MECs themselves, or indirectly by uptake of antigens released from MECs by thymic dendritic cells (DCs) (**Figure 14.1**). Differentiating T-cells that recognize these antigens are then removed primarily by apoptotic clonal deletion, although some may survive by adopting alternative fates that have regulatory rather than autoreactive properties. These mechanisms thus prevent the autoimmune attack of peripheral organs. There is a clear match between the antigens that are ectopically expressed under the dictates of AIRE and the specific antigenic targets that manifest in its absence. Hence, it is evident that AIRE plays an important role in prevention of autoimmunity by regulating the thymic transcription of genes encoding peripheral tissue antigens, thereby controlling thymocyte tolerization.

Does negative selection occur in the B-cell compartment?

Similar to T-cells, developing B-cells in the bone marrow undergo a series of proliferative expansion and apoptotic contraction events to shape the final B-cell repertoire. During the

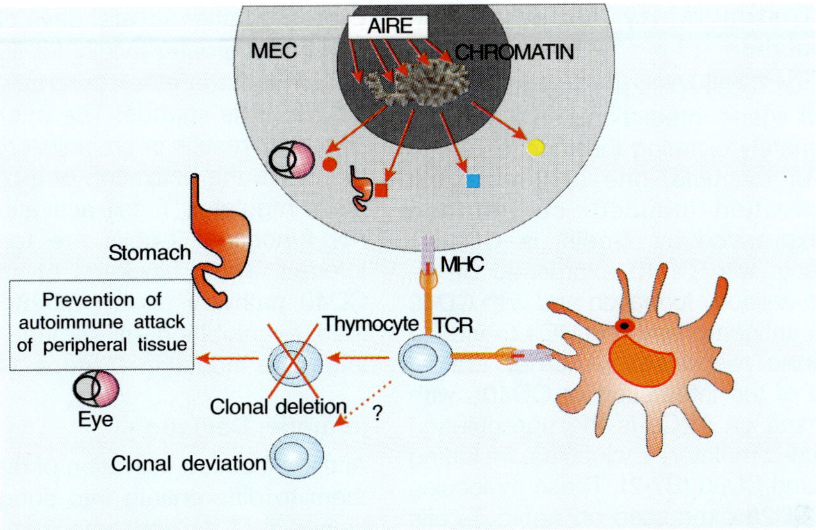

Fig. 14.1: AIRE–from transcriptional regulation to tolerance induction (Source: Mathis D, Benoist C. Nat Rev Immunol 2007;7:645-50)

process of maturation, immunoglobulin (Ig) gene rearrangement starting at the pro-B stage generates the B-cell receptor (BCR) and the survival of developing lymphocytes is promoted by IL-7, which is crucial at the pro-B/pre-B juncture. Subsequent to successive gene rearrangements at the heavy- and light-chain Ig loci, a process of selection occurs. B-cells that fail to generate a productive BCR, due to adoptive Ig gene rearrangements, are eliminated by apoptosis. At the other end of the spectrum, B-cells that express BCRs directed against self-antigens are eliminated by apoptosis or undergo receptor editing to acquire new antigen specificity.

PERIPHERAL REGULATION

Activation of mature T-cells requires multiple signals. The binding of the T cell's antigen receptor to an HLA–peptide complex activates only one signal. The others, termed costimulatory signals play a very important role in regulating immune response. In addition, the selection within thymus allows some self reactive T-cells to enter periphery, where they have the potential to become pathogenic effector cells. The peripheral regulatory mechanisms fine-tune the self-reactive T cell repertoire and suppress pathogenic autoimmunity in the periphery.

Regulatory Mechanisms Intrinsic to Antigen Activation

Antigen is at the centre of the immunoregulatory process since immune responses wane as antigen concentration decreases. Intrinsic mechanisms induced when the T cell receptor engages MHC-antigen-peptide complexes are a major point of control over the magnitude and class of immune responses. One level of control resides at the initial clonal activation of the T cell receptor itself by MHC-peptide complexes. The functional consequences of T cell signaling are dependent on the affinity and duration of binding of the TCRs with MHC-peptide complexes. For example, there is a threshold of affinity necessary for optimal activation and differentiation of T-cells, whereas triggering of very high-affinity TCRs can induce apoptotic pathways leading to activation-induced cell death (AICD).

Role of Co-stimulatory Molecules in Immune-regulation

During the initial T cell-MHC-peptide interaction, other receptor ligand interactions also become pivotal in ultimately dictating the functional fate of T-cells. For example, one of the earliest antigen activation–induced cell-surface molecules expressed by T-cells is CD40L. CD40L interacts with CD40 expressed on B-cells to induce antibody formation and with CD40 expressed on antigen-presenting DCs to induce cellular immune responses. Another critical consequence of the interaction of CD40L with CD40 expressed on APCs is the upregulation of other key co-stimulatory molecules, including CD80 (B7-1) and CD86 (B7-2). These molecules interact with CD28 expressed on naïve T-cells to provide the costimulatory signal required for optimal activation of T-cells. Binding of CD28 receptors on T-cells by accessory cell B7 molecules results in dramatic enhancement of IL-2 production by T-cells stimulated through their TCR. The importance of this CD28-B7 interaction is further underscored by the findings that CD28-deficient naïve T-cells are unable to produce IL-2 in response to TCR stimulation. The non-bone marrow-derived tissues, in spite of expressing self antigen-MHC complexes, are unable to activate naïve self-reactive T-cells due to absence of B7 molecules. In addition, TCR signaling in the absence of CD28-B7 interaction not only fails to elicit IL-2 production but also results in a long-lasting state of unresponsiveness to subsequent antigen stimulation (clonal anergy). Once anergy is induced, unresponsive T-cells remain viable but fail to proliferate in response to antigen stimulation because of transcriptional defect in IL-2 production. This defect appears to be caused by the failure of a critical inducible transcription factor to bind to its target sequence within the IL-2 gene enhancer.

Cytotoxic T-lymphocyte–Associated Antigen 4 (CTLA-4)

CTLA-4 molecule is homologous to CD28, but is not detectable on resting T-cells. It is expressed after several days of T cell activation and has a greater avidity for B7 molecules than CD28 and therefore favorably competes with CD28 for its ligands. The interaction of CTLA-4 with B7 results in an inhibitory signal (believed to involve the activation of a phosphatase) that down-regulates T cell activation. The resulting non-functional T-cells are termed anergic or tolerant. Thus, blockade of either the CD40L/CD40 pathway or the CD28/B7 pathway can lead to inhibition of immune responses and tolerance induction (**Figure 14.2**).

Immune Deviation

Antigen-induced activation of helper cells causes them to differentiate into subgroups of type 1 helper T (T_H1) and type 2 helper (T_H2) cells. T_H1 cells produce interferon-γ (IFN-γ), interleukin-2 (IL-2) and tumor necrosis factor β (TNF-β), and give rise to a cell-mediated immune response protective against intracellular pathogens and viruses, but these cells have also been implicated in organ-specific autoimmune diseases. T_H2 cells produce IL-4, IL-5 and IL-13 and activate mast cells and eosinophils, thereby eradicating helminths and other extracellular parasites, but in addition these cells are mediators of allergic and atopic manifestations. T_H1 and T_H2-specific cytokines can augment the growth or differentiation of their respective subset, and additionally may inhibit the development of the opposing subset.

The differentiation program for these T helper cell subsets can be influenced by a number of factors, including the dose and form of antigen, the antigen-presenting cell and/or co-stimulatory molecules; however, the dominant regulators of T helper cell differentiation are undoubtedly cytokines. The development of T_H1 cells from an antigenically naïve CD4+ T-cell precursor is driven by IL-12 produced by macrophages and dendritic cells. T_H1 commitment is enhanced by IFN-γ, which upregulates the IL-12 receptor while inhibiting the growth of T_H2 cells. On the other hand, IL-4 induces T_H2 development. IL-4 also downregulates IL-12 receptor expression on

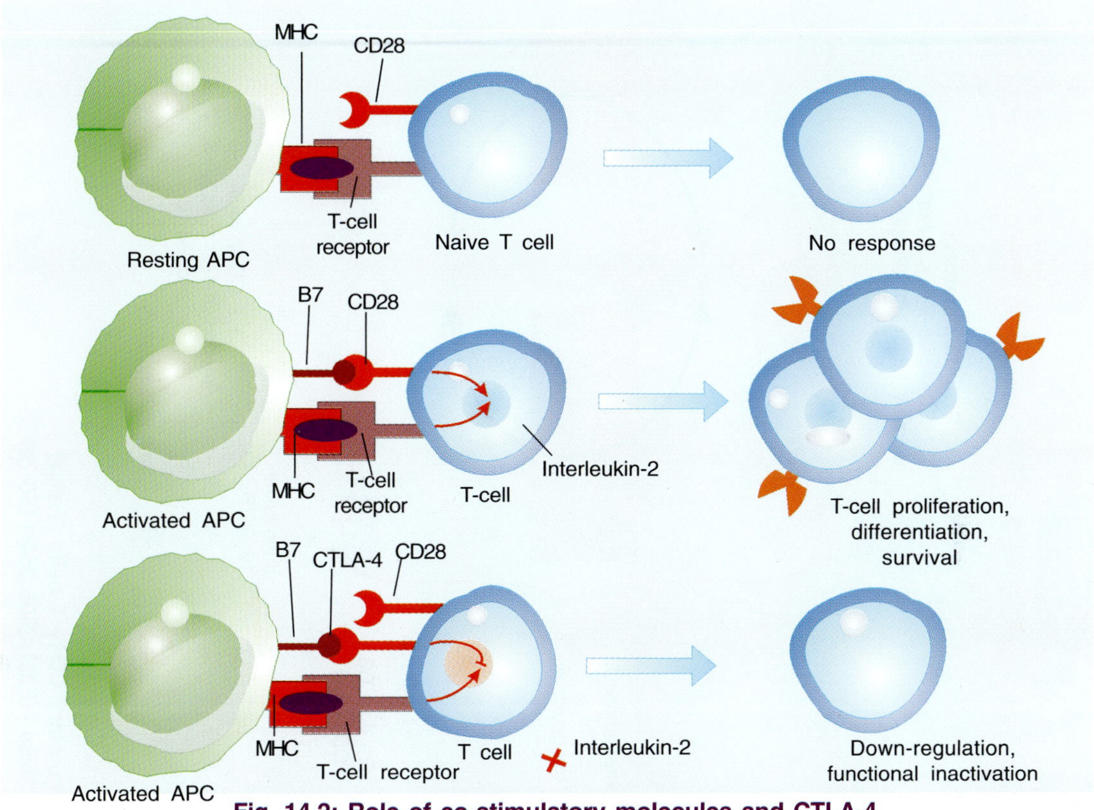

Fig. 14.2: Role of co-stimulatory molecules and CTLA-4 (Source: Sharpe *et al.* NEJM 2006;355:973-75)

developing cells thereby facilitating their commitment to the T_H2 lineage. Thus, a specific genetic program results in the differentiation towards either the T_H1 or the T_H2 lineage. The molecular mechanisms of such immune deviations have been elicited in recent past with studies evaluating role of various transcription factors in modulating the cytokine milieu. T-bet (T-box expressed in T-cells), a novel T_H1-specific transcription factor, controls the expression of the hallmark T_H1 cytokine–IFN-γ. Two T_H2-specific transcription factors, c-Maf and GATA-3, have been described. c-Maf augments the induction of IL-4 by transactivation of the IL-4 promoter. GATA-3 plays a dominant role because it can induce a wide range of T_H2-specific cytokines in developing and committed T_H1 cells, and GATA-3 can also inhibit the production of IFN-γ.

Other cytokine secreting subgroups of CD4+ cells, termed "Type 1 regulatory T (Tr1)" or "Th3 cells", secrete the immunosuppressive cytokines IL-10, TGF-β or both. The emergence of T_H1, T_H2, and other cytokine-secreting T-cells after antigen activation has a major role in regulating T cell functions. All these cytokine-secreting T-cells constitute a set of conventional T-cells that exert regulatory functions on immune response to both self and foreign antigens. They are specifically activated by antigen but mediate suppression non-specifically through their cytokines. Collectively, these cells, by controlling the magnitude and class of immune response, constitute to the non-specific inhibition of pathogenic autoimmunity (**Figure 14.3**).

Activation Induced Cell Death (AICD)

AICD is an important mechanism for the

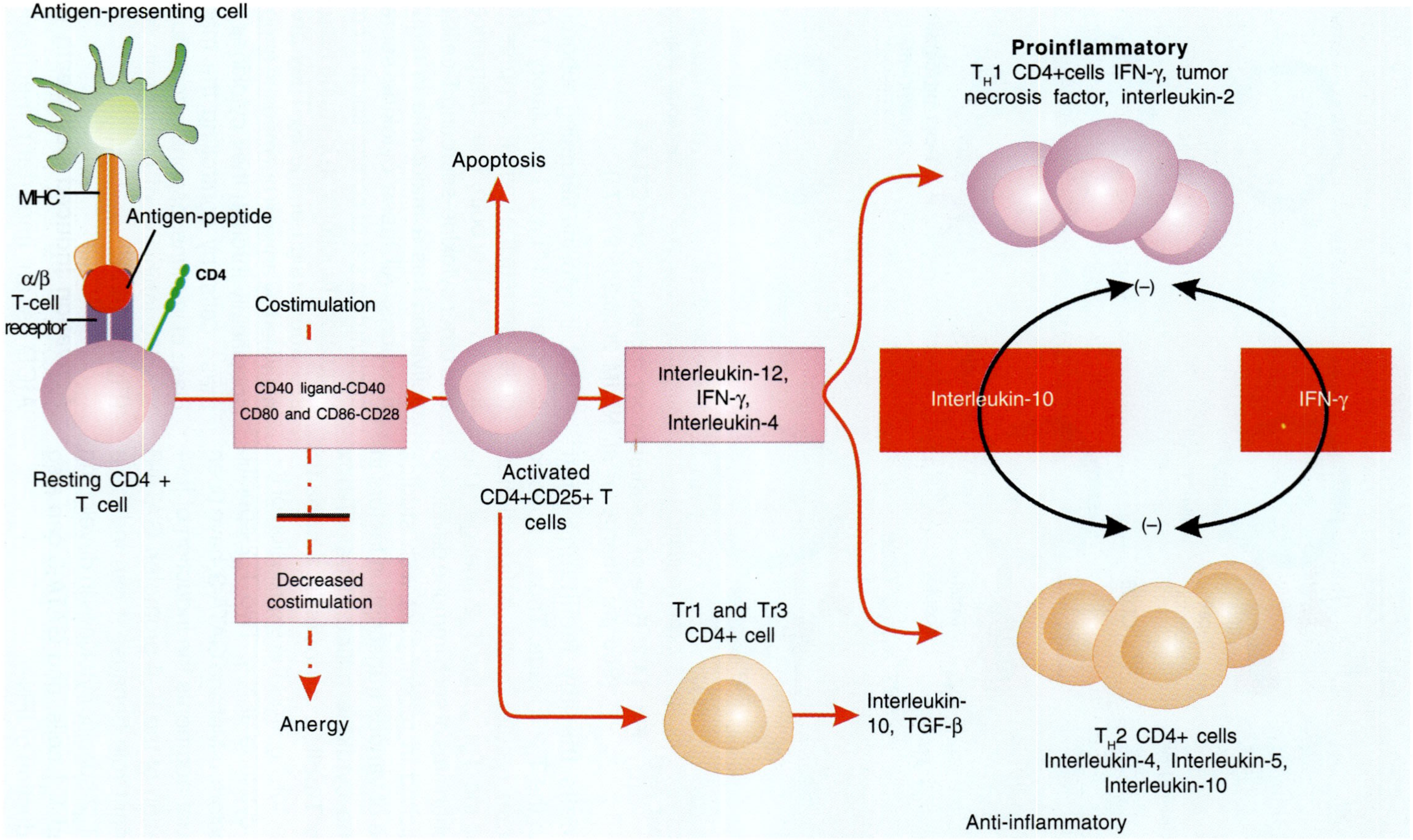

Fig. 14.3: Role of regulatory CD4+ T cells (Tregs) (Source: Jiang and Chess NEJM 2006;354:1166-76)

maintenance of T cell homeostasis. The active death mechanism involves apoptosis of mature T-cells in response to antigen stimulation. However, activation per se does not directly cause cell death; instead, death induction requires antigenic re-stimulation of activated T-cells, that is, reengagement after the initial activation. The presence of repeated or continuously high amounts of antigen is a powerful stimulus for IL-2 induced cell cycling and proliferation. Exponential T-cell expansion is prevented by a simple and specific feedback loop in which a fraction of the re-stimulated cells undergo apoptosis by production of death ligands which engage specific death receptors in the tumor necrosis factor-receptor (TNFR) superfamily. Current evidence suggests that Fas ligand (FasL) as well as TNF are the key death ligands that mediate this process in mature T-cells. Ligation of Fas with FasL induces trimerization of the Fas receptor, wherein the adaptor protein, Fas-associated death domain protein (FADD), binds to the trimerized Fas cytoplasmic region through the interaction of the respective death domains. Pro-caspase-8 [also called FADD-like IL-1β-converting enzyme (FLICE)] is then recruited to FADD through binding of the death effector domains (DEDs), which in turn induces self-activation of caspase-8. The Fas receptor, FADD and pro-caspase-8 form a functional death-inducing signaling complex (DISC). The activated caspase-8 is released into the cytosol where it results in activation of a caspase cascade that initiates apoptosis (**Figure 14.4**).

This process of apoptosis is antigen specific, and linked with TCR engagement leading to IL-2 production and cell-cycle progression. IL-2 is not only a T cell growth factor, but also sensitizes T-cells to AICD. One important role of IL-2 in mediating the susceptibility of T-cells to AICD is upregulating FasL expression. AICD also plays a role in clonal deletion of thymocytes, however the

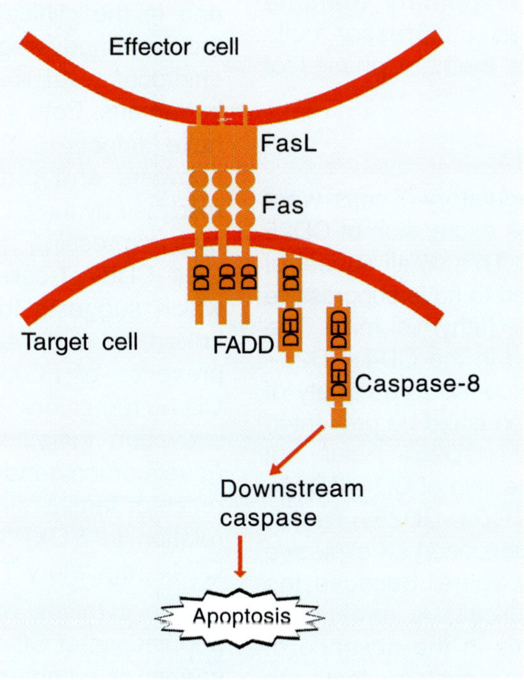

Fig. 14.4: Fas-FasL mediated apoptosis
(Source: Zhang J, Xu X and Liu Y Cellular and Molecular Immunology 2004;1:186-92)

mechanisms does not seem to involve the death ligands.

Regulatory/Suppressor T-cells

These are distinct subsets of T-cells which control the outgrowth of potentially pathogenic antigen-reactive T-cells and may play potentially important clinical roles in preventing and treating immune-mediated disease. There is emerging evidence that these cells consist of a heterogeneous population of T-cells and belong to subgroups of CD4+, CD8+, and natural killer T-cells. Each of these subgroups has a distinct effector mechanism and act at a different stage of immune response. Natural killer T-cells and specialized CD4+ regulatory T-cells are "natural suppressor cells" and are present before the activation of T-cells by antigen. These cells act primarily during the early phases of innate or primary immune responses or both. In contrast, CD8+ T suppressor cells differentiate into effector cells during the primary immune response and function as suppressor cells during the secondary and memory phases of immunity.

CD4+ Regulatory T Cells

The specialized CD4+ regulatory T-cells were initially characterized by the expression of CD25 molecule on their surface. This small subset of CD4+CD25+ cells was found to have suppressive function by studies on nude (athymic) mice. The transfer of T-cells depleted in the CD4+CD25+ population into athymic mice led to a variety of autoimmune diseases, which could be prevented by injection of purified CD4+CD25+ T-cells but not CD4+CD25- T-cells. The field of CD4+CD25+ regulatory T-cells termed "CD4+CD25+ Tregs", was thus born and has experienced an explosive growth over the past few years. Because the number of CD4+CD25+ T-cells is remarkably constant in normal animals in the absence of perturbation of the immune system, they are referred to as "naturally occurring" or "endogenous" T suppressor cells. However, the idea that these cells are a distinct lineage is complicated by the fact that the CD25 molecule, originally used to identify these cells, is the α chain of the IL-2 receptor, which is expressed on virtually all T-cells during antigen-induced activation. Later, certain experiments revealed that besides CD4+CD25+ T-cells, certain CD4+CD25- T-cells were also involved in regulatory functions and suppression of autoimmunity. This suggests that CD25 is not the essential feature of CD4+ regulatory cells. Further efforts to characterize these CD4+ regulatory cells led to the discovery of a transcription factor called FOXP3, which is a member of the fork head family of DNA-binding transcription factors, and is highly expressed in CD4+ regulatory cells, irrespective of CD25 expression. Importantly, mutational defects in the *FOXP3* gene result in the fatal autoimmune and inflammatory disorder of the scurfy mouse and in the clinical and molecular features of the immunodysregulation, polyendocrinopathy, enteropathy, X-linked syndrome (IPEX syndrome) in humans. Both scurfy mice and IPEX patients have defects in T cell activation and reduced numbers and reduced suppressor functions mediated by the CD4+CD25+ T-cells. In FOXP3–over expressing mice, both CD4+CD25– and CD4–CD8+ T-cells show suppressive activity, which suggests that expression of FOXP3 is linked to suppressor functions. Therefore, presence of FOXP3, and not CD25, defines CD4+ regulatory T-cells. Some other surface activation molecules like, CTLA-4 and GITR (glucocorticoid-induced tumor necrosis factor receptor family-related gene) when analyzed in relation to FOXP3, refine the identification of CD4+ regulatory T-cells.

The cytokine profiles found in the various populations of CD4+ suppressor cells include a variety of combinations of the already known immunoregulatory cytokines (i.e., IL-10, TGF-β,

IL-4, and IFN-γ). For example, there are CD4+ CD45*Rb* low activated suppressor cells that secrete large quantities of either IL-10 and IL-4 (termed Tr1 cells) and other CD4+CD45*Rb* low suppressor T-cells that secrete large quantities of TGF-β (termed T_H3 cells).

The effector phase of CD4+ regulatory T cell-mediated suppression does not seem to involve the T-cell receptor and antigen presentation by MHC molecules (i.e., MHC restriction). Besides, the secretion of above mentioned cytokines, the suppression depends, at least in part, on cell contact, but the surface molecules involved in the contact are unknown. IL-10 secretion by Tregs needs a special mention, as it seems not only to inhibit T_H1 responses via its inhibitory action on dendritic cells and macrophages, but also inhibits the development of T_H1 and T_H2 responses (**Figure 14.5**).

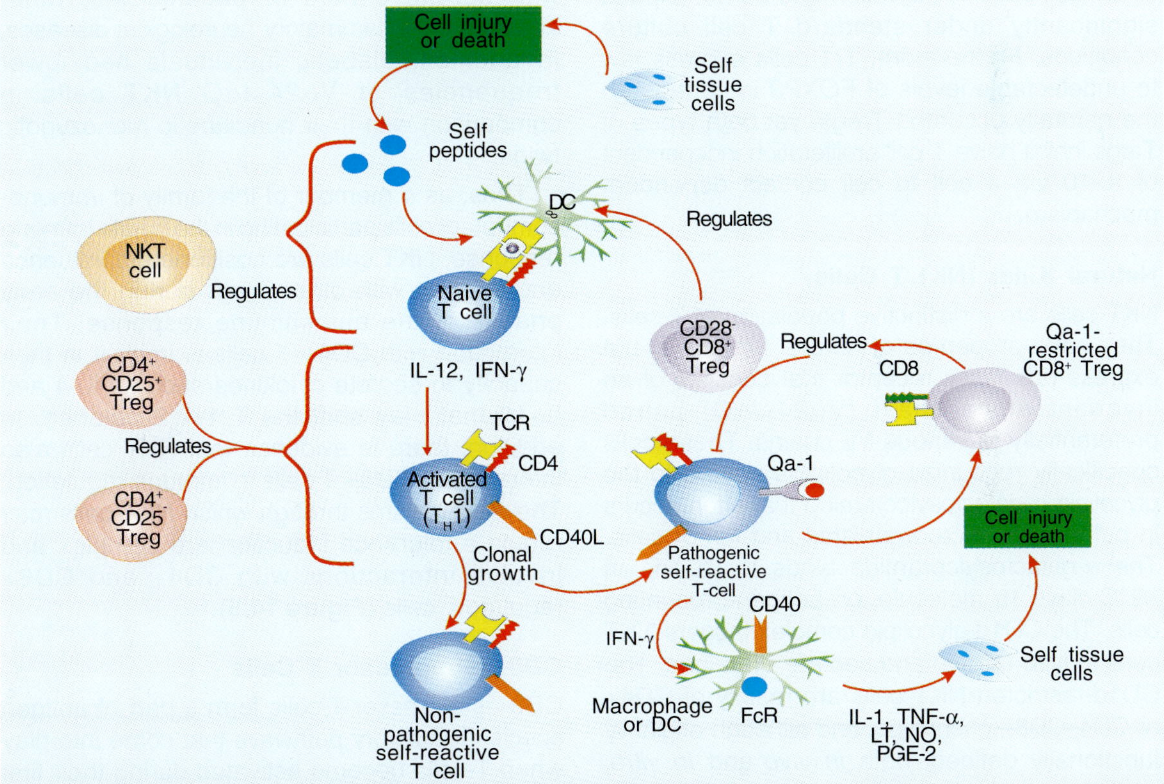

Fig. 14.5: Tregs control the peripheral induction and clonal outgrowth of antigen-reactive T cells. This illustration shows various pathways of immunoregulation mediated by suppressor subsets of NKT, CD4+ and CD8+ T cell subsets. Each of the regulatory T cell subsets expresses distinct receptors, employs different effector mechanisms, and functions predominately at different stages during the course of the peripheral immune response. The NKT and CD4+CD25+ regulatory cells are "natural suppressor cells"; they are present prior to antigen activation and primarily function during the early "innate" and/or primary adaptive immune responses. In contrast, the CD8+ regulatory cells are induced to differentiate into suppressor effector cells during the primary immune response, and they function as effector-suppressor cells predominately during the secondary and memory phases of immunity (Source: Jiang H, Chess L. J Clin Invest 2004;114:1198-208)

T Regulatory 1 (Tr1)

Tr1 cells, also called IL-10 Tregs by some, are a distinct category of IL-10-producing suppressive CD4+ cells. Tr1 cells can be induced under particular experimental conditions of antigenic stimulation *in vitro* and *in vivo* and in natural infection *in vivo*. IL-10 itself is a major factor for the induction of suppressive IL-10-producing T-cells. Most of these cells produce high levels of IL-10, TGF-β, moderate amounts of IFN-γ and IL-5, but no IL-2 or IL-4. Tr1 cells proliferate poorly after polyclonal TCR-mediated or antigen-specific activation and do not expand significantly under standard T cell culture conditions. Furthermore, Tr1 cells express low to undetectable levels of FOXP3 in contrast to the naturally occurring Tregs, yet both types of Tregs inhibit naive T cell proliferation independent of IL-10 via a cell to cell contact dependent mechanism.

Natural Killer (NK) T Cells

NKT cells are a distinctive population of T-cells. They have properties of natural killer cells but express α/β T cell receptor that consists of an invariant alpha chain (Vα24-JαQ) paired preferentially to various Vβ chains. These cells specifically recognize glycolipids related to the glycolipid α-galactosylceramide that often occurs in pathogenic microorganisms and tumor cells. The α-galactosylceramide binds to CD1d, an MHC class 1b molecule, on antigen-presenting cells. The CD1d-glycolipid complex triggers NKT cells to lyse targets and secrete cytokines. The CD1d-restricted NKT cells are mainly of CD4+ or CD4–CD8– phenotype, and although originally functionally defined, both *in vivo* and *in vitro*, by their capacity to lyse a variety of tumor cells, they were later found also to be involved in the regulation of autoimmune diseases. These *in vivo* roles in immune responses are thought to be linked to the fact that following TCR antigen triggering *in vivo*, NKT cells were observed to develop augmented killer cell activity and secrete large amounts of cytokines, including IL-4 and IFN-γ, as well as TGF-β and IL-10, known to be involved in the activation of cell types important in mediating both innate immunity and T_H2-type adaptive immunity. As a consequence, NKT cells have been shown to influence the course of autoimmune disease in a variety of animal models. A reduction in number or altered function of NKT cells has also been correlated with autoimmune disease in humans. In patients with multiple sclerosis who are in relapse or remission, the frequency of Vα24-JαQ NKT cells is reduced in comparison with normal donors or patients with other autoimmune/inflammatory neurological diseases. In addition, diabetic individuals had lower frequencies of Vα24-JαQ NKT cells in comparison with their nondiabetic monozygotic twins.

Thus, as a member of the family of immunocompetent cells participating in the innate immune response, NKT cells are positioned to influence and interact with other Tregs during the early phases of the autoimmune response. Their interaction with CD4+ T cells is implicit in their capacity to secrete cytokines such as IL-4 and IL-10 that may shift the T_H1-T_H2 balance. In addition, there is evidence that NKT cells also interact with CD8+ T cells in immune regulation. The mechanisms through which NKT cells may regulate tolerance induction are complex and involve interactions with CD4+ and CD8+ regulatory cells (**Figure 14.5**).

CD8+ Suppressor T Cells

CD8+ suppressor T-cells form a part of antigen specific regulatory pathways that come into play when T-cells become activated during their first encounter with conventional self or foreign antigens. It is initiated by the activation of naive CD4+ T-cells during the primary immune response, in which the TCRs on CD4+ T-cells interact with MHC class II–peptide complexes presented by conventional APCs. This initial interaction induces the surface expression of activation-dependent MHC class1b molecule

(Qa-1 in mice and HLA-E in humans)–self-peptide complexes which is not observed in resting T-cells. These activation-dependent Qa-1–self-peptide complex serve as both the inducer and target structures recognized by TCR αβ on regulatory CD8+ T cells. Thus, the Qa-1–self-peptide complex expressed by activated CD4+ T cells triggers TCR αβ on regulatory CD8+ T cells. These CD8+ T cells then differentiate into effector cells, which in turn suppress CD4+ T cells expressing the same target Qa-1–self-peptide complex. This suppression is linked to specific antigen activation of CD4+ T cells, and as a consequence the peptides bound by Qa-1 will likely be those induced by antigen activation (**Figure 14.5**). Whether they represent specific peptides derived from the CD4+ T cell TCR (TCR Vβ or Vα peptides) or peptides derived from activation molecules induced by antigen triggering is not known. The mechanism of effecting suppression of the CD4+ T cells by the Qa-1–restricted CD8+ T cells has not been definitively delineated; however, the consequences of TCR triggering of CD8+ T cell precursors may be conventional and involve differentiation into specific CTLs that lyse target cells and/or secrete lymphokines that downregulate the target cells.

Antibody-Mediated Immune Regulation

Passive transfer of antibodies into a naïve animal often prevents the priming of that animal with a subsequent injection of antigen. High-affinity antibodies are more effective than low-affinity ones. Some of this effect is due to formation and clearance of antigen-antibody complexes. Antibody production could be regulated by other antibodies that recognized unique idiotypic determinants in the V regions of the first antibody. These are called "Idiotype networks". The antigen binding site (formed by the light and heavy chain variable domains) of an antibody molecule has a characteristic structure or conformation which can be recognized by anti-idiotypic antibodies. When a foreign antigen enters the body, the idiotypes of responding clones of lymphocyte are expanded and anti-idiotypic responses are triggered that shut off the antigen-specific (idiotype-expressing) lymphocytes. Complementary interactions between idiotypes and anti-idiotypes reach a steady state at which the immune system is at homeostasis.

Besides, regulatory lymphocytes, many other cells may play a suppressive role to control immune response depending on site and type of antigen. Dendritic cells, forming the link between innate and acquired immunity, are of a particular interest. The discovery of pathogen-associated molecular patterns and toll-like receptors provides the mechanistic basis for dendritic cell recognition of specific pathogens and induction of appropriate innate and adaptive immune responses. Only recently has insight been gained into how dendritic cells contribute to establishing and/or maintaining immunological tolerance to self. Soluble and cellular mediators have been reported to effectively regulate the function of dendritic cells by inducing several outcomes ranging from non-inflammatory dendritic cells that lack the ability to induce T lymphocyte activation to dendritic cells that actively suppress T lymphocyte responses. The other important subset of cells is the γδ T-cells. In contrast to αβ T-cells, γδ T-cells show less TCR diversity, are particularly enriched at epithelial surfaces and appear to respond to self-molecules that signal potential danger or cellular stress. In addition, various subsets of γδ T-cells have shown antitumor and immune regulatory activities.

Immune regulation is carried out in an integrated manner by distinct suppressor T-cells subsets that are superimposed on intrinsic homeostatic control mechanisms. Understanding the precise interplay between these intrinsic and suppressor mechanisms will undoubtedly be reveal the immunopathogenesis of a variety of diseases associated with abnormalities in immune regulation. Scientists and clinicians have spent the better part of the past century attempting to manipulate the immune system. These efforts have primarily focused upon induction of immunity to pathogens. Currently, a major emphasis is on the development of effective immunotherapies, by clinical induction of suppressor mechanisms, for the prevention and/or suppression of proinflammatory responses associated with immunological diseases like autoimmunity and also in transplantation.

At this time you should know the following:

1. Definition of immune regulation.
2. "Central" mechanism of immune regulation:
   - Role of AIRE gene.
   - Negative and positive selection of T-cells in thymus.
3. "Peripheral" mechanisms of immune regulation:
   - Mechanisms intrinsic to antigen activation.
   - Role of co-stimulatory molecules like CD40 and CD40L, CD28, CD80, CD86 and CTLA-4.
   - Immune deviation.
   - Activation induced cell death.
   - Role of CD4+ regulatory T-cells, NK cells, CD8+ suppressor T-cells.
   - Antibody mediated immune regulation.

Further Reading

Fundamental Immunology by William E Paul, 5th Edition.

15

CHAPTER

MHC: Genetics and Role in Transplantation

(Dr. Poonam Elhence docpoonam@yahoo.co.in)

OBJECTIVES

1. To review structure, organization and inheritance of MHC genes.
2. To learn about the expression, function and interaction of class I and class II MHC molecules.
3. To outline the role of MHC in immune functions and disease.
4. To learn techniques for detection of MHC molecules.
5. To provide a brief overview of the genetic basis of transplantation.

INTRODUCTION

Survival depends on the ability of the immune system to recognize various foreign particles **(antigens)** and to mount an immune response against them. In adaptive immune responses, antigen recognition takes place by immunoglobulins present on the B lymphocytes and by antigen-specific T cell receptors (TCR) present on the T lymphocytes. As opposed to **immunoglobulins** which **directly encounter** and interact with intact antigens or pathogens and their products in the extracellular spaces of the body, **T-cells recognize only those antigens** which **have been processed and are presented on the surface of the body's own cells**. These foreign antigens can be either intracellular (such as viruses or intracellular bacteria which replicate within the cells) or those which have been taken up by the cell from extracellular fluids via endocytotic mechanisms. These infected cells display foreign peptides/antigenic fragment on their cell surface and hence, T-cells can detect the presence of intracellular pathogens.

When disease associated proteins occur in a cell, they are broken down into smaller fragments by unfolding and digestion by the proteolytic machinery of the cell. Cellular proteins bind to these antigen fragments and translocate them to the surface of the cell where these cell protein-antigen complexes are **"presented"** to the defense mechanisms of the body. These transport molecules are called the **"MHC proteins"**. Once formed, the complex of antigenic peptide and MHC is generally very stable (half life~ 24 hours). In the absence of peptide, class I heavy chains of the MHC associated with β2–microglobulin are very unstable and dissociate rapidly.

MHC proteins and their associated molecules are fundamental in the process of presentation of foreign or non-foreign antigens bound by the MHC. These antigens are constantly being presented to the circulating T-lymphocytes for inspection by their T-cell receptors (TCR). Without this presentation, other aspects of the immune response cannot occur. Receptors on T-lymphocytes interact with the antigen-MHC complex, triggering both cellular and humoral responses.

Composition and Organization of MHC Genes

MHC complex is a cluster of genes located on the short arm of chromosome 6 at 6p21.31 in humans that codes for proteins unique to each individual and has both immunological and non-immunological functions. It was originally named the MHC because of its role in tissue rejection following transplantation studies carried out in mice by Peter A. Issac Gorer.[1] In mouse, the MHC genes are known as the **H-2 genes** and are present on chromosome 17. It is also referred to as **human leukocyte antigen** (HLA) system in humans as it was first detected on human leukocytes or white blood cells from different individuals. HLA proteins are present on the surface of most of the body's cells and are important in helping the immune system to distinguish "self" from "non-self" molecules. It spans over 3,500 kilobases depending on the haplotype and comprises three regions: class I, class II and class III (**Figure 15.1**).The class I and class II antigens are expressed on cells and tissues whereas class III antigens are associated with proteins in serum and other body fluids.

The human class I molecules include HLA-A, HLA-B and HLA-C. Class II molecules include HLA-DR, HLA-DQ and HLA-DP. Class III molecules or the non-HLA region includes complement components (C2,C4 and BF), P450 21-hydroxylase (Cyp21), heat shock proteins 70 (Hsp 70) and tumour necrosis factor (TNF) (**Figure 15.2**).

The map order of genes within the MHC is HLA-A,-C,-B,-DR,-DQ,-DP, with HLA-A being distal to the centromere. The GLO1 locus marks the centromeric boundary of the MHC. Each of the HLA subregion (HLA-A,B,C, DR, DQ and DP) encodes a minimum of one cell surface glycoprotein.

Expression and Function of Class I HLA Molecules

MHC molecules act as cell surface markers enabling the infected cells to signal both helper and cytotoxic T lymphocytes.HLA class I molecules are expressed on almost all nucleated cell surfaces and platelets. These are not expressed on brain cells, sperm cells and muscle cells. Their levels vary extensively and are highest on lymphoid cells. They bind

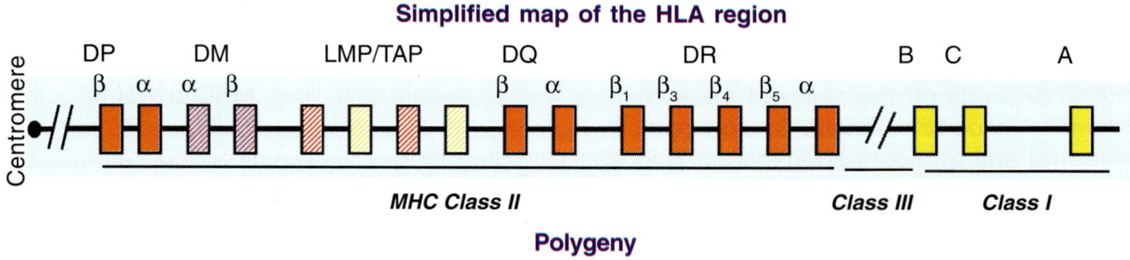

Fig. 15.1: Class I: 3 types HLA-A, HLA-B, HLA-C (sometimes called class Ia genes). Class II: 3 types HLA-DP HLA DQ, HLA DR. 3 extra DRβ genes in some individuals can allow 3 extra HLA-DR molecules. (Modified from www.le.ac.uk/microbiology/website)

MHC class	I			II			III	
Region	A	B	C	DP	DQ	DR	C4, C2, BF	
Gene products	HLA-A	HLA-B	HLA-C	DP αβ	DQ αβ	DR αβ	C' proteins	TNF-α TNF-β

Fig. 15.2: MHC class and gene products (Modified from Immunology, Chapter 7, 5th Edition by Kuby *et al.*)

peptides from intracellular or endogenous proteins which can be either self-proteins, an abnormal protein (tumour antigen) or foreign substances such as viral peptides (**Figure 15.3**), bacterial products, protozoa etc which have penetrated the cell and display antigen to CD8+ T lymphocytes/Cytotoxic T lymphocytes (CTLs) in **cellular immunity** and are particularly important in organ and tissue rejection following transplantation. Class I genes can be **up-regulated** by γ-IFN and TNF and can be **suppressed** or down regulated by viral infections (HIV), malignancies etc.

CTLs possess both CD8 molecules and T-cell receptors (TCR) on their surfaces. These TCRs on CTLs recognize peptides complexed with class I molecules as foreign leading to the **activation** of CTLs. Granules of activated CD8 killer cells contain a pore-forming protein called **perforin**. This process involves the formation of pores in the plasma membrane of target cells and also the initiation of programmed cell death by different pathways and leads to destruction of target cells and pathogens (**Figure 15.4**). Killer cells are specific for both the virus peptide and the host MHC class I.

Class I MHC associates with β-2 microglobulin which is a non-variable protein component coded by a gene on chromosome 15. In the absence of β-2 microglobulin, class I antigens will not be expressed on the cell surface. Such individuals with defective β-2 microglobulin gene have a deficiency of cytotoxic T lymphocytes as they do not express any class I antigen.

Expression and Function of Class II HLA Molecules

Unlike class I HLA molecules, expression of class II antigens is more selective.

MHC class II molecule expression is restricted to **antigen presenting cells** (APCs). These are

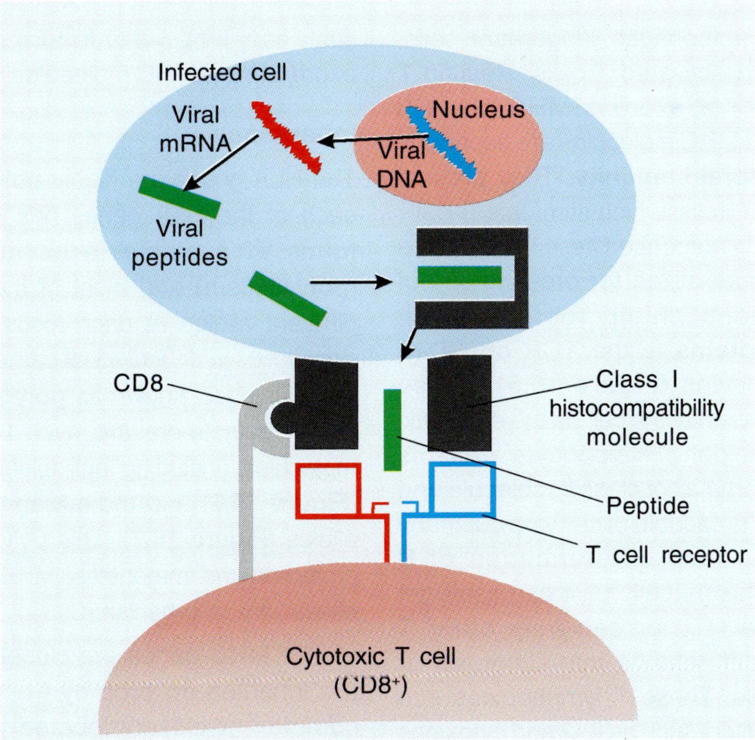

Fig. 15.3: Presentation of viral peptides by class I MHC molecule to CD8+ T-cell (Modified from: *http://users.rcn.com/jkimball.ma.ultranet/BiologyPages/H/HLA*)

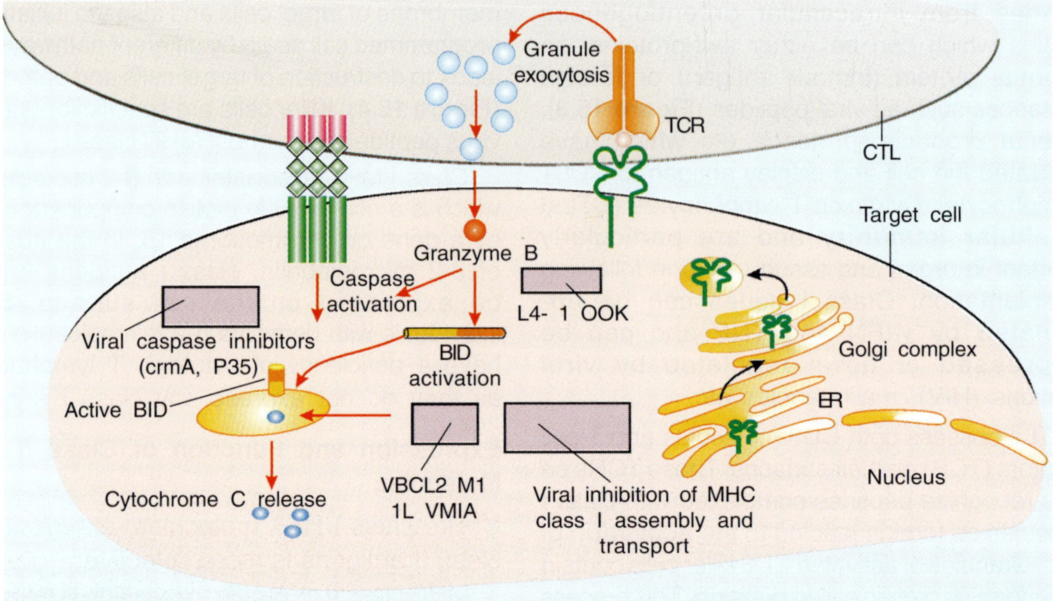

Fig. 15.4: Mechanism of T-cell mediated killing (Barry and Bleackly Nat Rev Immunol 2:401-9, 2002)

B lymphocytes, macrophages, langerhans cells, dendritic cells and activated T-cells. Resting T lymphocytes do not express MHC class II molecules. Class II MHC molecules are especially important in **humoral immunity**. They present antigen to helper T-cells, which stimulate B-cells to elicit an antibody response.Class II molecules are functionally specialized for presentation of antigenic peptides chiefly derived from **extracellular proteins** to the TCR on **CD4+** helper T lymphocytes (**Figure 15.5**). These exogenous antigens enter the cell via the endocytic pathway. Each helper T lymphocyte which is activated by the complex of class II molecule and the bound antigen is capable of carrying out many functions. It can help differentiation of B lymphocytes to plasma cells or it can itself get transformed into CTL or can help other T lymphocytes to differentiate into Cytotoxic or Suppressor T-cells. These T lymphocytes can produce growth factors such as IL-2 and cytokines such as γ-IFN. γ-IFN in turn causes increased expression of MHC molecules on the target cells.

Inheritance

The HLA genes are highly **polymorphic**, that is, each of the HLA genes has multiple alleles or forms at a single locus in the population **(polyallelism)** and most of the individuals have different alleles at each locus. Duplication of a gene locus in an individual can also occur resulting in multiple loci known as **polygeny**. According to recent data, there are over 1400 MHC class I molecules (including null alleles, synonyms etc) (**Figure 15.6**) and more than 800 MHC class II alleles (**Figure 15.7**). This polymorphism confers protection and immense survival advantage against diverse micro-organisms.

The MHC genes are closely linked and they are inherited **en bloc** by the offspring. Such a complex of closely located genes which are

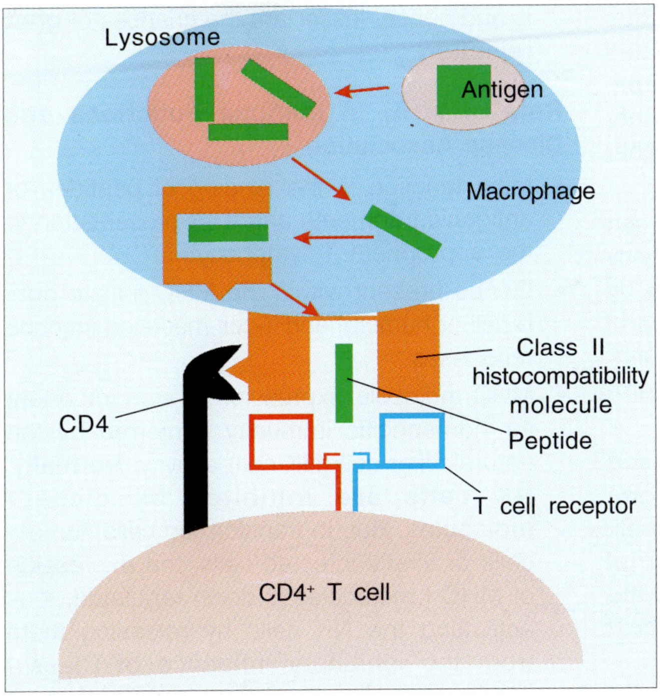

Fig. 15.5: Presentation of viral antigenic peptides by class II MHC molecule to CD4+ T-cell
(Modified from: *http://users.rcn.com/jkimball.ma.ultranet/BiologyPages/H/HLA*)

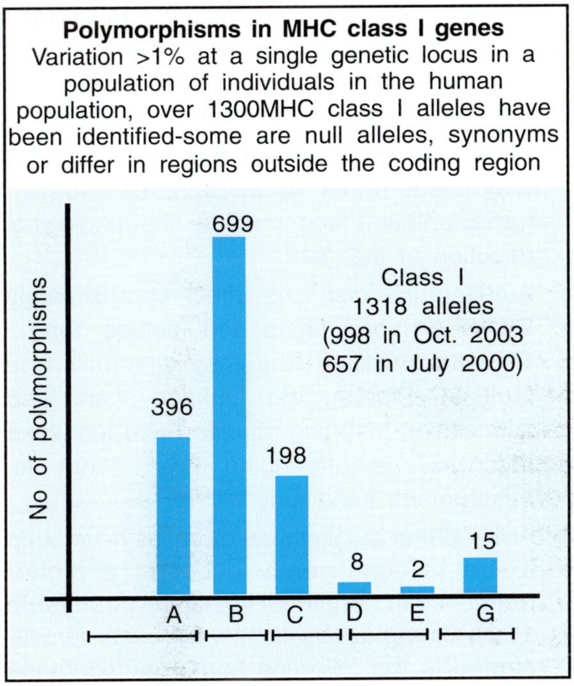

Fig. 15.6: Polymorphism in MHC class I genes
(Source of Figure: www.anthonynolan.org.uk/HIG.)

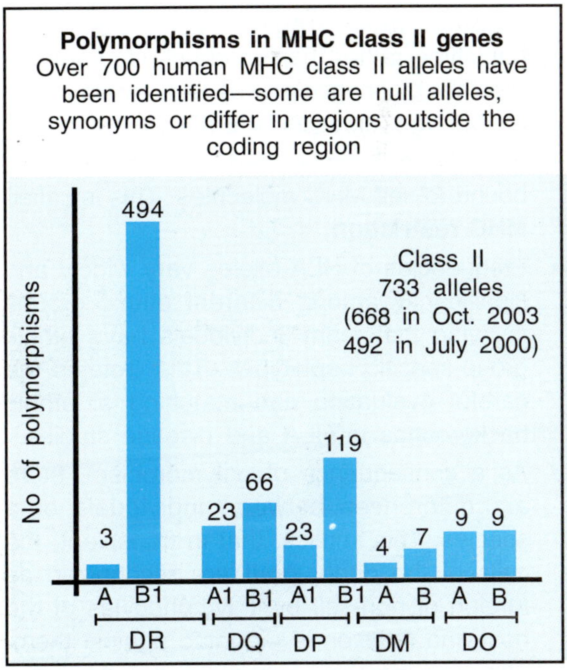

Fig. 15.7: Polymorphism in MHC Class II genes
(Source of Figure: www.anthonynolan.org.uk/HIG.)

present on one of the pair of homologous chromosomes and are almost always segregated en bloc to the offspring is called a **haplotype**. Two MHC haplotypes, one acquired from either parent, are present in each individual, one on either chromosome 6.

- In spite of close linkage, **cross over** can occur and has been reported. The frequency of crossing over of genes is controlled by the distance separating those genes and some characteristics of the intervening DNA strand. This cross over results in vast heterogeneity in a given population.
- These genes are **codominantly expressed** i.e., both maternal and paternal gene products are expressed in the same cell. Generally, by convention, the paternal haplotypes are designated a and b, and the maternal haplotypes are designated c and d.
- Certain alleles tend to occur or cluster together more frequently on the same haplotype rather than randomly segregating together by chance alone. This is referred to as **linkage disequilibrium** (LD).
- An antigen is recognized only as a peptide bound to self MHC molecules. This is called **MHC restriction**.
- Frequencies of HLA alleles vary widely and significantly among different ethnic groups implying that many individuals have ethnic group-specific haplotypes. This dictates the careful evaluation and matching of ethnic backgrounds in HLA and disease studies.
- As a consequence of polymorphism, there are differences between individuals of a species. This implies, that in transplant, the cells of the donor graft are recognized as foreign or non-self by T lymphocytes of the host and reaction is mounted against them. The more matching genes between the donor and recipient, the better compatibility there is and hence, lesser are the chances of **graft rejection**.

Role of MHC in Immune Functions and Disease Association

- Main function is the binding of peptides or antigenic fragments and their presentation to the appropriate T lymphocytes.
- Genes present within the MHC initiate both B-cell or humoral and T-cell mediated immune responses.
- MHC molecule expression is also important for non-specific immunity conferred by the natural killer cell (NK cell) activity. **Normally, NK cells are inhibited by class I molecules**. But, in transformed cells, tumour cells or virally infected cells, the expression of MHC I molecules is down regulated, thus activating the NK cells by releasing them from the inhibitory influence of Class I molecules. Hence, these transformed or infected cells become susceptible to NK cell-mediated killing (**Figure 15.8**). Tumours that lose expression of all MHC class I molecules are more likely to be killed by NK cells.
- Molecules encoded by the MHC are the major obstacles to successful allograft transplantation and mediate immunological rejection of the graft.
- Autoimmune diseases affect approximately 5% of the population and include Type I Diabetes mellitus, Rheumatoid arthritis and Multiple sclerosis etc. Linkage scans and association-mapping studies have identified the MHC as influencing most, if not all, autoimmune conditions.[2,3]
- A number of autoimmune diseases have been found to consistently occur at a higher frequency in certain MHC haplotypes (**Table 15.1**). Strong associations have been demonstrated in the following human autoimmune diseases:

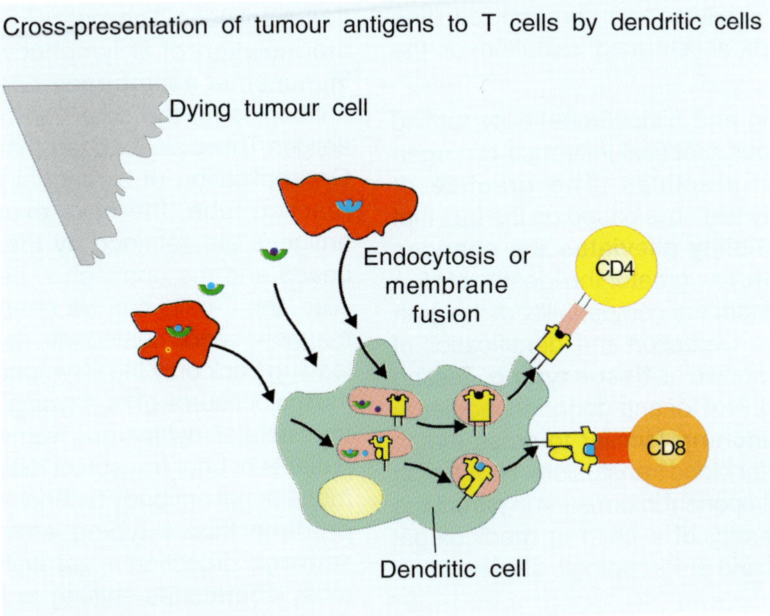

Fig. 15.8: Presentation of tumour antigens in the context of MHC (Modified from: The Immune System by Peter Parham, 2nd Edition)

Table 15.1: Disease association with MHC and relative risk

Disease	***Association with HLA***	***Relative Risk***
Ankylosing Spondylitis (AS)	HLA-B 27	90-100
Type I Diabetes Mellitus (IDDM)	HLA-DR3 and DR-4	Both combined:20-40
Rheumatoid Arthritis (RA)	HLA-DR4	3-6
Pemphigus Vulgaris	HLA-DR4, HLA-DQ8	15
Gluten Sensitive Enteropathy (GSE)	HLA-DR 5/7	5-10
Goodpasture syndrome	HLA-DR2	15-18
Multiple Sclerosis	HLA-DR2	3
Reiter's disease	HLA-B27	37
Myasthenia Gravis	HLA-DR3	2-3

Modified from: Robbins Textbook of Pathology, 6th edition, Cellular and Molecular Immunology, 6th Edition by Abbas *et al.*

- The clinical significance of the MHC is highlighted in organ transplantation in which cells and tissues are transplanted for the treatment of a wide range of conditions such as End Stage Renal Disease (ESRD), chronic liver disease, certain leukemias, severe thalassemia etc. However, reaction of the recipient against alloantigens of the graft results in graft rejection and is the major hurdle in organ transplantation. The survival time of a graft is determined by the immune mechanisms involved and the nature of the graft (xenograft is rejected much faster as compared to an allograft).

Techniques for the Detection of MHC Molecules

Exposure to HLA antigens can occur as a result of previous blood transfusions, prior organ grafts or multiple pregnancies. Formation of specific antibodies to these antigens is known as **sensitization**. Reexposure to these antigens on a new allograft can produce rapid immune responses, both cellular and humoral resulting in hyperacute or accelerated rejection of the graft.

HLA matching and histocompatibility testing have an enormous practical influence on organ transplantation practices. The practice of histocompatibility testing is based on the fact that **greater compatibility alleviates the chances of graft rejection.** The greater the identity of HLA antigens, the greater the compatibility of the graft with the recipient. Detection and identification of HLA antigens is known as **tissue typing**. Testing serum of the recipient for anti-donor antibodies is called **cross-matching** (similar to cross match procedure done for blood transfusion). HLA typing can also provide important information in parentage (determine paternity of a child in medicolegal cases), forensic and anthropologic studies.

Cell Isolation

- Lymphocytes are the preferred cell type for HLA typing, antibody screening and cross-matching. They are harvested from whole peripheral blood (**PBL**-peripheral blood lymphocytes) by buoyant density gradient separation (Ficoll-Hypaque centrifugation).
- A solution of Ficoll-Hypaque is layered underneath the whole blood, and the tube is centrifuged.
- Red blood cells being denser go to the bottom of the tube, mononuclear cells are less dense and are found in the middle layer in the tube underneath the platelets which are present in the buffy coat layer.
- The mononuclear cells are removed and washed and their volume adjusted to $2x10^6$ cells/mL. Adequate precautions to prevent contamination of the prepared suspension by platelets and red blood cells must be taken.

Tissue typing for class II HLA antigens is performed on lymphocyte preparations which have been enriched for B lymphocytes. Special isolation procedures are required for obtaining B lymphocytes as PBL are comprised of about 80% resting T lymphocytes which do not express Class II HLA antigens. The most widely used method for the isolation of B lymphocytes is the use of immunomagnetic beads coated with anti-DR antibodies for the detection of class II HLA-DR antigen. These plastic beads have a magnetic core. On application of a magnet to the side of the reaction tube, the cells expressing HLA-DR antigens are retained by the immunomagnetic beads and the unattached cells are discarded. Also, the T-cells can be removed by binding to magnetic beads coated with anti-T-cell antibodies, leaving back only the B lymphocytes. Previously, the major source of HLA typing antisera was either from sera of multiparous women, multitransfused patients or prior transplant recipients. Nowadays, monoclonal antibody technology is being used to produce tissue typing antisera. The use of serologic detection is gradually decreasing with most laboratories shifting to PCR (Polymerase Chain Reaction) for HLA typing.

1. **Serologic detection** of class I and class II molecules by the **complement-dependent lymphocyte microcytotoxicity assay**. HLA typing for the HLA-A,-B,-C,-DR,-DQ specificities is performed. HLA-DP is not usually defined by serology.
   - 1 µL of cells is added to each well of a microtiter tissue-typing plate which has predispensed panel of HLA typing sera, each containing alloantibodies to specific HLA antigens. If a certain MHC cell is present, the antibodies will bind to it, forming an antigen-antibody complex.
   - After incubation, 5µL of rabbit complement is added to each well and incubated for an hour. If an antigen-antibody complex is present, complement will be activated and will destroy the cells with an antigen-antibody complex.
   - After incubation, formalin is added to fix the cells and stop the complement reaction. A vital dye called Eosin Y is added. The live cells exclude the dye and appear bright and refractile. The dead cells take up the dye and appear dark.

- Cells are examined under a phase contrast microscope and cells that are pink are positive. Each well is scored by visual inspection and the percentage of dead cells per well is noted.
- If 50% or more of the cells are stained, they are considered positive for that HLA antigen.

2. ***Cellular detection of class II molecules:*** By **mixed leukocyte culture** (MLC). MLC test is also known as **mixed lymphocyte reaction** (MLR).When the lymphocytes of 2 HLA non-identical persons are mixed in tissue culture, the cells are stimulated. They enlarge, synthesize DNA (**transformation**) and proliferate chiefly due to differences in class II HLA antigens. On the other hand, cells from HLA-identical persons do not get stimulated and remain quiescent. This reactivity may reflect the *in vivo* process of graft rejection. The more the immunogenic differences, the greater the cellular response. The most compatible donor shows the least cellular response.
3. ***Molecular-biologic methods:*** DNA typing of HLA alleles: Variations that exist in the exact sequences of nucleotides of genomic DNA have been detected by various methods like: RFLP (Restriction Fragment Length Polymorphism), PCR (Polymerase Chain Reaction) etc. Example: more than 7 variants of HLA B27 and more than 14 variants of HLA DR 4 etc. have been sequenced. Matching for the **splits (subtypes)** of HLA antigens may be more significant for graft outcome than matching only the generic HLA antigens.

TRANSPLANTATION

Historical Background

Alexis Carrel is known as the founding father of experimental organ transplantation. In 1905, Carrel and Guthrie performed the first cardiac transplantation in animals at the University of Chicago. The work of Carrel and Charles Guthrie described in *The Transplantation of Veins and Organs* served as the foundation of vascular surgery and organ transplantation.[4]

1935—First human kidney transplant in Russia with immediate graft rejection and death of the recipient.

1950's—First successful human kidney transplant between identical twins in Boston.

1960's –First successful liver transplant in 1967 in Denver, first successful heart transplant in 1968 in South Africa.

Commonly used Terms

Transplantation: The act of moving of cells, organs, tissues from one site to another.

Graft: The transplanted organ.

Donor: Person from whom graft is taken.

Recipient (host): Person who gets the graft.

Rejection: When the recipient recognizes graft as foreign and destroys it.

Autograft/Autologous: Tissue from one site to another in the **same individual**.

Isograft/Syngenic: Between **identical** twins or same strains of mice.

Allograft/homograft/allogenic: Between genetically different individuals, but of the **same species**.

Xenograft/Heterograft: Transplant between members of **different species**.

Histocompatible: When grafts are antigenically similar to the host and do not induce rejection.

Histoincompatible: When grafts are antigenically different from host and induce rejection.

Transplantable Organs

- Kidney
- Cornea
- Skin
- Bone marrow
- Liver
- Pancreas
- Heart
- Lung
- Intestine

Types of Donors

- Deceased/Cadaveric donors
- Living donors-related or unrelated

Principles of Transplantation

- Transplantation can be classified according to either:
  a. The **genetic relationship** between the donor and recipient; or
  b. The **anatomical site** of the implantation.
- On genetic basis, grafts may be categorized as autografts, isografts, allografts and xenografts.
- Based on the site of implantation, the transplantation can be described as either **orthotopic** or **heterotopic**. Orthotopic transplantation implies donor tissue implanted in the anatomically correct position in the recipient; heterotopic transplantation refers to the placement of implant in the recipient at a site different from the normal anatomical position.
- An **immunocompetent** recipient recognizes foreign antigens on allogenic grafts and mounts an immune response against those antigens resulting in rejection. This is called **Host-versus-graft rejection**.
- In contrast to this, if an immunocompromised recipient is exposed to foreign immunocompetent donor T-cells, these T-cells recognize the tissues of the recipient as foreign and cause a life threatening inflammatory reaction called **Graft-versus-host disease** (GVHD).

Antigens which Determine Rejection of Grafts

Many antigens determine compatibility or rejection. These are:

1. **MHC antigens** are the most important and are responsible for the most vigorous allograft rejection. Early experimental research on allogenic transplantation in mice found a chromosomal region where non-identity always led to very rapid rejection of the transplanted tissue.[5] This region was termed the **MHC**.
2. **ABO antigens** are also important. These are glycosphingolipids expressed on red blood cells, endothelial cells, and many other cell types.
3. **Minor Histocompatibility antigens (Minor H Ags):** Rejection of grafts exchanged between MHC-matched individuals is ascribed to T-cell-mediated immune responses caused by incompatibility of minor histocompatibility antigens.[6] Minor H Ags are naturally processed peptide fragments derived from normal cellular proteins presented by MHC molecules.[7] They are perceived as foreign during allogeneic transplantation because of naturally occurring polymorphisms that either alter amino acid residues within a self-peptide or determine whether proteins that give rise to the minor H Ags are expressed or not.[8]

How do T Lymphocytes Recognize the Cells to be Killed?

The T lymphocytes of the recipient recognize the MHC by two different pathways. The direct pathway initiates $CD8^+$ cytotoxic T-cells by interaction of human leukocyte antigen (HLA); the indirect pathway activates $CD4^+$ helper T-cells and leads to a delayed-type hypersensitivity response, cell-mediated toxicity, and alloantibody production.

1. ***Direct pathway of recognition:*** T-cell recognizes **unprocessed** allogeneic MHC molecule on graft APCs. It is the major pathway involved in **acute *rejection***.
   a. Recipient T lymphocytes recognize donor HLA molecules on the surface of donor APCs. The initiation of graft rejection involves encounter of recipient T-cells with **donor APCs** either in the graft, or after the donor APCs have migrated to the draining lymph nodes of the recipient. Donor APCs express many class I and class II HLA molecules, and they have costimulatory molecules (B7-1 and B7-2) which are essential for T-cell activation.

b. Recipient CD8+ T lymphocytes recognize donor class I HLA molecules, and differentiate into mature CTLs which kill the donor graft cells.

c. Recipient CD4+ T lymphocytes recognize donor class II HLA molecules, and differentiate into TH1 cells. These secrete cytokines which cause proliferation and maturation of B-cells and CD 8+ T lymphocytes and also cause damage by a delayed hypersensitivity reaction (DTH).

2. ***Indirect pathway of recognition:*** T-cell recognizes **processed** peptide of allogeneic MHC molecule **bound to self MHC molecule** on **recipient APCs**. It is the major pathway involved in **chronic** rejection:

   a. Recipient APCs process graft MHC molecules and exhibit them on their own MHC molecules. These donor HLA molecules are recognized by the recipient T lymphocytes as foreign. Recipient CD4+ T lymphocytes enter the graft and recognize antigens being displayed by recipient APCs which have also entered the graft.

   b. Recipient CD4+ T lymphocytes recognize donor class II HLA molecules, and differentiate into TH1 cells which secrete cytokines leading to proliferation and maturation of B-cells and CD8+ T lymphocytes. They also cause damage by a delayed hypersensitivity reaction (DTH).

Histocompatibility Testing

It consists of three tests (**Table 15.2**):

1. Antigen typing (tissue typing)
2. Screening of the recipient for Class I and Class II HLA antibodies: The recipient serum must be tested against a panel of cells of known HLA phenotype for specific anti-HLA antibodies. The panel of cells usually contains the most frequent HLA antigens.This is termed **screening**.
3. Lymphocyte cross match (compatibility): Detection of preformed anti-donor antibodies in the recipients serum by reaction of donor cells and recipient serum.

Rejection of Allogenic Grafts

Rejection of an allograft is an adaptive immune response.[9] The genes responsible for immunologic reactions leading to graft rejection were termed **histocompatibility genes**. Peter Gorer established that the major histocompatibility locus is **antigene II**, and thus named the locus **histocompatibility II (H-2)**.[1] Further work by Jean Dausset led to the knowledge that MHC genes are required for the presentation of peptide antigens to T-cell receptors, and they play a vital role in transplantation immunology.[10] Rolf Zinkernagel and Peter Doherty stated that the role of the MHC is to signal changes in self to the immune system.[11,12]

Any two individuals, except for identical twins, will express a few HLA proteins as the HLA system is highly complex and polymorphic. Therefore, every recipient recognizes allogenic antigens and mounts an immune response against a few of these antigens present in the grafted tissue. This forms the basis of **graft rejection**. Rejection is a complex process involving several mechanisms. Example: involvement of lymphocytes, involvement of specific and increasing response etc.

First set donor tissue rejection is a primary adaptive immune response and is slow (naive). **Second set donor tissue rejection** involves memory antigen, host T and B lymphocytes and is fast (exhibits memory) especially if the graft is taken from the same donor. Thus, once a graft is rejected by a recipient, a second graft from the same donor will be rejected much more rapidly.

Stages of Graft Rejection

Sensitization Stage: When migration of donor APCs occurs from graft to draining regional

Table 15.2: Serologic and cellular methods used in histocompatibility testing. Modified from: (Basic and Clinical Immunology, 8th Edition by Daniel P. Stites, Abba I. Terr, Tristram G. Parslow)

Test	*Method*	*Time taken*	*Test type*	*Application*
Tissue typing	Complement – dependent lymphocytotoxicity	3 hours	Serologic	Identification of Class I and II HLA antigens
	MLC test	6 days	Cellular	Class II HLA antigen compatibility
Cross-matching	PBL cross-match (Allogenic)	3 hours	Serologic	Detection of preformed donor specific antibodies against separated donor T and B cells in the recipients' serum
	CML Test (Direct Cell Mediated Lympholysis)	4 hours	Cellular	Detection of anti-donor CTL
	Flow cytometry	3-4 hours	Serologic	Detection of very weak and non-cytotoxic anti-donor antibodies, (more sensitive and objective)
	Autologous cross-match for the detection of antibodies	3-4 hours	Serologic	To distinguish non-specific anti-lymphocyte antibodies from the specific anti-donor antibodies by reacting recipient sera with separated recipient T and B cells
Antibody screening	For anti-Class I HLA antibodies	3 hours × 40 cells	Serologic	Identifies antibody specificity
	For anti-Class II HLA antibody	4 hours × no. of cells+ absorption time	Serologic	Identifies antibody specificity

lymph nodes of the host, the CD4+ and CD8+ T lymphocytes of host recognize the antigens expressed on the graft as foreign.

Effector stage: The most common effector mechanisms are:

1. **Cell mediated or cellular rejection:** CD4+T lymphocytes, CD8+ T lymphocytes, NK cells, activated macrophages and delayed type of hypersensitivity are chiefly involved in this.
2. **Antibody mediated rejection or humoral rejection:** involves antibody dependent cell mediated cytotoxicity (ADCC), complement

dependent cell mediated cytotoxicity and cytokines such as IL-1 and IL-2 etc.

Clinical Types of Rejection

Rejection remains the main stumbling block to long-term survival of organ allografts. Graft rejection reactions occur at different time intervals depending on different susceptibility of individual tissues to rejection and the immune responses involved (**Table 15.3**). The types of rejection are clinically classified as:

1. **Hyperacute rejection:**
   - When recipient has preexisting antibodies, either natural as in ABO or induced (anti-HLA).
   - Occurs within minutes to hours due to immediate reaction of antibodies and complement.
   - Target is vascular endothelium of the graft leading to intravascular thrombosis and ischaemic death of the graft.
   - Preformed antibodies (usually IgG) are seen in recipients of blood transfusions, patients with previous organ transplant and multiparous women who develop antibodies against paternal HLA antigens shed by the foetus.
   - It is extremely rare these days as recipients are extensively tested for anti-HLA and anti-ABO antibodies against cells of the donor.
2. **Accelerated (Secondary or 2nd set) rejection:**
   - Almost similar to hyperacute rejection and is caused by antibodies which are formed immediately post-transplant.

Table 15.3: Different patterns of rejection

Type of rejection	*Time taken*	*Cause*	*Microscopic features*
Hyperacute	Minutes-hours	Preformed high titre anti-donor antibodies which bind to donor endothelial antigens and complement	Intravascular thrombosis, ischemic necrosis of the graft
Accelerated	Days	Reactivation of sensitized T-cells	
Acute	Days-weeks	Primary activation of T-cells	Massive infiltration of the graft by macrophages and lymphocytes, microvascular endothelialitis
Chronic	Months-years	Multitude of causes: Recurrence of disease, many minor histocompatibility antigens, cross-reactive antibodies, immune complexes etc	Progressive occlusion of vessels and fibrosis as a result of proliferation of intimal smooth muscle cells leading to progressive loss of graft function

- Transplantation of a second graft, from the same donor who donated the first graft (graft shares a significant number of antigenic determinants with the first one) results in a rapid rejection, within 2 to 5 days. This is due to presence of T lymphocytes sensitized during the 1st graft rejection.
- It is mediated by induction of CTLs, immediate production of lymphokines and activation of monocytes and macrophages.

3. Acute (Primary or 1st set) rejection:

- Follows the first grafting of a foreign transplant.
- Clinically appears at >10 days post-transplant and can occur anytime thereafter.
- It is primarily a cellular rejection mediated by T-cells.
- Massive infiltration of the graft by macrophages and lymphocytes results in decreased graft function.

4. Chronic rejection:

- Some grafts survive for a long time. Then, all of a sudden, they start to exhibit signs of rejection.
- Occurs months to years after transplant.
- Gradual, steady and progressive loss of graft function.
- Progressive occlusion of vessels.
- Occurs as a result of both cellular and humoral mechanisms.
- In spite of immunosuppression, it is difficult to prevent and difficult to treat.

Example: Allogenic bone marrow and stem cell transplantation may result in either: Hyperacute rejection (1-7 days), acute rejection (7-10 days) and/or chronic rejection (100 days – 5 years) and GVHD. Graft-versus-host disease occurs not only when there is a mismatch of a major MHC class I or class II antigen but also in the context of disparities between minor H antigens. Graft-versus-host disease is a common complication in recipients of bone marrow transplants from HLA-identical siblings, who typically differ from each other in many polymorphic proteins encoded by genes unlinked to the MHC.

GVHD: Graft-Versus-Host-Disease

GVHD is the opposite of graft rejection. It is one of the major complications of allogenic bone marrow or stem cell transplantation used for the treatment of certain leukemias, lymphomas, severe thalassemia etc. Prior to transplantation for leukemia, the recipient's bone marrow is first destroyed by aggressive cytotoxic therapy. After bone marrow transplantation, the mature donor T lymphocytes recognize the tissues of the recipient as foreign, causing a severe life threatening inflammatory reaction called GVHD characterized by maculopapular rashes on palms and soles, bullae, pruritus, increased bilirubin and increased transaminase enzyme levels, fever, malaise, pneumonitis, joint pains, diarrhoea, weight loss, abdominal pain, vomiting etc.

Essential components required for GVHD are an **immunoincompetent host**, infusion of **competent donor T-cells** and **HLA disparity** between host and donor.

Mixed Leukocyte Chimerism

- Coexistence and survival of leukocytes from both the donor and the recipient within one person.
- Chimerism can be demonstrated in all graft types.
- Mechanism of successful engraftment is ascribed to 'reciprocal clonal exhaustion, followed by peripheral clonal deletion' of lymphocytes.

Pregnancy

The fetus is an allograft which is not rejected by the mother in spite of carrying one haplotype from the father along with other foreign antigens.

Methods to Enhance Graft Survival

Till date, the most successful transplantation programs have been with kidneys and corneas. However, other organs are being transplanted with increasing frequency and success which can be attributed to a better understanding of immunological mechanisms and development of more effective immunosuppressive regimens. Example: Cyclosporin A, FK-506 (tacrolimus) etc. These above mentioned agents block T-cell proliferation and T-cell cytokine production by inhibiting activation of the NFAT transcription factor. In recipients of allogenic bone marrow transplantation for the treatment of leukemia, malignant cells must first be eradicated by aggressive therapy.

New immunosuppressive agents that have been approved include sirolimus, rapamycin, daclizumab, basiliximab, anti-CD3 monoclonal antibody, anti-IL-2 receptor antibody and antithymocyte globulin (Thymoglobulin).

At this time you should know the following:

1. Location and composition of the various classes of MHC molecules.
2. The expression, function and inheritance of MHC molecules.
3. The role of MHC in immune functions , disease and transplantation.
4. Histocompatibility testing.
5. Transplantation and rejection mechanisms.
6. GVHD.

Further Reading

1. Immunology, 5th edition by Richard A Goldsby, Thomas J Kindt, Barbara A Osborne, Janis Kuby. WH Freeman and Co., 2003. Chapter 7: Major Histocompatibility Complex (pp161-182), Chapter 21; Transplantation Immunology (pp479-498).
2. The Immune System, 2nd edition by Peter Parham, Garland Science, 2005.
3. http://users.rcn.com/jkimball.ma.ultranet/BiologyPages/H/HLA.
4. Roitt's Essential Immunology (5th edition) by Ivan M. Roitt.
5. Robbins Textbook of Pathology, 6th edition.
6. Cellular and Molecular Immunology, 6th edition by Abul K Abbas, Andrew H Lichtman and Shiv Pillai (Section II: Chapter 6), (Section V: Chapter 16).
7. Basic and Clinical Immunology, 8th edition by Daniel P Stites, Abba I.Terr, Tristram G Parslow-(Chapter 16-Histocompatibility testing by Beth W Colombe).
8. Gebe JA, Swanson E, Kwok WW. HLA class II peptide-binding and autoimmunity. Tissue Antigens.2002; 59:78-87[Pubmed].
9. Singer DS, Mozez E, Kirshner S, Kohn LD. Role of MHC class I molecules in autoimmune disease. Crit Rev Immunol 1997;17:463-468 [Pubmed].
10. Barry and Bleackly. Mechanism of T-cell mediated killing. Nat Rev Immunol 2002;2: 401-9.
11. www.anthonynolan.org.uk/HIG.
12. www.le.ac.uk/microbiology/website/Topic%204%20MHC.ppt by Dr.Colin RA Hewitt.

References

1. Gorer PA. The genetic and antigenic basis of tumour transplantation. Journal of Pathology and Bacteriology 1937;44:691-697.
2. Gebe JA, Swanson E, Kwok WW. HLA class II peptide-binding and autoimmunity. Tissue Antigens 2002; 59(2):78-87.
3. Singer DS, Mozez E, Kirshner S, Kohn LD. Role of MHC class I molecules in autoimmune disease. Crit Rev Immunol 1997;17(5-6):463-468.
4. The transplantation of veins and organs. Alexis Carrel and Charles Guthrie. American Medicine, Philadelphia, 1905.
5. Little CC, Tyzzer EE (1916). Further experimental studies on the inheritance of susceptibility to a transplantable tumor, carcinoma (JWA) of the Japanese waltzing mouse. J Med Res 33, 393-453.

6. Loveland B,E Simpson. The non-MHC transplantation antigens: Neither weak nor minor. *Immunol.* Today 1986; 7:223.
7. Wallny HJ, HG Rammensee. Identification of classical minor histocompatibility antigen as cell-derived peptide. *Nature* 1990; 343:275.
8. Roopenian DCE Simpson 2000. *Minor Histocompatibility Antigens: From the Laboratory to the Clinic 185*. Landes Bioscience, Georgetown, TX.
9. Medawar, PB (1945).The behavior and fate of skin allografts and skin homografts in rabbits. J.Anat 78,176-199.
10. Dausset J Iso-leuco-anticorps. Acta Haematologica 1959;20:156-166.
11. Zinkernagel RM (Nov 1997). "The Nobel Lectures in Immunology. Cellular Immune recognition and the biological role of major transplantation antigens". Scand J Immunol. 46(5):421-36.
12. Doherty PC (Dec 1997). "The Nobel Lectures in Immunology. Cell mediated immunity in virus infections". Scand J Immunol 46(6):527-40.

16
CHAPTER

Tolerance and Autoimmunity

(Dr. Vinay Bharat and Dr. B K Gupta anchitbharat@hotmail.com)

OBJECTIVES

1. To understand the concept and significance of tolerance.
2. To understand the factors that determine induction of tolerance.
3. To understand the mechanism of tolerance induction.
4. To discuss the concepts of autoimmunity and disease.
5. To discuss the features of major autoimmune diseases.
6. To discuss the theories on etiology of autoimmune disease.

INTRODUCTION

Tolerance refers to specific immunological non-reactivity to an antigen. The immune system has a challenging task of distinguishing foreign versus self antigens. While strong immunity against foreign antigens including pathogens is critical for preventing lethal infections, it is important that the immune system maintains tolerance against self antigens. Lack of self tolerance would lead to autoimmunity.

The mechanisms that lead to self tolerance are intriguing and can broadly be classified as "central" and "peripheral". Here, we discuss the basic mechanisms underlying induction of self-tolerance as well some common autoimmune diseases that result as a loss of self-tolerance.

Central Mechanisms

Antigen specificity of lymphocytes is a result of random recombination of gene segments coding for the variable regions of immunoglobulins in B-cells and T-cell receptors in T-cells. Following expression of these antigenic receptors on lymphocytes, the next step is evaluation of the receptor specificity and affinity. Both specificity and affinity of the antigenic receptors determines whether the lymphocyte would develop further or die without maturation.

Central tolerogenic mechanisms take place in the central lymphoid organs like the thymus and bone marrow. The B-cells undergo maturation in the bone marrow while T-cells migrate to the thymus. Following expression of antigenic receptors on cell surface, lymphocytes interact with self-antigens in the respective environment (B-cells in bone marrow stromal cells and T-cells in the thymus). Lymphocytes that bind weakly with self-antigens receive a signal that enables them to survive (positive selection). The positive selection of T-cells in the thymus is especially critical. It is noteworthy that both the nature of MHC and the MHC bound antigen (self versus foreign) determine the reactivity of T-cells. T-cells that do not react at all to self-MHC bound peptides would be functionless. Therefore, positive selection allows maturation of T-cells that would also react to foreign peptides bound to self-MHC, although the initial selecting peptides are self-derived.

In contrast, lymphocytes that bind strongly with self-antigens have autoimmune potential. Such lymphocytes undergo mechanism that lead to self-tolerance like deletion, receptor editing, or anergy (negative selection). Interestingly, while developing (immature) lymphocytes undergo inactivation by strong signals through their antigenic receptors, mature lymphocytes get activated by the same signals. Lymphocytes that escape such interactions and do not receive any signal from their antigen receptor also undergo cell death by default. The negative selection process has been widely studied in the context of thymus. The antigens that mediate negative selection are expressed abundantly on the epithelial cells of the thymus. A transcription factor called "Autoimmune Regulator (AIRE)" has been shown to be crucial for the expression of self antigens in the thymus. Loss of the AIRE gene causes the rare but severe autoimmune disorder called APECED (autoimmune polyendocrinopathy).

Peripheral Mechanisms

The immune system has unique mechanisms to prevent lymphocytes emerging into the periphery from inducing autoimmunity. Most self-antigens are expressed abundantly on the cell surface. These can undergo strong ligation with antigenic receptors on lymphocytes. Immature lymphocytes are especially sensitive to strong signals and undergo inactivation or death as a consequence of strong signals. Another important check point is the innate immune system. When a lymphocyte encounters an antigen in the absence of activation markers or co-stimulatory molecules present on the innate immune system including the antigen presenting cells, it gets inactivated or anergized.

Despite these protective mechanisms, autoimmunity can still develop. First, not all self-antigens are expressed in the central lymphoid tissues. Lymphocytes with specificities against such "sequestered" or "cryptic" self-antigens would escape the negative selection and leak out in the periphery. Cellular immunity against a foreign antigen can also spread to additional epitopes within the parent or related self proteins, so called intramolecular and intermolecular epitope spreading respectively. An inflammatory milieu can lead to the release of previously "cryptic" determinants on self-antigens and neo-antigens that may trigger autoimmunity. Furthermore, during inflammation, up-regulation of MHC and associated co-stimulatory molecules, along with resultant infiltration by new antigen presenting cells can lead to the lowering of T-cell activation threshold, thereby priming autoreactive T-cells. Therefore, the peripheral tolerance provides a backup for the prevention of autoimmunity.

Anergy: Auto-reactive T-cells when exposed to antigenic peptides (signal 1) in the absence of co-stimulatory molecules including B7-1 or B7-2 (signal 2) become anergic (nonresponsive) to the antigen. Also, B-cells when exposed to large amounts of soluble antigen down-regulate their surface IgM and become anergic. These cells also up-regulate the Fas molecules on their surface. An interaction of these B-cells with Fas-ligand bearing cells results in their death via apoptosis.

In the resting state, the antigen presenting cells constantly sample self antigens derived the host tissues. Any T lymphocytes with antigenic receptors specific for the self antigens interact with the antigen presenting cells. However, they receive only signal 1 in the form of cognate antigen but no signal 2 (co-stimulatory molecules) that are required for full activation of the T lymphocytes.

Deletion: Functionally immature cells of a clone when encounter antigen undergo a programmed cell death (apoptosis). Just like the negative selection in the central lymphoid tissues, elimination of autoreactive lymphocytes by apoptosis has also been demonstrated in the periphery (deletion). When mature lymphocytes react with autoantigens in the absence of costimulatory molecules in the periphery, they can undergo apoptosis. In addition, repeated stimulation of mature lymphocytes by self-antigens leads to a process called activation-induced cell death (AICD). Repeated activation of lymphocytes leads to upregulation of Fas and FasL. Ligation of FasL with Fas on the same of adjacent cell induce apoptosis of the lymphocytes.

Ignorance: T-cells reactive to self-antigen not represented in the thymus will mature and migrate to the periphery, but they may never encounter the appropriate antigen because it is sequestered in inaccessible tissues. Such cells may die out for lack of stimulus. Auto-reactive B-cells that escape deletion may not find the antigen or the specific T-cell help and hence not be activated and die out.

Receptor editing: B-cells which encounter large amounts of soluble antigen, as they do in the body, and bind to this antigen with very low affinity become activated to re-express their RAG1 and RAG2 genes. These genes cause them to undergo DNA (VDJ/VJ) recombination and thus change their idiotype (specificity).

Anti-idiotype antibody: Some anti-idiotype antibodies produced experimentally have been demonstrated to inhibit immune response to specific antigens. Such anti-idiotype antibodies are produced during the development of tolerance and have been demonstrated in tolerant animals. These antibodies may prevent the receptor from combining with antigen.

Cellular regulation: Recently, T cell-mediated modulation of immune system has emerged as a crucial pathway in the suppression of autoimmunity in the periphery. Gershon and Kondo coined the term "suppressor T-cells" in early 1970s. However, due to lack of specific "suppressor T cell" markers, the enthusiasm in this field subsided. Sakaguchi *et al.* in 1995 demonstrated that a subset of CD_4^+ T cells characterized by constitutive expression of CD25 (IL-2 receptor alpha chain) was critical in maintaining immunological self-tolerance in the periphery. Further studies demonstrated that "FOXP3", a transcriptional factor, is essential for the development of these CD4+CD25+ regulatory T-cells. In addition, it serves as a unique marker for these regulatory T-cells. These CD4+CD25+ FOXP3+T-cells have been shown to suppress both CD8+ and CD4+ T cells in the periphery. Other subsets of regulatory T-cells such as CD8+CD28, TCR+CD4-CD8-, NK T cells, and myeloid suppressor T-cells have also been described.

AUTOIMMUNITY

Introduction

Autoimmunity can be defined as breakdown of mechanisms responsible for self-tolerance leading to an immune response against autoantigens.

Both antibodies and lymphocytes can be involved in autoimmunity. At least 1-2% of the population is estimated to suffer from autoimmune disorders. Nevertheless, we do not know the exact etiology of most autoimmune disorders. This is because, in humans, autoimmune disorders are multifactorial and frequently the self-antigens involved in the pathogenesis are unknown.

Etiology of Autoimmunity Disease

Studies in mice and observations in humans suggest a genetic predisposition for autoimmune diseases. Association between certain HLA types and autoimmune diseases has been noted (HLA: B8, B27, DR2, DR3, DR4, DR5 etc.).

The exact etiology of autoimmune diseases is not known. However, various theories have been offered. These include sequestered antigen, escape of auto-reactive clones, loss of regulatory cells, cross-reactive antigens including exogenous antigens (pathogens) and altered self antigens (chemical and viral infections).

Sequestered antigen: Lymphoid cells may not be exposed to some self-antigens during their differentiation, because they may be late-developing antigens or may be confined to specialized organs (e.g., testes, brain, eye, etc.). A release of antigens from these organs, resulting from accidental traumatic injury or surgery, can result in the stimulation of an immune response and initiation of an autoimmune disease.

Escape of auto-reactive clones: The negative selection in the thymus may not be fully functional to eliminate self reactive cells. Not all self antigens may be represented in the thymus or certain antigens may not be properly processed and presented.

Cross-reactive antigens: Antigens on certain pathogens may have determinants which cross-react with self antigens and an immune response against these determinants may lead to effector cells or antibodies against tissue antigens. Post streptococcal nephritis and carditis, anticardiolipin antibodies during syphilis and association between Klebsiella and ankylosing spondylitis are examples of such cross-reactivity.

Diagnosis

Diagnosis of autoimmune diseases is based on symptoms and detection of antibodies (and/or very rarely T-cells) reactive against antigens of tissues and cells involved. Antibodies against cell/tissue-associated antigens are detected by immunofluorescence. Antibodies against soluble antigens are normally detected by ELISA or radioimmunoassay (see table above). In some cases, a biological/biochemical assay may be used (e.g., Graves' diseases, pernicious anemia).

Treatment

Anti-inflammatory (corticosteroid) and immunosuppressive drug therapy is the present method of treating autoimmune diseases. Immunosuppressive drugs include cycophosphamide (Cytoxan) and cyclosporine (Neoral and Sandimmune). Future treatments may include more sophisticated methods based on modern understanding of the immune system (e.g., anti-idiotype antibodies, antigen peptides, anti-IL2 receptor antibodies, anti-CD4 antibodies, anti-TCR antibodies, etc.).

General Classification

Autoimmune diseases are generally classified on the basis of the organ or tissue involved. These diseases may fall in an organ-specific category in which the immune response is directed against antigen(s) associated within a target organ or a systemic category in many tissues of the body are affected. Some of the common organ-specific and systemic autoimmune diseases are presented in **Table 16.1**.

At this time you should know the following:

1. Possible mechanisms of tolerance induction to self.
2. Role of antigen and host components in tolerance induction.
3. Different autoimmune diseases and organs/antigens involved in these conditions.
4. Type of immunologic tests normally used to diagnose different autoimmune diseases.
5. Possible etiology of autoimmune diseases and the major experimental models.

Table 16.1: Common autoimmune disorders

A. ORGAN SPECIFIC

Disease	***Target organ***	***Etiology (Antibodies against)***
Hashimoto's thyroiditis	Thyroid	Thyroglobulin, thyroid peroxidase
Primary myxedema	Thyroid	Cytoplasmic
Graves' disease	Thyroid	TSH receptor
Pernicious anemia	Red cells	Intrinsic factor (IF), Gastric parietal cell
Addison's disease	Adrenal	Adrenal cells
Insulin dependent juvenile diabetes	Pancreas	Pancreatic islet β cells
Myasthenia Graves	Muscle	Muscle, acetyl choline receptor
Goodpasture's syndrome	Kidney, lung	Renal and lung basement membrane
Pemphigus	Skin	Desmosomes
Pemphigoid	Skin	Skin basement membrane
Vitiligo	Skin	Melanocytes
Phacogenic uveitis	Lens	Lens protein
Autoimmune hemolytic anemia	Red cells	Red cells
Idiopathic thrombocytopenic purpura	Platelets	Platelets
Primary biliary cirrhosis	Liver	Mitochondria

B. SYSTEMIC

Disease	***Target***
Systemic lupus erythematosus	Skin, kidney, joints, etc.
Ankylosing spondylitis	Vertebrae
Rheumatoid arthritis	Connective tissue
Multiple sclerosis	White matter (Brain)
Scleroderma	Neclei, heart, lung, GIT, kidney,
Sjögren's syndrome	Salivary gland, liver, kidney, thyroid

Further Reading

1. Roitt's Essential Immunology: Delves, Martin, Burton and Roitt.
2. Cellular and Molecular Immunology: Abbas, Lichtman, Pillai.
3. Janeway's Immunobiology: Murphy, Travers, Walport.

17

CHAPTER

Hypersensitivity Reactions

(Dr. S C Parija subhashparija@yahoo.co.in)

OBJECTIVES

1. To understand the hypersensitivity reactions and their classification.
2. To know the diseases associated with hypersensitivity reactions.
3. To understand the mechanisms of damage in hypersensitivity reactions.
4. To know the methods for diagnosing conditions due to hypersensitivity.
5. To know the modes of treating disease due to hypersensitivity and their rationale.

INTRODUCTION

Immune responses are usually protective. They generally trigger a number of effector molecules which eliminate the antigen through local inflammatory reactions without damaging the host's tissue. Sometimes, the immune responses may cause tissue injury and disease in a host. Such dysregulated responses result in hypersensitivity. The immune system capable of causing tissue injury and disease in a host through an inappropriate response was recognized in the early 20th century by Paul Portier and Charles Richet.

The term 'Hypersensitivity' refers to the injurious consequences in the sensitized host, following contact with specific antigens. In the protective processes of immunity, the focus of attention is the antigen whereas; hypersensitivity is an exaggerated form of immunity resulting in tissue damage.

Classification

Traditional classification systems divided hypersensitivity reactions into immediate or delayed type, depending on the time required by the sensitized host to develop clinical manifestations on contact with the antigen.

Immediate hypersensitivity reactions are B cell or antibody mediated. These show clinical symptoms within minutes or hours of contact with the antigen. Anaphylactic reactions, atopy, antibody mediated cell damage, arthus phenomenon and serum sickness are the various immediate hypersensitivity reactions.

Delayed hypersensitivity reactions are T cell mediated reactions which appear days after contact with the antigen, usually through intradermal contact. Typical examples are contact dermatitis and tuberculin reactions.

P.G.H. Gell and R.R.A. Coombs (1963) divided hypersensitivity reactions into four types: type I, type II, type III and type IV, based on the mechanisms involved and time taken for the reaction. Although this classification has helped to identify differences in pathogenic immune mechanisms and the tissue damage characteristics in various hypersensitivity reactions, it may be remembered that a particular clinical condition may often involve a complex interplay of all these four categories. Various immune mechanisms and pathologic lesions in different types of hypersensitivity reactions are summarized in the **Table 17.1.**

Table 17.1: Mechanisms and pathologic lesions in different types of hypersensitivity reactions

Type	*Disorder*	*Immune mechanisms*	*Pathologic lesions*
Type I—IgE mediated hypersensitivity	Localized anaphylaxis like eczema; systemic anaphylaxis like bronchial asthma, food allergy	Production of IgE antibody→ Ag induces cross-linking of IgE bound to mast cells and basophils with release of vasoactive amines and other mediators; recruitment of inflammatory cells (late-phase reaction)	Vascular dilatation, edema, smooth muscle contraction, mucus production, inflammation
Type II—Antibody mediated cytotoxic hypersensitivity	Autoimmune hemolytic anemia; Goodpasture's syndrome	Production of IgG, IgM → binds to antigen on target cell or tissue→ Phagocytosis or lysis of target cell by activated complement or Fc receptors; recruitment of leukocytes	Cell lysis; inflammation
Type III—Immune complex mediated hypersensitivity	Systemic lupus erythematosus; some forms of glomerulonephritis; serum sickness; Arthus reaction	Deposition of antigen antibody complexes→ complement activation→ recruitment of leukocytes by complement products and Fc receptors →release of enzymes and other toxic molecules	Necrotizing vasculitis (fibrinoid necrosis), inflammation
Type IV—Cell mediated hypersensitivity	Contact dermatitis; multiple sclerosis; type I diabetes, transplant rejection, tuberculin test	Activated T lymphocytes→ i. Release of cytokines and macrophage activation; ii. T cell mediated cytotoxicity	Perivascular cellular infiltrates; edema, cell destruction, granuloma formation

Type I Hypersensitivity (IgE dependent) Reaction

Type I (immediate) hypersensitivity is a rapid and IgE antibody-mast cell mediated reaction that occurs in a person sensitized earlier with the antigen and on re-exposure to the same antigen. These antigens which induce immediate type I hypersensitivity reactions are also known as allergens. These common allergens are listed in the **Table 17.2**.

It may range from minor urticarial rash, conjunctivitis, and rhinorrhea to life-threatening anaphylaxis with respiratory distress secondary to bronchospasm and hemodynamic instability.

Anaphylaxis

It is an IgE mediated reaction and occurs due to the action of histamine and other vaso active amines. Sensitization with the antigen occurs in the initial exposure. Though it occurs more effectively when introduced parenterally, introduction through any route can cause sensitization. An interval of 2-3 weeks is seen between the sensitizing and shocking dose. The shocking antigen should be similar or show immunological correlation with the sensitizing antigen.

Mechanism of Anaphylaxis

Immediate hypersensitivity is mediated by IgE. The primary cellular component in this hypersensitivity is mast cell or basophil. The reaction is amplified and/or modified by platelets, neutrophils and eosinophils.

Type I reaction involves production of IgE in response to the concerned antigen (allergens). IgE has high affinity for receptor on mast cells and basophils. A subsequent exposure to the same allergen cross links the cell-bound IgE and triggers the release of various pharmacologically active substances. Importantly, mast cell degranulation is preceded by increased Ca^{++} influx. Substances which increase cytoplasmic Ca^{++} promote degranulation, whereas agents that deplete cytoplasmic Ca^{++} suppress degranulation.

The pre-formed mast cell mediators includes histamines and tetrapeptides. These cause a rapid increase in vascular permeability, smooth muscle contraction that lead to most of the manifestations observed during anaphylaxis such as stridor, bronchospasm, vasodilation, vasogenic edema and hypotension. The reaction is amplified by (PAF) which causes platelet aggregation and release of histamine, heparin and vasoactive amines. The mast cell mediators that are subsequently produced, like leukotrienes and prostaglandins also lead to the recruitment of inflammatory cells including neutrophils-over several hours. The latter is called the late phase reaction.

Table 17.2: Common allergens associated with type I hypersensitivity

Proteins	***Foods***	***Insects***	***Drugs***
1. Foreign serum	1. Nuts	1. Bee venom	1. Penicillin
2. Vaccines	2. Seafood	2. Wasp venom	2. Sulfonamides
	3. Egg	3. Ant venom	3. Local anaesthetics
Pollens	4. Peas, beans	4. Cockroach calyx	4. Salicylates
1. Rye grass	5. Milk	5. Dust mites	
2. Ragweed			**Others**
3. Timothy grass			1. Mold spores
4. Birch trees			2. Animal hair

Eosinophil chemotactic factor of anaphylaxis (ECF-A) and neutrophil chemotactic factors are two factors that mediate the late phase reaction. Cyclic nucleotides appear to play a significant role in the modulation of immediate hypersensitivity reaction, although their exact function is ill understood. Substances which alter cAMP and cGMP levels significantly alter the allergic symptoms. Thus, substances that increase intracellular cAMP seem to relieve allergic symptoms, particularly bronchopulmonary ones, and are used therapeutically. Conversely, agents that decrease cAMP or stimulate cGMP aggravate these allergic conditions. Relationship between allergic symptoms and cyclic-nucleotides is summarized in **Table 17.3.**

Mast cells may also be triggered by other stimuli such as exercise, emotional stress, chemicals (e.g., photographic developing medium, calcium ionophores, codeine, etc.), anaphylatoxins (e.g., C4a, C3a, C5a, etc.). These reactions mediated by agents without IgE-allergen interaction are not hypersensitivity reactions, although they produce the same symptoms.

Cutaneous anaphylaxis: It is a localized hypersensitivity reaction that manifests in the form of a wheal and flare. It occurs in sensitized individuals when, an antigen is injected into the skin to which a person is sensitive. The wheal and flare response forms the basis of the skin test which is used to determine the sensitivity of the person to various allergens.

Prausnitz-Kustner Reaction

Prausnitz and Kustner demonstrated the transmission of IgE mediated hypersensitivity by injecting serum from an allergic person containing IgE antibodies into a nonallergic individual. In an experiment that they carried out on themselves, Kustner's serum, which was allergic to certain species of cooked fish, was injected into Prausnitz who was not hypersensitive to the same. This was followed 24 hours later by intracutaneous injection of cooked fish to which Kustner was sensitive into Prausnitz. A wheal and flare was seen within 20 minutes in Prausnitz, thereby showing the transmission of hyper sensitivity to cooked fish from Kustner to Prausnitz.

Atopy

Hereditary human allergic states which develop after re-exposure of allergen is called atopy. There are evidence of HLA (A2) association with atopy. Examples include hay fever, allergic asthma and atopic dermatitis.

Diagnostic tests for immediate hypersensitivity include skin (prick and intradermal) tests, measurement of total IgE and specific IgE antibodies against the suspected allergens. Total

Table 17.3: Relationship between allergic symptoms and cyclic-nucleotides

Lowering of cyclic-AMP	*Elevation of cyclic-AMP*
Stimulation of α-adrenergic receptor (nor-epinephrine, phenyl-epinephrine) Or Blocking of β-adrenergic receptor (propranolol)	Stimulation of β-adrenergic receptor (epinephrine, isoproterenol) Blocking of α-adrenergic receptor (phenoxybenzamine) Inhibition of phosphodiesterase (theophylline) Binding of histamine-2 or PGE to their receptors
Elevation of cyclic-GMP	
Stimulation of γ-cholinergic receptor (acetylcholine, carbachol)	
WORSENING OF SYMPTOMS	**IMPROVEMENT OF SYMPTOMS**

IgE and specific IgE antibodies are measured by a modification of enzyme immunoassay (ELISA). Increased IgE levels are indicative of atopic condition, although IgE may be elevated in some nonatopic diseases (e.g., myelomas, helminthic infection, etc.).

Symptomatic treatment is achieved with antihistamines which block histamine receptors. Chromolyn sodium inhibits mast cell degranulation, probably, by inhibiting Ca^{++} influx. Late onset allergic symptoms, particularly bronchoconstriction which is mediated by leukotrienes, are treated with leukotriene receptor blockers (Singulair, Accolate) or inhibitors of cyclooxygenase pathway (Zilentoin). Symptomatic, although shortterm relief from bronchoconstriction is provided by bronchodilators (inhalants) such as isoproterenol derivatives (Terbutaline, Albuterol). Theophylline which elevates cAMP by inhibiting cAMP-phosphodiesterase and inhibits intracellular Ca^{++} release is also used to relieve bronchopulmonary symptoms.

Hyposensitization (desensitization) is another treatment modality which is successful in a number of allergies, particularly against insect venoms and pollen dust. The mechanism is unclear but there is a correlation between appearance of IgG (blocking) antibodies and relief of symptoms.

Type II Hypersensitivity Reaction

These reactions involve antibody mediated cell destruction. It is also known as 'cytotoxic hypersensitivity' and may affect a variety of organs and tissues. The antigens are normally endogenous, although exogenous chemicals (haptens) which can attach to cell membranes can also cause type II hypersensitivity reaction. Drug-induced hemolytic anemia, granulocytopenia and thrombocytopenia are such examples. The reaction time is minutes to hours.

Following two mechanisms are responsible for type II hypersensitivity reactions:

1. *Complement mediated cytotoxicity:* Complements are activated following binding of antibodies to the cell membrane. The classical pathway is activated which lyses the cell through membrane attack complex (MAC). Activation of the complement cascade leads to formation of C3a and C5a fragments, which are chemotactic for phagocytes. Thus the phagocytic response ensues.
2. *Antibody dependent cell mediated cytotoxicity (ADDC):* In this mechanism Fc portion of IgG and IgM interact with the Fc receptor on NK cells leading to lysis of target cells. This lysis does not involve phagocytes or complements.

Combination with antibodies may sometimes cause stimulation as seen in long acting thyroid stimulator (LATS). Such a reaction is often called type V Hypersensitivity reaction. Target antigen, mechanism of disease and clinic-pathological conditions of type II hypersensitivity reactions are listed in **Table 17.4**.

Diagnostic tests include detection of circulating antibody against tissue antigens involved and the presence of antibody and complement in the lesion by immuno-fluorescence. The staining pattern is normally smooth and linear such as that seen in Goodpasteur's nephritis involving renal and lung basement membrane; and pemphigus vulgaris involving skin intercellular protein, desmosome.

Treatment consists of anti-inflammatory and immunosuppressive drugs.

Type III Hypersensitivity Reaction

This condition is also known as 'immune complex hypersensitivity'. This reaction is mediated by the formation of soluble immune complexes and subsequent activation of complement. Under normal circumstances, the combination of an antibody with an antigen leads to the formation of immune complexes

Table 17.4: Target antigen, mechanism of disease and clinic-pathological conditions of type II hypersensitivity reactions

Disease	*Target antigen*	*Mechanism of disease*	*Clinico-pathologic manifestations*
Autoimmune hemolytic anemia	Erythocyte membrane proteins (Rh blood group antigens, I antigen	Opsonization and phagocytosis of erythrocytes	Hemolysis, anemia
Autoimmune thrombocytopenic purpura	Platelet membrane proteins (gpllb:IIIa integrin)	Opsonization and phagocytosis of platelets	Bleeding
Pemphigus vulgaris	Proteins in intercellular junctions of epidermal cells (epidermal cadherin)	Antibody-mediated activation of protease, disruption of intracellular adhesions	Skin vesicles (bullae)
Vasculitis caused by ANCA	Neutrophil granule proteins, presumably released from activated neutrophils	Neutrophil degranulation and inflammation	Vasculitis
Goodpasture's syndrome	Noncollagenous protein in basement membranes of kidney glomeruli and lung alveoli	Complement and Fc receptors mediated inflammation	Nephritis, lung hemorrhage
Acute rheumatic fever	Streptococcal cell wall antigen, antibody cross-reacts with myocardial antigen	Inflammation, macrophage activation	Myocarditis, arthritis
Myasthenia gravis	Acetylcholine receptor	Antibody inhibits acetylcholine binding, down-modulates receptors	Muscle weakness, paralysis
Graves' disease (hyperthyroidism)	TSH receptors	Antibody-mediated stimulation of TSH receptor	Hyperthyroidism
Insulin-resistant diabetes	Insulin receptor	Antibody inhibits binding of insulin	Hyperglycemia, ketoacidosis
Pernicious anemia	Intrinsic factors of gastric parietal cells	Neutralization of intrinsic factors, decreased absorption of Vitamin B_{12}	Abnormal erthropoiesis, anemia

which facilitate the clearing of antigen by phagocytic cells. Large complexes can be cleared by macrophages but they have difficulty in binding to small immune complexes for clearance. These immune complexes insert themselves into small blood vessels, joints and glomeruli; causing symptoms.The severity of the reaction is determined by the amount and distribution of immune complexes formed, as well as the ratio of antigen to antibody. Mild local type III reactions occur at the site of injection if the complex components are in equivalence or slight excess e.g. Arthus reactions. When the antigen is in excess, large number of soluble complexes are formed which can circulate causing serum sickness or get deposited in different organs.

Arthus Reaction

It is a localised type III hypersensitivity reaction. This reaction is called 'Arthus reaction' because, Arthus who observed an intense local reaction of edema, hemorrhagic necrosis and induration in rabbits who were injected repeatedly by normal horse serum subcutaneously first observed the reaction. The reaction never occurred with the initial doses but latter injections led to this reaction. The lesion primarily contains neutrophils and deposits of immune complexes and complement. Macrophages infiltrating in later stages may be involved in the healing process.

Serum Sickness

It is a systemic form of type III hypersensitivity reaction. This reaction develops in individuals who have received a high dose of antigen as seen in administration of horse antitoxin against tetanus, diphtheria etc. The clinical features develop 7-12 days later with fever, lymphadenopathy, splenomegaly, arthritis, glomerulonephritis, endocarditis, vasculitis, urticarial rash, abdominal pain, nausea etc. These features are a result of systemic soluble complexes, which get deposited in various organs of the body like skin, joints, kidney and heart. These complexes can fix complement leading to tissue damage and inflammation. The symptoms resolve in a week once the immune complexes are removed from the circulation.

The lesion contains primarily neutrophils and deposits of immune complexes and complement. Macrophages infiltrating in later stages may be involved in the healing process. The affinity of antibody and size of immune complexes are important in production of disease and determining the tissue involved. Diagnosis involves examination of tissue biopsies for deposits of immunoglobulin and complement by immunofluorescence. The immunofluorescent staining in type III hypersensitivity is granular (as opposed to linear in type II: Goodpasture). Presence of immune complexes in serum and depletion in complement level are also diagnostic. Polyethylene glycol mediated turbidity (nephelometry), binding of C1q and Raji cell test are utilized to detect immune complexes. Treatment includes anti-inflammatory agents.

Target antigen, disease and clinic-pathological conditions of type III hypersensitivity reactions are listed in the **Table 17.5**.

Type IV Hypersensitivity Reaction

It is also known as 'cell mediated or delayed type hypersensitivity'. The reaction is brought about by sensitized T lymphocytes and macrophages. The classical example of this hypersensitivity is tuberculin (Mantoux) reaction, which peaks 48 hours after the injection of antigen (PPD or old tuberculin). The lesion is characterized by induration and erythema.

Type IV hypersensitivity is involved in the pathogenesis of many autoimmune and infectious diseases (tuberculosis, leprosy, blastomycosis, histoplasmosis, toxoplasmosis, leishmaniasis, etc.) and granuloma due to infections and foreign antigens. Another form of

Table 17.5: Target antigen, mechanism of disease and clinic-pathological conditions of type III hypersensitivity reactions		
Disease	***Antigen involved***	***Clinicopathologic manifestations***
Systemic lupus erythematous	DNA, nucleoproteins, others	Nephritis, arthritis, vasculitis
Polyarteritis nodosa	Hepatitis B virus surface antigen (in some causes)	Vasculitis
Poststreptococcal glomerulonephritis	Streptococcal cell wall antigen(s); may be "planted" in glomerular basement membrane	Nephritis
Acute glomerulonephritis	Bacterial antigens (*Treponema*); parasite antigens (malaria parasites, schistosomes); tumor antigens	Nephritis
Reactive arthritis	Bacterial antigens (*Yersinia*)	Acute arthritis
Arthus reaction	Various foreign proteins	Cutaneous vasculitis
Serum sickness	Various proteins, e.g., foreign serum (anti-thymocyte globulin)	Arthritis, vasculitis nephritis

delayed hypersensitivity is contact dermatitis (poison ivy, chemicals, heavy metals, etc.) in which the lesions are more papular. Type IV hypersensitivity can be classified into three categories depending on the time of onset and clinical and histological presentation as described in **Table 17.6**.

Mechanisms of damage in delayed hypersensitivity include T lymphocytes and monocytes and/or macrophages. Cytotoxic T cells (Tc) cause direct damage whereas helper T (T_H1) cells secrete cytokines, which activate cytotoxic T cells and recruit and activate monocytes and macrophages, which cause the bulk of the damage. The delayed hypersensitivity lesions mainly contain monocytes and a few T cells. Major lymphokines involved in delayed hypersensitivity reaction include monocyte chemotactic factor, interleukin-2, interferon-γ, TNF α/β etc.

Table 17.6: Delayed hypersensitivity reactions				
Type	***Reaction time***	***Clinical appearance***	***Histology***	***Antigen and site***
Contact dermatitis	48-72 hr	Eczema	Lymphocytes, followed by macrophages; edema of epidermis	Epidermal (organic chemicals, poison ivy, heavy metals)
Tuberculin reaction	48-72 hr	Local induration	Lymphocytes, monocytes, macrophages	Intradermal tuber-(culin, lepromin tests)
Granuloma	21-28 days	Hardening	Macrophages, epitheloid and giant cells, fibrosis	Persistent antigen or foreign body presence (tuberculosis, leprosy)

Intracellular pathogens and contact antigens that induce type IV hypersensitivity reaction are listed in the **Table 17.7**. Diseases associated with type IV hypersensitivity reactions are summarized in the **Table 17.8**.

Diagnostic tests *in vivo* include delayed cutaneous reaction (e.g., Mantoux test) and patch test (for contact dermatitis).

In vitro tests for delayed hypersensitivity include mitogenic response, lymphocytotoxicity and IL-2 production. Corticosteroids and other immunosuppressive agents are used in treatment.

Table 17.9 compares different types of hypersensitivity reactions.

At this time you should know the following:

1. Distinctions between different types of hypersensitivity.
2. Mechanisms of immune-mediated damages.
3. Examples of different types of hypersensitivity and overlap amongst them.
4. Diagnostic test for hypersensitivity diseases and treatments.

Table 17.7: Intracellular pathogens and contact antigens that induce type IV hypersensitivity

Intracellular bacteria	*Intracellular viruses*	*Intracellular fungi*	*Intracellular parasite*	*Contact antigens*
1. *Mycobacterium tuberculosis*	1. Herpes simplex	1. *Pneumocystis jiroveci*	1. *Leishmania spp*	1. Picryl chloride
2. *Mycobacterium leprae*	2. Variola	2. *Candida albicans*		2. Hair dyes
3. *Listeria monocytogenes*	3. Measles	3. *Histoplasma capsulatum*		3. Nickel salts
4. *Brucella abortus*		4. *Cryptococcus neoformans*		4. Poison ivy 5. Poison oak

Table 17.8: Diseases with type IV hypersensitivity reaction

Disease	*Target antigen*	*Effects*
Diabetes mellitus type 1	Pancreatic beta cell proteins (possibly insulin, Glutamate decarboxylase)	• Insulitis • Beta cell destruction
Multiple sclerosis	Oligodendrocyte proteins (myelin basic protein, proteolipid protein)	• Demyelinating disease • Perivascular inflammation • Paralysis • Ocular lesions
Crohn's disease	Unknown	• Chronic inflammation of ileum and colon
Some peripheral neuropathies	Schwann cell antigen	• Neuritis • Paralysis

Table 17.9: Comparison of different types of hypersensitivity reactions

Characteristics	*Type-I (anaphylactic)*	*Type-II (cytotoxic)*	*Type-III (immune complex)*	*Type-IV (delayed type)*
Antibody	IgE	IgG, IgM	IgG, IgM	None
Antigen	Exogenous	Cell surface	Soluble	Tissues and organs
Response time	15-30 minutes	Minutes-hours	3-8 hours	48-72 hours
Appearance	Wheal and flare	Lysis and necrosis	Erythema and edema, necrosis	Erythema and induration
Histology	Basophils and eosinophil	Antibody and complement	Complement and neutrophils	Monocytes and lymphocytes
Transferred with	Antibody	Antibody	Antibody	T-cells
Examples	Allergic asthma, hay fever	Erythroblastosis fetalis, Goodpasture's nephritis	SLE, farmer's lung disease	Tuberculin test, poison ivy, granuloma

Further Reading

1. Cohen DE, Brancaccio RR, Soter NA. Diagnostic tests for type IV or delayed hypersensitivity reactions. *Clin Allergy Immunol* 2000;15:287-305.
2. Fadal RG. IgE-mediated hypersensitivity reactions. *Otolaryngol Head Neck Surg.* 1993 Sep;109(3 Pt 2):565-78.
3. Parija SC. Hypersensitivity. In: Textbook of Microbiology and Immunology. New Delhi, 2009:155-161.
4. Rajan TV. The Gell–Coombs classification of hypersensitivity reactions: A re-interpretation. *Trends in Immunology,* Volume 24, Issue 7, July 2003, 376-379.
5. Thomas K, Barbara O, Richard G. Hypersensitive Reactions. Kuby Immunology. London: W H Freeman 2011: 361-388.
6. Virella G. Hypersensitivity reactions. *Immunol Ser* 1993;58:329-41.
7. Virella G. Hypersensitivity reactions. In: Gabriel Virella, editor. Medical Immunology, New York: Marcel Dekker 2001: 397-410.
8. Weiss RB. Hypersensitivity reactions. *Semin Oncol* 1992 Oct;19(5):458-77.

18

CHAPTER

Immune System and Tumor Immunology

(Dr. Najmul Islam and Dr. Jawed Iqbal nxi7@hotmail.com)

OBJECTIVES

To discuss tumor immunology in following heads:

1. Introduction.
2. Relationship between antigen recognition and immune system.
3. Antibodies.
4. Cytotoxic and helper T-cells.
5. Tumors are immunogenic.
6. Tumor antigens.
7. Immunity and tumor growth.
8. Immunotherapeutic strategies.
9. Tumor immunoediting.

IMMUNE SYSTEM–DEFENSE SYSTEM OF HUMANS

Introduction

The discipline of immunology grew out from the observation that individuals who had recovered from certain infectious diseases were thereafter protected from that disease. The term 'immunity' has been derived from the Latin word "immunis"—thereby meaning exempt. Thus, immunity means the state of protection or exemption from infectious diseases. It may be worth mentioning that the phenomena of immunity can be traced back to 430 B.C. where it is reported that only those individuals who had recovered from plague can nurse the sick ones, as they would not contract the disease a second time. However, it took around more than 2000 years to understand the concept of immunity and in turn, utilize it successfully into a medically effective practice.

A vast network of molecules and cells comprise the immune system, having a single goal – to distinguish between self and non-self. The primary function of the immune system is to provide protection to the host against microorganisms like viruses, bacteria and parasites. The beauty of immune system lies in the fact that it possesses a remarkable property of having the ability to scan continuously countless number of molecular units, and in turn, instantly recognizes and consequently initiates the destruction of foreign molecules.

Functionally, an immune response is a two type of sequentially related activities. They are:

a. Immune recognition; and
b. Immune response: Immune recognition is a phenomenon that possesses a remarkable property of specificity i.e. the immune system possesses the quality to recognize even subtle chemical differences that distinguishes one pathogen from the other. Thus, only after accurate recognition, an immune response is elicited, which is of two types–an effector immune response and memory immune response.

Once the foreign molecules or pathogens are recognized by the immune system, then immediately, the immune system prepares a list of molecules and cells that will participate in eliminating or neutralizing the foreign molecule. Such a phenomenon is known as effector immune response. It is the first step in pathogen elimination. In this way, the system is able to convert the initial recognition event into different effector responses, which in turn, are essential for elimination of foreign molecules.

After encountering effector response, the later exposure of host to the same foreign organism results in the induction of memory immune response, which is characterized by a rapid and intense response that serves to eliminate the foreign organism and prevent the host from disease.

Immunity can be natural or artificial, innate or acquired—adaptive, and either active or passive.

- Active natural (contact with infection): Develops slowly, is long term, and antigen specific.
- Active artificial (immunization): Develops slowly, lasts for several years, and is specific to the antigen for which the immunization was given.
- Passive natural (transplacental—mother to child): Develops immediately, is temporary, and affects all antigens to which the mother has immunity.
- Passive artificial (injection of gamma globulin): Develops immediately, is temporary, and affects all antigens to which the donor has immunity.

TUMOR IMMUNOLOGY

The immune system has three primary roles in the prevention of tumors. First, the immune system can protect the host from virus-induced tumors by eliminating or suppressing viral infections. Second, the timely elimination of pathogens and prompt resolution of inflammation can prevent the establishment of an inflammatory environment conducive to tumorigenesis. Third, the immune system can specifically identify and eliminate tumor cells on the basis of their expression of tumor-specific antigens or molecules induced by cellular stress. A wide spectrum of lines of evidences argue for a pivotal role of the immune system in endogenous defense against tumor cells in a process termed *"immune surveillance"*.

The first line of defense against both microbes as well as tumor cells is constituted by the so called non-specific or innate immune system, which comprises granulocytes, macrophages and natural killer (NK) cells as its effector cells. With respect to immune surveillance against tumors, the key role in recognition and elimination of newly arising cancer cells, is played by macrophages and NK-cells. Whereas the direct antitumor activity of NK-cells is restricted to certain types of tumor cells, activated macrophages are able to specifically recognize and selectively destroy a wide spectrum of different tumor cell types in a still quite incompletely understood reaction termed Macrophage-mediated Tumor Cytotoxicity (MTC). In addition, these cells, together with the so called dendritic cells, via the process of antigen presentation, serve as a crucial link between innate and acquired immunity, the second part of our immune system, which is constituted by antigen-specific T and B lymphocytes. In fact, it has become clear only recently, that macrophages and dendritic cells actually control the induction of specific, T-lymphocyte-mediated immune responses and thus also govern specific immunity against tumor antigens, which is essential for final, long term eradication of tumor cells in the body.

Yet, despite these immune defense mechanisms against tumor cells and despite their principal antigenicity many tumors grow progressively and spread through the body apparently more or less unrestricted by the immune system, eventually resulting in death of the host. This is due to the suppression of immune functions exerted by the tumor, again primarily involving the control of macrophage activity both at the step of tumor cytotoxicity as well as antigen presentation, finally leading to specific immunological tolerance for the tumor cells and tumor progression.

Given this central role of macrophages both in endogenous tumor defense and tumor progression, the main focus of various research projects is the further elucidation of the molecular and cellular mechanisms involved in MTC and their consequences for induction of specific antitumor immune responses as well as the biological signal circuits controlling these reactions, as a prerequisite for therapeutical application and manipulation of these mechanisms in the treatment of human cancer.

Malignant tumors develop by stepwise accumulation of genetic defects. This process of malignant transformation includes inactivation of genes that negatively regulate growth (tumor suppression genes) and activation of genes that promote cell growth and independent proliferation (oncogenes). A cell can replicate endless and grow without control, only when a threshold of genetic defects has been reached–independent of regulatory processes. These events happen through structural changes, such as deletions, mutations, or amplification of DNA leading to destruction or copying of critical genes, or by changes in gene regulation, such as methylation. Hereby, the expression of the affected gene is changed quantitatively.

Relationship between Antigen Recognition and Immune System

Immunotherapy for cancer is essentially the stimulation of the immune system via a variety of reagents such as vaccines, infusion of T-cells, or cytokines. These reagents act through one of several mechanisms:

1. By stimulating the antitumor response, either by increasing the number of effector cells or by producing one or more soluble mediators such as lymphokines;
2. By decreasing suppressor mechanisms;
3. By altering tumor cells to increase their immunogenicity and make them more susceptible to immunologic defenses; and
4. By improving tolerance to cytotoxic drugs or radiotherapy, such as stimulating bone marrow function with granulocyte colony-stimulating factor (G-CSF).

The basic premise of immunotherapy for cancer, then, is to stimulate the immune system in some way to treat and even prevent cancer. Historical data show that the immune system clearly plays a role in cancer progression. For example, immunosuppression is associated with cancer development. In fact, cancer is 100 times more likely to occur in people who take immunosuppressive medications (e.g., for organ transplant or rheumatic disease) than in people with normal immune function.

Lymphoma, skin, and cervical cancer are just a few types of cancer that have been associated with immunosuppression. Patients who have undergone renal transplantation have an estimated 3 to 5 times higher overall incidence of malignancy in long-term follow-up than in the general population, and this is felt to be due in part to long-term immunosuppression. Conversely, heightened antitumor activity of the immune system has been suggested in the many reports of spontaneous cancer regression.

Antibodies

Antibodies have been the focus of research in the past 20 years or so, as researchers discovered that antibodies recognize and respond to antigens produced by cancer cells. Antibodies are types of protein made by certain white blood cells—B-cells—in response to a foreign substance. Each antibody binds to a specific antigen. The more specific the antibody, the greater the strength of the antibody-antigen bond. All antibodies are composed of light and heavy polypeptide chains. The number of chains may vary considerably, but at a minimum there are two of each type. Every heavy chain is paralleled by a light chain at one of its ends.

Fc receptors on the heavy chain regions confer antibody function.

Antibodies protect the body against invading agents in one of two ways:

1. By direct attack on the invader; and
2. By activation of the complement system, which has multiple means of destroying invading cells. Direct attack is accomplished by agglutination, precipitation, neutralization, or lysis. Agglutination involves binding in a clump multiple large particles with antigens on their surfaces (e.g., bacteria or red blood cells). The antigen-antibody bonding can also create a molecular complex so large that it is rendered insoluble, and precipitates (e.g., tetanus toxin). Neutralization occurs when the antibodies simply cover the toxic sites of the antigen. Lysis involves very potent antibodies capable of directly attacking cell membranes, thus rupturing the cell.

The direct attack of antibodies on antigens is not usually sufficient to completely protect the body. The major protective efforts of antibodies take place through the amplifying effects of the "complement" system, a collection of about 20 different proteins. Many of these proteins are enzyme precursors that are normally inactive, but can be activated by the antigen-antibody reaction. When an antibody binds with an antigen, a specific reactive site on the antibody is activated. This site binds with a molecule of the complement system and sets into motion a cascade of reactions. A single antibody-antigen combination can activate many molecules of the complement system, which in turn activate increasing amounts of enzymes. In this manner an amplified reaction occurs. The multiple end products formed help prevent damage by the invaders.

Antibodies have also been shown to kill cells by blocking growth mechanisms, particularly in cancer cells. Growth factor proteins such as HER-2/neu can become over expressed after the gene that encodes the protein is amplified. Antibodies specific for HER-2/neu bind to the molecule on the surface of the cell. Binding antibody may also block the growth signal.

Monoclonal antibody therapies that specifically target growth factor receptors have resulted in some significant clinical responses. The researchers have a good understanding of the potential immunologic function of monoclonal antibodies, but their main application may be their potential to alter the biology of the proteins they target.

Cytotoxic and Helper T-cells

Another focus of immunotherapy for cancer is the role of the T-cells. T-cells are either cytotoxic (CD8+) or helpers (CD4+). Unlike antibodies, which react to intact proteins only, the CD8+ T-cells react to peptide antigens expressed on the surface of a cell. Peptide antigens are proteins that have been digested by the cell, and presented as protein fragments or peptides displayed in the MHC. The peptide and the MHC together attract T-cells. CD8+ T-cells are specific for class I MHC molecules, while CD4+ T-cells are specific for class II MHC molecules.

After attaching to the MHC-peptide complex expressed on a cell, the CD8+ T-cell destroys the cell by perforating its membrane with enzymes or by triggering an apoptotic or self-destructive pathway. The CD8+ T-cell will then move to another cell expressing the same MHC-peptide complex, and destroy it as well. In this manner cytotoxic T-cells can kill many invasive cells. Ideally, CD8+ T-cells could engender a very specific and robust response against tumor cells.

One of the biggest breakthroughs in tumor immunotherapy in the past several years has been our increased understanding of the role of helper T-cells. The helper T, or CD4+ T-cell, is the major regulator of virtually all immune system activities. These cells form a series of protein mediators called lymphokines that act on other cells of the immune system and on bone marrow. Some of the most important lymphokines secreted by the helper T-cells include interleukin-2, interleukin-3, interleukin-4, interleukin-5, interleukin-6, granulocyte-monocyte colony stimulating factor (GM-CSF), and interferon-gamma. Without these lymphokines, the remainder of the immune system does not function as effectively as it would with the appropriate cytokine environment.

Like the CD8+ T-cells, CD4+ T-cells also recognize MHC-peptide complexes in the context of class II MHC. CD4+T-cells augment the immune response by secreting cytokines that stimulate either a cytotoxic T-cell response (T_H1 helper T-cells) or an antibody response (T_H2 helper T-cells). These cytokines can initiate B-cells to produce antibodies, or enhance CD8+ T-cell production. The function of the CD4+ T-cell depends upon the type of antigen it recognizes, and the type of immune response required.

Lymphokines produced by helper T-cells also regulate macrophage response. The lymphokines slow or stop the migration of macrophages after they have been engaged, allowing macrophages to accumulate at the site. These lymphokines also stimulate more efficient phagocytosis, so they can destroy rapidly increasing numbers of toxins.

The helper T-cell amplifies itself by secretion of lymphokines, particularly interleukin-2. This action enhances the helper cell response, as well as the entire immune system's response, to foreign antigens.

Tumors are Immunogenic

Tumors are now established to be immunogenic. The most exciting aspect of stimulating an endogenous immune response, however, is the potential to initiate long-term immunologic memory. This represents a dramatic shift in how cancer is treated. If we can focus this type of immunologic memory, targeting immunogenic proteins involved in malignant transformations, we may be able to prevent relapse. Of course, relapse is one of the major problems in long-term survival of cancer patients. Some patients can initially respond to chemotherapy, surgery, or radiation therapy, but tumors may recur.

Tumor Antigens

As a matter of fact, antigens are foreign substances recognized by and targeted for destruction by the cells of the immune system. When cells become cancerous they produce new, unfamiliar antigens. The immune system may recognize these antigens as foreign, and contain or even destroy the cancer cells. However, the immune responses elicited by tumor antigens are not robust. Most tumor antigens are "self" proteins, rendering them weakly immunogenic. Our immune systems tolerate self-proteins, and tolerance is a major mechanism by which cancer can evade immune recognition.

Many tumor antigens have been defined in terms of multiple solid tumors: MAGE 1, 2, and 3, defined by immunity; MART-1/Melan-A, gp100, carcinoembryonic antigen (CEA), HER-2, mucins (i.e., MUC-1), prostate-specific antigen (PSA), and prostatic acid phosphatase (PAP) are just a short list. Viral proteins–hepatitis B (HBV), Epstein-Barr (EBV), and human papilloma (HPV) – are important in the development of hepatocellular carcinoma, lymphoma, and cervical cancer, respectively. Even proteins as ubiquitous as p53, glycosylate proteins, and carbohydrates are tumor antigens. Some immune-based therapies targeting these tumor antigens are in phase III studies assessing whether immunizing against these antigens affects overall survival.

Many of these proteins are shared between multiple tumor types, and with molecular and cellular techniques investigators have defined more than 500 tumor antigens. These antigens have been elucidated by virtue of the fact that they elicit an immune response in patients who have cancer, but not in volunteer blood donors or people who do not have cancer. For instance, the blood of patients with cancer of the colon, breast, pancreas, bladder, ovary, or cervix may have high levels of CEA, and actually is used to help detect the presence of cancer. PSA levels may be high in men with benign prostate enlargement, but are typically much higher in men with prostate cancer.

The question now is why, if tumors are immunogenic, do cancers grow? Thus, despite an immune response is elicited, yet what prevents the immune response from obliterating the cancer. One explanation is that in patients with cancer, the immune response is simply not robust enough. Researchers have evaluated the endogenous HER-2/neu specific antibody response in patients with colorectal cancer. This protein is over expressed in approximately 20% of human adenocarcinomas, and is a defined tumor antigen in breast cancer. HER-2/neu antibodies (titer > or = 1:100) were detected in 14% (8/57) of patients with colorectal cancer compared to none of the control population (0/200). Detection of HER-2/neu specific antibodies in the patient population was significantly associated with HER-2/neu protein overexpression in the patients' tumor ($p < 0.01$). Nearly half (46%) of the patients with HER-2/neu over expressing tumors (6/13) and 5% of HER-2/neu negative tumors (2/44) had detectable HER-2/neu specific antibodies.

Immunity and Tumor Growth

The antibody responses to HER-2/neu generated by tumor over expression is logs lower than what would be expected from an infectious disease vaccine. One might postulate that this difference is due to cancer-mediated immune suppression. Yet their response to tetanus vaccines was similar to that of the control population. While the cancer patients could respond quite actively to a foreign antigen vaccine, they did not respond so well to an endogenous vaccination of HER-2/neu over expression.

This model suggests an insufficient response to the oncogenic protein. The cytokine environment does not allow amplification of helper T-cells to occur. Several studies have examined the phenotype of these cells found at the tumor site, and found they are not functional. They are not generating a T_H1 or T_H2 response, and secreting low levels of cytokines. Antigen-presenting cells, critical to stimulating T-cell activity, are also not functional. Either immune receptor molecules have been down regulated or the most potent antigen-presenting cells are absent from the tumor site.

As tumors grow, they secrete immunosuppressant factors. This immunomodulatory effect occurs directly, by viral proteins binding to immune receptor molecules and thus preventing their expression on the surface of the virally infected cell, or by tumors secreting factors that downregulates immune activation. Many of the genes that encode chemokines and cytokines that would normally allow the immune system to function are lost in those cells, as they become anaplastic tumors.

As previously stated, one of the essential things to understand about human tumor antigens is that they are self-antigens. Unlike viral proteins, they are derived from otherwise normal cells whose biologic function has been altered in such a way that they no longer respond to the body's normal mechanisms for controlling cell growth and reproduction. They may be qualitatively distinct in that they are over expressed, but they are simply cell cycle regulatory proteins gone awry. The immune system is designed to protect "self", and we now recognize this is a major mechanism by which tumors escape immunization. Many of the newer immunotherapeutic strategies focus on getting the immune system to recognize tumors as dangerous, mount a full-fledged attack, and eradicate the cancerous cells.

Immunotherapeutic Strategies

The phenomena of immunotherapy are generally thought of as conferring either passive or active immunity. Passive immunity supplies the immune response – antibodies, cytotoxic T-cells – rather than activating the immune system directly. These approaches have met with some success, albeit short-lived. Any element infused this way has a half-life, so for the effect to continue the infusion must be repeated. Since the immune system is not engaged, the attack may not be full-fledged. For example, when we infuse cytotoxic T-cells we do not see the expansion *in vivo* with helper T-cells.

On the other hand, active immunity may be the ideal of immunotherapy. What researchers have tried to achieve with active immunity is an endogenous immune response, where the immune system is primed to recognize the tumor as foreign. This approach has not been successful in patients with widespread disease, as their immune systems are unable to mount a sufficient response. In the past several years, efforts have focused on using active immune therapies in patients with minimal disease. However, workers have seen that the immune system can be quite functional despite advanced stage cancer when the patient has been treated to maximal response. That is, the cancer patient can be vaccinated.

The future of immunotherapy holds two specific challenges. First one needs to discover antigenic formulations that target multiple antigens. Monovalent vaccines, which target a single protein, may not supply the long-term immunity necessary to prevent relapse. Single-antigen vaccines may have a role in advanced disease, if the targeted antigen is critical to tumor growth. Clinically useful tumor vaccines will have to immunize against multiple immunogenic proteins, targeting the important proteins involved in malignant transformation.

Researchers also need to determine a therapeutically effective range for antitumor protection. Furthermore, workers are strongly beginning to think in terms of T-cell precursor frequencies specific to different types of disease status. Precursor frequency defines the level at which immunity is conferred. For example, protective immunity against hepatitis B may occur at 1 in 10,000 T-cells. In infections such as influenza precursor frequency during the active flu infection can get to 1 in 50 or 100 T-cells specific for influenza. At this point, workers do not know what precursor frequency would be necessary to have an effect on cancer. What levels confer immunity in patients with clinically undetectable disease–those who have been cured by chemotherapy but are at high risk for relapse? Where should we set the bar for patients with localized disease, or uncontrolled advanced stage disease?

Thus, as a matter of fact, immunotherapy for cancer is in a state of transition. It is clear that different strategies will benefit different patient populations. Because the struggle is between immune control and tumor escape, the best strategies to combat cancer will need to attack on multiple fronts. Most of our efforts now are focused on making self more immunogenic using immune system activators, supplying antigen-presenting cells, or actually predigesting some of these tumor antigen proteins into immunogenic peptides to thwart all tumor-evading mechanisms. Ultimately, an achievable goal may be a durable anti-tumor immune response that can be maintained throughout the patient's lifespan.

Tumor Immunoediting

It's an interesting phenomenon that despite tumor immune surveillance, tumors do develop in the presence of a functioning immune system, and therefore the updated concept of tumor immunoediting is a more complete explanation for the role of the immune system in tumor development. The tumor immunoediting concept is divided into three phases, designated as (a) elimination (b) equilibrium and (c) escape.

The elimination phase of cancer immunoediting is exactly the same process described in the initial theory of tumor immune surveillance, whereby the immune system detects and eliminates tumor cells that have developed as a result of failed intrinsic tumor suppressor mechanisms. The elimination phase can be complete, when all tumor cells are cleared, or incomplete, when only a portion of tumor cells is eliminated. In the case of partial tumor elimination, the theory of immunoediting is that a temporary state of equilibrium can then develop between the immune system and the developing tumor. During this period it is envisaged that tumor cells either remain dormant or continue to evolve, accumulating further changes (such as DNA mutations or changes in gene expression) that can modulate the tumor-specific antigens and stress-induced antigens that they express. As this process continues, the immune system exerts a selective pressure by eliminating susceptible tumor clones where possible. The pressure exerted by the immune system during this phase is sufficient to control tumor progression, but eventually, if the immune response still fails to completely eliminate the tumor, the process results in the selection of tumor cell variants that are able to resist, avoid, or suppress the antitumor immune response, leading to the escape phase. During the escape phase the immune system is no longer able to contain tumor growth, and a progressively growing tumor results. This new concept of cancer immunoediting is a more satisfactory interpretation of various clinical and experimental data, which implicate a protective role for the immune system in tumor control.

Human cancer immunoediting: As is the case for mouse studies, varying evidence has been gathered supporting each of the distinct phases of human tumor immunoediting. The phenomenon of spontaneously regressing melanoma lesions accompanied by the clonal expansion of T-cells is presently the strongest evidence for the elimination phase of cancer immunoediting in humans. Generally speaking, however, cases of spontaneous tumor regression are rare, and it is presently unknown why regression is most common in melanoma. Spontaneous tumor regression accompanied by lymphocyte infiltration has also been noted for a number of other tumor types, including basal cell carcinoma, malignant lymphoma, Merkel cell carcinoma, mesothelioma, lung carcinoma, and congenital fibrosarcoma; however, the role of the lymphocyte infiltrate in tumor regression has not been established in these cases, and doing so is likely to be difficult due to the rarity with which such cases are observed.

Clinical evidence suggests that tumors can remain dormant in patients for many years, and cases of relapse after long periods (at least 10 years) of tumor remission have been noted, making immune control with subsequent escape an intriguing possibility in these cases. In a similar vein, cases of transmission of tumors from organ donor to recipient have also been noted. In such cases, it is possible that the tumor was being held under control by an immunologic mechanism in the donor and that transplantation of the organ into an immunosuppressed host allowed tumor outgrowth. Once again, although this is consistent with the theory of tumor immunoediting, other explanations for the growth of donor-derived malignancies are possible, such as alterations in tumor oncogene expression from a common cancer stem cell.

The escape phase is the best characterized of the three in both mice and humans. For example, the growth of melanomas clearly results in the priming of a tumor-specific immune response, even though this response is often insufficient to completely eliminate tumors. Similarly, the antitumor immune response seen in patients with paraneoplastic autoimmune syndromes indicates that an ongoing immune response is, in many cases, insufficient to control tumor growth, even when it is sufficient to destroy normal self-tissues. How tumors escape immune control is now an active area of research, and the number of escape mechanisms reported is ever increasing.

Note: An attempt has been made to concisely compile from literature available in various books and reviews including e-information's available on net, about the knowledge of immune system and tumor immunology in this chapter. Prior to any writing, it is to be specifically pointed out that concepts as well as credit about the contents of this chapter is solely of the original contributors from where this material has been taken and not to this author. This author has only tried to compile the scattered information in a concise manner, which in turn, may be of immense help to students and interested readers.

At this time you should know the following:

1. Tumor immunology, relationship between antigen recognition and immune system, antibodies, cytotoxic and helper T-cells, tumors are immunogenic.
2. Tumor antigens, immunity and tumor growth, immunotherapeutic strategies and tumor immunoediting.

Further Reading

1. Fundamentals of Biochemistry by AC Deb, Tenth Edition; New Central Book Agency (P) Ltd; (2011) (ISBN: 81-7381-144-x).
2. Cellular and Molecular Immunology by Abul K Abbas, Andrew H Lichtman, Jordan S. Pober, Fourth Edition; WB Saunders (2000); (ISBN: 0721682332).
3. Textbook of Medical Biochemistry by MN Chatterjea and R Shinde, Seventh Edition; Jaypee Brothers, Medical Publishers (P) Ltd. (2007); (ISBN: 81-8448-134-9).
4. Medical Biochemistry by NV Bhagavan, Fourth Edition, Academic Press (2004) (ISBN: 81-8147-322-1).
5. Immunology: Understanding the immune system by Klaus D Elgert; John Wiley and Sons, (2009). (ISBN: 0470081570).
6. Roitt's Essential Immunology by Ivan M. Roitt and Peter J. Delves, Tenth Edition; Blackwell Publishing (2001), (ISBN: 0-632-05902-8).

19

CHAPTER

Immunodeficiency

(Dr. Rajinder Chawla chawlarn@cmcludhiana.in)

OBJECTIVES

1. To know the characteristics of immunodeficiency disorders.
2. To learn the genetic and secondary causes of immunodeficiency.
3. To learn the types of primary immunodeficiency disorders and their pathogenesis.
4. To understand the causes of secondary immunodeficiency.
5. To learn the laboratory investigations for diagnosing these disorders.

INTRODUCTION

As discussed in the previous chapters, the immune system is made up of lymphoid tissue in the body, that includes the thymus, lymph nodes, tonsils, parts of the spleen and gastrointestinal tract and bone marrow.

Lymphocytes (the specialized white blood cells that provide acquired immunity) are produced or become mature in various lymphoid tissues. Lymphocytes are divided into 2 groups: T lymphocytes and B lymphocytes which provide the two arms of the immune defense system of an organism, i.e., Cellular and Humoral immunity.

- T lymphocytes are the vehicles of cellular immunity. They transform into sensitized lymphocytes that directly attack antigens.
- B lymphocytes are the instruments of humoral immunity. They produce highly specific proteins, the immunoglobulins, commonly known as 'Antibodies', that attach to the antigen and trigger a number of biological responses like phagocytosis, opsonization and complement fixation. The B lymphocytes also secrete a number of active molecules like complement that potentiate the immune destruction of the antigens and invading organisms.

Immune system disorders occur when the immune response is inappropriate (excessive or lacking) or is targeted against the organism's own molecules (Autoimmunity). Immunodeficiency disorders reflect the inadequacy of the immune system to fight tumors or invading organisms. The immunodeficiency state, as the name implies, is associated with a deficient force to fight against the foreign substances or organisms like bacteria or viruses. Therefore, immuno-deficiency causes persistent or recurrent infections, severe infections by organisms that are normally mild, incomplete recovery from illness or poor response to treatment, and an increased incidence of carcinogenesis.

Immunodeficiency disorders may affect any part of the immune system. Most commonly, this involves decreased functioning of T or B lymphocytes (or both), or deficient antibody production.

Causes of Immunodeficiency

The genesis of immunodeficiency can be divided into three groups:

a. ***The genetic or congenital (inherited) defects:*** The genes responsible for the synthesis of immunoglobulins, if defective, can cause congenital immunodeficiency disorders of antibody production (B lymphocyte abnormalities), which include hypogammaglobulinemia (lack of one or more specific antibodies) and agammaglobulinemia (lack of all or most antibody production), which results in frequent severe infections and is often fatal.

b. ***Acquired immunodeficiency:*** A disease that affects the immune system e.g., HIV (Human Immunodeficiency Virus) infection and AIDS (acquired immunodeficiency syndrome) can result in impaired immuno-surveillance leading to the increased susceptibility to opportunistic infections. Bacterial, viral, protozoal and fungal infections may lead to B-cell, T-cell, PMN and macrophage deficiencies.

c. ***Immunosuppression:*** A number of drugs can suppress the immune system, e.g., corticosteroids or other immunosuppressant medications. These medications are prescribed to keep the immune system in check in patients with autoimmune disorders or those who have undergone organ transplantation. Immunosuppression is also seen in cancer patients after chemotherapy, because the chemotherapy often kills the rapidly multiplying cells and hence reduces the number of white blood cells available to fight infection.

d. ***Other causes of immunodeficiency:*** Apart from the above, other causes of immunodeficiency include *malnutrition*, particularly with lack of protein, and many *cancers*. Those who have had a *splenectomy,* face a higher risk of infection from certain encapsulated bacteria that the spleen would normally help fight. Patients with *diabetes mellitus* are also at higher risk for certain infections. *Increasing age* also reduces the effectiveness of the immune system to some degree. Immune system tissues (particularly lymphoid tissue such as the thymus) shrink, and there is also reduced lymphocyte number and activity.

Some immunodeficiency disorders are mild and result in occasional illness. Others are severe and may be fatal. Immunosuppression that results from medications is often reversible once the medication is stopped.

1. CONGENITAL IMMUNODEFICIENCY DISORDERS

The inherited immunodeficiency disorders due to the dysfunctional or absent gene(s) are the basis of about 70 types of congenital immunodeficiency disorders. Since these disorders manifest at the time of birth, they are known as the **primary immunodeficiencies**. About 50,000 new cases are diagnosed in the United States each year. The genetic defect may be reflected in the reduced numbers or malfunction of B lymphocytes, T lymphocytes, or both. Some of these disorders also occur in the innate immune system.

The genetic causes of the immunodeficiency disorders can be best understood by considering the normal development of the immune system (**Figure 19.1**) and the cell collaborations necessary to generate an effective immune response. Lymphocytes are derived from hematopoietic stem cells that reside in the fetal liver and bone marrow. These cells proceed through an orderly sequence of maturation even in the absence of any antigens. Early in differentiation, gene rearrangements occur which commit the cell to either T-cell or B-cell differentiation. Further development of T-cells occurs in the thymus gland, whereas, B-cell development occurs in the bone marrow. Once functionally mature cells have developed, the

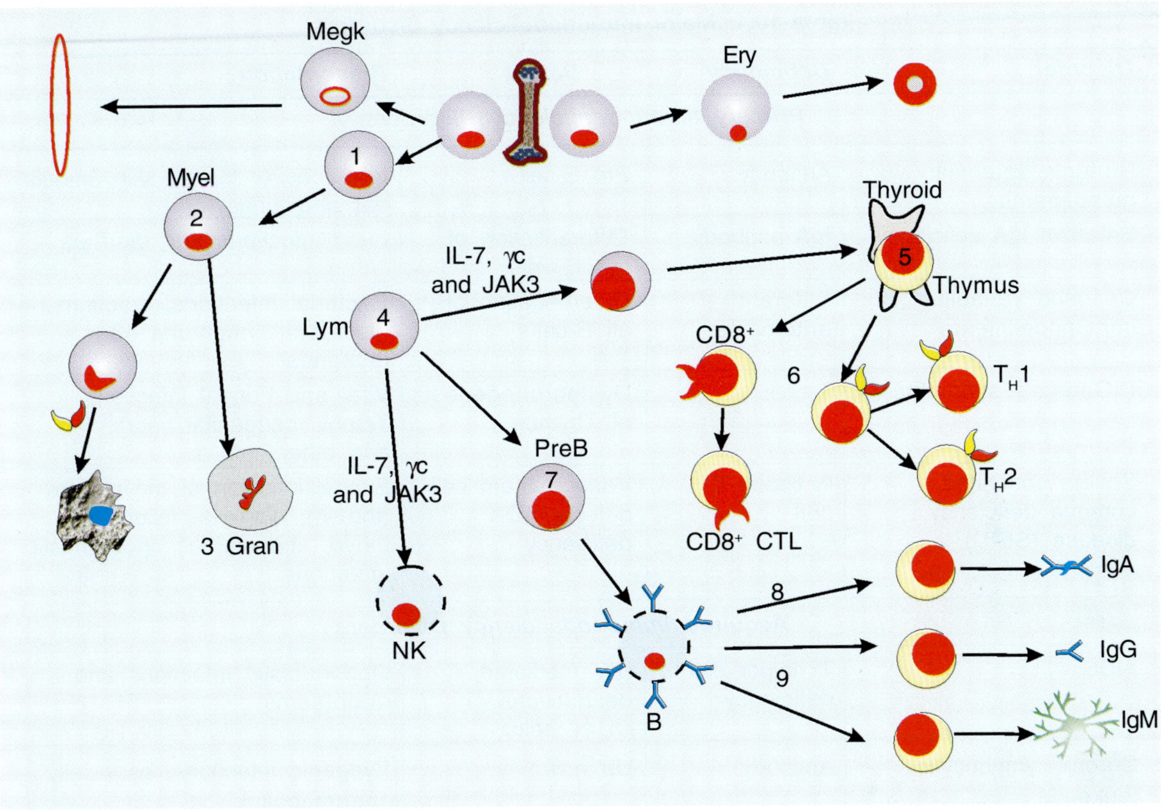

Fig. 19.1: Defects in the hematopoietic system that cause different immunodeficiency diseases

1. Reticular dysgenesis, 2. Cyclic neutropenia, 3. Chronic granulomatous disease, 4. Severe combined immunodeficiency, 5. DiGeorge syndrome and Bare Leucocyte syndrome, 6. Abnormal T-Cell function, 7. X-linked infantile (Bruton's) hypogammaglobulinemia, 8. Selective immunoglobulin deficiencies, 9. Hyper IgM immunodeficiency.

generation of a normal immune response depends upon collaboration between antigen-presenting cells, T helper cells, and T, B and NK effector cells. These interactions are tightly regulated by specific and nonspecific regulatory cells. Products (cytokines) released from these cells modulate the immune response. It is also important to note that cell-cell interactions depend upon the participation of cell surface molecules including the T-cell receptor and surface immunoglobulins, antigen-binding proteins (HLA class I and II antigens), adhesion molecules (LFA-1, LFA-3, ICAM-1) and their ligands which promote efficient binding between cells. **Table 19.1** lists the major immunodeficiency disorders.

Table 19.1: Major immunodeficiency disorders

Disorder	*Deficiency*	*Defect*	*Presentation*
		Primary Immunodeficiency Disorders	
Bruton's agamma globulinemia	Antibody	Pre B-cell	Infections of throat, skin, middle ear and lungs
Selective IgA deficiency	IgA antibody	Differentiation of IgA B-cells	Lung infections and diarrhea
Common variable immunodeficiency	Different antibodies	Differentiation of all B-cells	Bacterial infections, autoimmune disorders, lymphoma and leukemia
DiGeorge's syndrome	T-cells	Dysmorphogenesis of Thymus	Viral and Fungal infections, Tetany, congenital heart and other defects
Severe combined immuno deficiency disease (SCID)	Antibody T cell	Various Stem cell defects, ADA deficiency	Fungal infection of the mouth (thrush), diarrhea, failure to thrive, and serious opportunistic infections
		Acquired Immunodeficiency Disorders	
AIDS	T helper cell deficiency	HIV mediated destructions of CD4+ cells	Opportunistic infections and neoplasms
Chronic lymphocytic leukemia	Antibody	Unknown	Pyogenic infections, especially pneumococci

B LYMPHOCYTE DEFICIENCIES

B-cell development requires the presence of a B-cell-specific tyrosine kinase (Bruton's tyrosine kinase [Btk]). After antigen activation, B-cells differentiate into immunoglobulin-producing plasma cells. The B-cell response to polysaccharide antigens is T-cell-independent, however, for certain other antigens, the T-cell signals of antibody isotype switching in B-cells are mediated by specific cell-surface receptors, such as the CD40 antigen (on B-cells) and the corresponding CD40 ligand on T-cells. Additional binding of cytokines to specific receptors on B-cell surfaces triggers intracellular signaling cascades that lead to immunoglobulin synthesis.

The deficiency of either the cytokine release/interaction or downstream signaling pathway for immunoglobulin synthesis, can lead to impaired

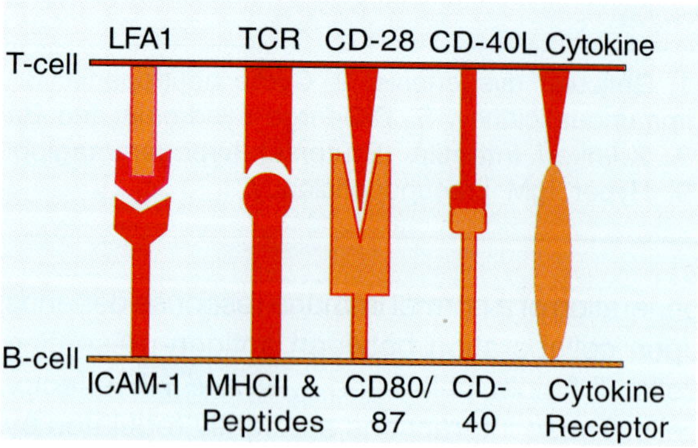

Fig. 19.2: The signaling interaction between T-cells and B-cells

LFA1 : Leucocyte function associated antigen.
ICAM : Intracellular Cell Adhesion molecule.
MHC : Major Histocompatibility Complex.

synthesis of antibodies, thus decreasing the plasma immunoglobulin levels.

Bruton's agammaglobulinemia: This X-linked (recessive) inherited disorder is characterized by a decrease or absence of B lymphocytes, and therefore a decreased ability to make antibodies. Since the defect is on the X-chromosome, the agammaglobinemia is more common in males; but the females homozygous for the mutated gene might also manifest the disorder. The heterozygous females are asymptomatic carriers. People with this disorder are particularly susceptible to infections of the throat, skin, middle ear and lungs. However, patients who receive gamma globulin injections may live upto 40 years and often die of lung infections.

IgA deficiency: The most common type of immunoglobulin deficiency is selective IgA deficiency, occurring in about one in every 500 white persons. Generally, the blood levels of other types of immunoglobulins are normal. Some patients with selective IgA deficiency experience no symptoms, while others have occasional lung infections and diarrhea. The subjects with selective IgA deficiency generally have a normal life span.

IgG and IgA deficiency: Another group of patients have a combined deficiency of IgG as well as IgA type of immunoglobulins. In these patients, IgM is found to be increased in plasma. People with this disorder tend to get severe bacterial infections.

Common variable immunodeficiency: Common variable immunodeficiency is the most common of the immunodeficiency disorders. In this disorder, the production of one or more of the immunoglobulin types is decreased and the antibody response to infections is impaired. It generally develops around the age of 10-20 years. The symptoms vary among affected people. Most people with this disorder have frequent infections, and some also experience anemia and rheumatoid arthritis. There is increased incidence of carcinogenesis in these patients. The patients have a normal total B lymphocyte count in plasma, although the number of B-cells carrying the membrane bound IgG antibodies is lower than normal. B-cells with IgG antibodies on their surface are capable of responding to microorganisms. The lack of IgG on the surface of the B-cells means that they are not prepared to fight infection. The T lymphocytes cell count is usually normal, although some cell signal components may be lacking.

The main symptom is recurring infections that tend to be chronic rather than acute. Patients may also develop diarrhea and, as a consequence of the diarrhea, do not absorb food efficiently. This can lead to malnourishment that can aggravate the disorder. Autoimmune disorders such as rheumatoid arthritis, thyroiditis, and systemic lupus erythromatosus and certain cancers such as lymphomas and leukemias may be associated with common variable immunodeficiency. Common variable immunodeficiency is treated with periodic injections of gamma globulin throughout life.

Diagnosis

The main diagnostic test that distinguishes common variable immunodeficiency from other immunodeficiency diseases is the low immunoglobulin level despite the normal B-cell count. The gammaglobulin band on paper electrophoresis appears to be less dense. The specific immunoglobulin deficiencies can be detected by immunodiffusion or ELISA using anti-IgG, anti-IgA and anti-IgM sera.

T LYMPHOCYTE DEFICIENCIES

Severe defects in the ability of T lymphocytes to mature result in impaired immune responses to infections with viruses, fungi, and certain types of bacteria. These infections are usually severe and can be fatal.

DiGeorge syndrome: DiGeorge syndrome is a T lymphocyte deficiency that starts during fetal development and is the result of a deletion in a particular gene. Children with DiGeorge syndrome either do not have a thymus or have an underdeveloped thymus. Since the thymus is a major organ that directs the production of T lymphocytes, these patients have very low numbers of T lymphocytes. They are susceptible to recurrent infections, and usually have physical abnormalities as well. For example, they may have low-set ears, a small receding jawbone and wide-spaced eyes. People with DiGeorge syndrome are particularly susceptible to viral and fungal infections.

The defect in thymic development results from a presumed failure of the neural crest mesenchyma to induce morphogenetic changes in the third pharyngeal pouch derived endoderm. The gene that is defective in the DiGeorge syndrome has been located to 22q11.

In some cases, no treatment is required for DiGeorge syndrome because T lymphocyte production improves on its own. Either an underdeveloped thymus begins to produce more T lymphocytes or organ sites other than the thymus compensate by producing more T lymphocytes.

Severe combined immunodeficiency: Some types of immunodeficiency disorders affect both B lymphocytes and T lymphocytes. The severe combined immunodeficiency disease (SCID) is caused by the defective development or function of these two types of lymphocytes. It results in impaired humoral and cellular immune responses. SCID is usually recognized during the first year of life. It tends to cause a fungal infection of the mouth (thrush), diarrhea, failure to thrive, and serious infections. If not treated with a bone marrow transplant, a person with SCID will generally die from infections before two years of age.

The molecular defect in X-linked SCID has been mapped to the 9p13 locus of the X-chromosome. The common γ chain (γc) of the IL-2, IL-4, IL-7, IL-9, and IL-15 receptors is encoded by an X-linked gene (located at Xq12-13.1). Defects in this gene lead to compromised T and NK cell development, but there is no defect in B-cell generation. This is the most common form of SCID, and a large variety of mutations have been discovered in γc. In man, IL-7 is required for T-cell development but is not critical for B-cell development. IL-15 is required for NK cell development and the combined loss of IL-7 and IL-15 derived signals leads to the failure of development of these lineages (**Figure 19.1**).

The disorder can also arise from deficiencies of the purine salvage pathway (deficiency of adenosine deaminase or purine-nucleoside phosphorylase, **Figure 19.3**) or X-linked traits that cause cytokine receptor defects. In addition, defects in signaling molecules (T-cell-receptor defects or deficiency of ZAP70 tyrosine kinase or Janus-associated kinase 3), loss of the major histocompatibility complex (MHC deficiency or bare lymphocyte syndrome), and rare cytokine deficiencies can lead to SCID.

Autosomal recessive SCID with JAK-3 deficiency: Mutations in an autosomal gene encoding the JAK3 kinase result in a very similar phenotype to that seen in X-linked SCID. This is not at all surprising since JAK-3 and γc are functionally linked (**Figure. 19.1**).

IL-7 plays a demonstrable role in B-cell development in the mouse but not in man, and this accounts for the differences in phenotype seen between the human disorders involving γc and Jak-3 and the corresponding knockout mice lines.

Autosomal recessive SCID with IL-7R deficiency: In a form of SCID in which there is a defect in T-cell development with normal numbers of B and NK cells, inherited mutations in the gene encoding the IL-7Ra chain have been described. This disease underscores the fact that in humans, IL-7Ra derived signals are not required for B-cell development, and that IL-7 is not required for NK cell development in mouse or man (although IL-15 is crucial).

Other autosomal recessive forms of SCID: Apart from the above, two autosomal recessive forms of SCID have been described in which B and T-cells are not seen. In one of these forms, mutations in Rag-1 or Rag-2 severely compromise V(D)J recombination. In the other, V(D)J recombination is compromised but no mutations have as yet been described in the Rag genes. Certain mutations in the Rag-1 and Rag-2 genes result in partially compromised V(D)J recombination and an unusual clinical phenotype described as **Omenn's syndrome**. The mutations in DNA ligase 1 have also been associated with

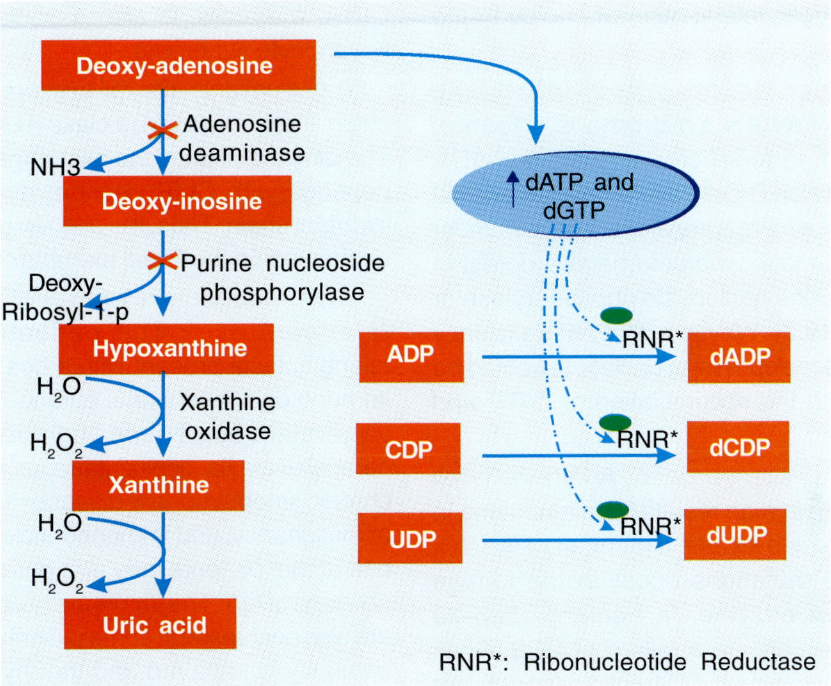

Fig. 19.3: Purine catabolism and the effect of adenosine deaminase and purine nucleoside phosphorylase on nucleotide synthesis

SCID phenotypes probably due to impaired V(D)J recombination.

Adenosine deaminase deficiency: A fairly common form of SCID occurs in infants with an inherited deficiency in adenosine deaminase or ADA. During the catabolism of purines to uric acid (**Figure 19.3**), ADA deaminates the purines (ATP, GTP, dATP and dGTP). Inosine, xanthosine and guanosine thus formed are degraded by the action of purine nucleoside phosphorylase or PNP and subsequently converted to uric acid by xanthine oxidase. Eight different mutant forms of ADA have been described in SCID patients, all of which compromise the active site of the enzyme. In the absence of functional ADA, deoxyadenosine is phosphorylated to produce very high levels of dATP. These high levels of dATP inhibit ribonucleotide reductase which is essential for dNTP synthesis. DNA synthesis and hence cell division is thereby blocked affecting all the rapidly dividing cells.

Patients with ADA deficiency have defects in the generation of T, B and NK cells suggesting a defect at the level of the putative common lymphoid progenitor, or in the early developmental stages of each of these three lineages. The defect appears to be largely confined to T-cell precursors, NK cell function is often unaffected in patients with ADA, and B-cell development may be minimally compromised. The manifestations of ADA deficiency may not be restricted to lymphoid cells – patients also exhibit rib cage and other skeletal abnormalities, presumably in response to toxic effects of dATP and the inhibition of proliferation of other cell types.

ADA is rapidly cleared from blood by liver, however, half life of ADA is increased to 5-7 days when it is covalently coupled to PEG (polyethylene glycol). These conjugates can be used to treat ADA deficiency fairly effectively. Preliminary attempts at gene therapy have yielded promising results, and it is very likely that this will prove to be the therapeutic intervention of choice in the near future.

Purine nucleoside phosphorylase deficiency: **Nezelof's syndrome** is a form of combined immunodeficiency just like ADA deficiency in which B-cell development is normal but T-cell development is impaired. A large number of patients with this syndrome have a defect in the enzyme purine nucleoside phosphorylase or PNP (**Figure 19.3**). Why exactly PNP deficiency targets T-cell development is unclear but could be associated with the accumulation of dATP and dGTP.

Mutations in Zap-70 gene: A form of T-cell deficiency seen in man results from mutations in the Zap-70 tyrosine kinase, a member of the Syk family. These mutations occur in the kinase domain of this enzyme. In humans, Zap-70 mutations result only in a failure of CD8 T cell development. However, CD4 cells although not deficient in patients with inherited defects in ZAP-70, cannot be readily activated. The activation of CD4 cells through binding with Lck has been proposed.

Bare lymphocyte syndrome: This syndrome is characterized by the deficiency of CD4 T-cells. The defect lies in the expression of MHC class II proteins. The failure to express HLA class II molecules in the thymic cortex during positive selection results in an absence of CD4 T cells. The patients with the Bare lymphocyte syndrome have inherited defects in transcriptional regulators of MHC class II (HLA DP, DQ, and DR) expression. Four regulatory genes are involved in this syndrome which are components of the multimeric RFX complex that regulates the expression of MHC class II, Ii, and HLA-DM genes. The activity of RFX depends on a co-activator 'CIITA' which is constitutively expressed in professional antigen presenting cells, but can also be induced by IFN-γ in certain cell types. The defective expression of CIITA, therefore, is also associated with Bare lymphocyte syndrome.

These patients also fail to express the invariant chain 'Ii' and HLA-DM, a class II like heterodimer. The dimer facilitates the exchange of the antigen peptides with CLIP peptide, derived from the invariant chain. Thus, the antigen peptides are not expressed on the T-cell membrane.

Immunodeficiency associated with ataxia telangiectasia: The patients with ataxia telangiectasia present with a host of neurologic, immunologic, endocrine, cutaneous and hepatic abnormalities. These include progressive cerebellar ataxia, oculocutaneous telangiectasias, chronic sinopulmonary disease, a high incidence of malignancy, and immunodeficiency. More than half of the patients may present with a selective absence of IgA. The immunoglobulins IgE and IgG are also decreased in some patients. Cell mediated immunity is impaired and the thymus has been noted to be hypoplastic.

The gene that is defective in ataxia telangiectasia is located on 11q22-23 and encodes a protein known as ataxia telangiectasia mutated-protein (ATM). This protein is a member of the PI-3 kinase family and is a dual serine/threonine protein kinase/lipid kinase. ATM is induced by DNA damage and may contribute to the induction of p53 and the induction of apoptosis, thus functioning as part of a cell cycle checkpoint (**Figure 19.4**). ATM can bind to p53 and phosphorylates it on serine-15, thus activating and stabilizing p53. P53, a transcription factor that is highly unstable (normal half-life is 30 minutes) becomes stable upon forming a complex with damaged DNA. The stabilized p53 activates transcription of proteins that are inhibitors of cell cyclins, CDKs. These inhibitors result in stoppage of the cell cycle and induction of DNA repair proteins to give time for repair. If the repair mechanisms fail, p53 induces proteins utilized by the cell to kill itself by apoptosis (**Figure 19.4**).

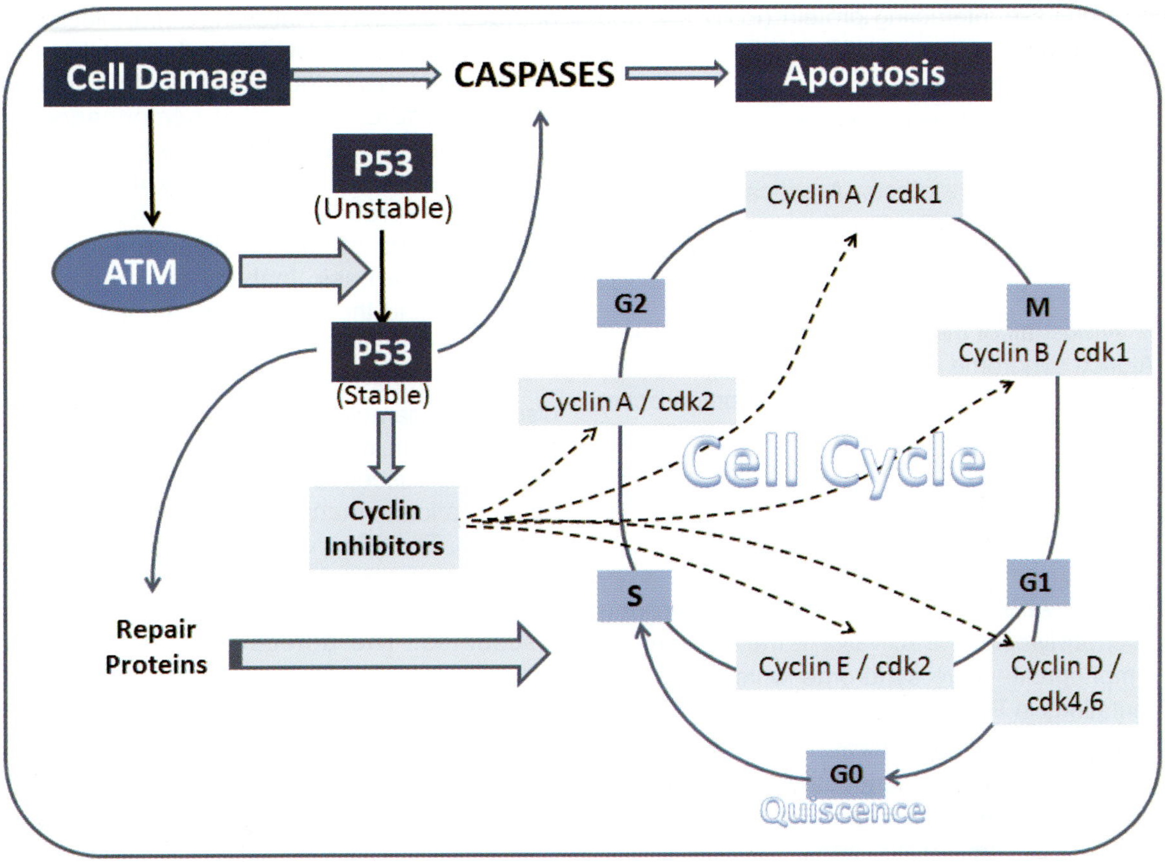

Fig. 19.4: ATM protein also appears to be important for the integrity of V(D)J recombination and hence ATM patients have an extremely high frequency of translocations in B and T lymphocytes. Association of ATM with cell cycle regulation may also be responsible for high incidence of cancer in these patients

DISORDERS OF ABERRANT LYMPHOCYTE ACTIVATION

Inappropriate activation of T lymphocytes also forms the basis of a number of immune disorders. The allergic and autoimmune disorders are examples but here we will discuss some specific immunodeficiency diseases where activation of T-cells has been implicated.

The Wiskott-Aldrich Syndrome: The Wiskott-Aldrich syndrome is an X-linked disease characterized by thrombocytopenia, defective platelet activation, pyogenic and opportunistic infections and eczema. IgM levels tend to be low, IgA and IgE levels are generally elevated and IgG levels are usually in the normal range. There is a failure to respond to microbial polysaccharide antigens due to defects in T-cells signaling and exoskeleton.

The X-linked gene that is defective in this disease encodes a protein which is known as WASP (Wiskott-Aldrich Syndrome Protein). WASP is a proline rich protein with multiple sites capable of interacting with SH3 domains. The WASP protein interacts with the Rho family small GTPase, Cdc42, with Src family kinases, with the Nck adaptor protein, with proline serine threonine phosphatase interacting protein (PSTPIP), and with a protein known as WIP (WASP interacting protein) among others.

Cdc42 is involved in actin rearrangements as are WIP and PSTPIP, thus these patients have T-cell exoskeleton defects. A critical function of Cdc42 and of WASP in T-cells is the formation of a polarized synapse like interface with antigen presenting cells.

Almost all of the defects seen in the Wiskott Aldrich syndrome can potentially be tied to the failure of WASP to help reorganize cortical actin. WASP also appears to be involved in B-cells triggered by T-independent polysaccharide antigens. Therefore, WASP patients have defective responses to polysaccharide antigens.

Autoimmune lymphoproliferative syndrome: Another very rare disorder involving aberrant lymphocyte activation is the autoimmune lymphoproliferative syndrome which is due to mutations in Fas.

Infants and young children with this disease present with lymphadenopathy, splenomegaly, and hypergammaglobulinemia. The lymphoid organs are overpopulated with $CD3^+$,$CD4^-$,$CD8^-$ T cells. In addition, common features of this syndrome include episodic autoimmune anemias, thrombocytopenia, autoantibody mediated neutropenias, and urticarial rashes. This syndrome closely mimics the phenotype of naturally occurring mutations in Fas and the Fas ligands involved in the process of apoptosis. The activated T-cells and self reactive B-cells, which normally are eliminated via Fas signals, proliferate and contribute to autoimmune manifestations. Fas is a trimeric protein, therefore, the mutations in Fas are generally observed in heterozygotes, and homozygous mutations are rare.

Disorders involving a post-infectious "accelerated phase": In some of the primary immunodeficiency disorders, an accelerated and uncontrolled end-state of T_H1 cell and macrophage activation is observed following a viral infection. A defect in NK cell activity is also frequently seen. Examples of this category include the Chediak-Higashi syndrome, familial hemophagocytic lymphohistiocytosis, partial albinism with immunodeficiency, and possibly the X-linked lymphoproliferative syndrome. The common feature in this otherwise diverse sub-set of diseases is a basic inability to counter viral infections, and the consequent triggering of an accelerated phase of T_H1 type T-cell activation.

The Chediak-Higashi syndrome (CHS): This disorder is characterized by partial cutaneous and ocular albinism, defective CTL and NK cell activity, increased susceptibility to infections, and the accumulation in many cells of large intracellular granules. There is a defect in granule discharge (accounting for the defects in CTLs and NK cells) and in the fusion of endosomes with primary lysosomes. The defective gene on human chromosome 1 has been identified and is believed to encode a cytosolic protein that is involved in a vesicular trafficking function during endocytosis and exocytosis. Most patients with CHS develop an accelerated phase which generally leads to death. During the accelerated phase, T-cells and macrophages are hyperactivated and there is increased synthesis of cytokines.

X-linked lymphoproliferative syndrome: In the X-linked lymphoproliferative (XLP) syndrome, also known as Duncan's syndrome, young boys are prone to succumb to Epstein-Barr virus (EBV) infections after entry into an accelerated phase. The causative gene on Xq25 encodes a small protein called SAP (for SLAM associated protein). SLAM is a member of Ig superfamily having only SH2 domain. The protein is present on activated T-cells (thymocytes), and some B-cells. Upon activation by homotypic interactions, it can induce lymphocyte proliferation, and facilitates the generation of T_H1 responses. This protein has a cytoplasmic tail that contains four potential tyrosine phosphorylation sites. The cytoplasmic tail of SLAM can potentially recruit a range of SH2 domain containing proteins, but the exact reason of immunodeficiency or uncontrolled B-cell proliferation following EBV infection is unclear. It is possible that the underlying defect is in a mechanism involved in viral clearance by T-cells, or may involve the dysregulation of proliferation in B-cells.

Omenn's syndrome: This is also a rare autosomal recessive disease in which the infants present with severe erythrodermia, alopecia, diarrhea and a failure to thrive. Large numbers of activated T-cells infiltrate the skin, the gut epithelium, and the lamina propria. There is a profound depletion of T and B lymphocytes in the blood and lymph nodes. The tissues show gross infiltrations of T-cells that appear to be generated from hyperproliferation of a few T-cell clones. The underlying defect in a number of families with Omenn's syndrome is an inherited missense mutation in the Rag-1 or Rag-2 gene that contributes to an incomplete V(D)J recombination. The generation of B and T-cells is blocked but a few T-cell clones escape the developmental block. Some of these T-cells undergo uncontrolled proliferation and result in a "T_H2" type accelerated phase disease with fatal consequences.

Some T-cell disorders present with characteristics that are specific and typical. For example, a child with Omenn's syndrome has lymphadenopathy, while a patient with DiGeorge syndrome may have craniofacial defects, hypocalcemic tetany, and cardiac defects. Features of ataxia-telangiectasia include progressive ataxia and oculocutaneous telangiectasia, whereas Wiskott-Aldrich syndrome presents with infections, eczema, and thrombocytopenia. Chronic mucocutaneous candidiasis syndrome presents with recurrent nail or mucous membrane involvement by candida as well as a polyendocrinopathy.

Phagocytic Defects

Phagocytic dysfunction is characterized clinically by recurrent abscesses, lymphadenitis, and periodontal disease. The causative organisms are more commonly gram-negative bacteria and include Staphylococcus aureus, Pseudomonas aeruginosa, and fungal pathogens (e.g., Aspergillus species).

Cyclic neutropenia: The disorder is characterized by decreased number of circulating neutrophils. The neutropenia lasts for about a week during which period the patients are at increased risk of infections. The neutrophil count improves in about a week but the bouts of neutropenia are observed at a regular cyclic interval of about 3-4 weeks. The defect appears to be due to poor regulation of neutrophil production.

Leukocyte adhesion deficiency (LAD): In this disorder, the leucocytes lack the complement receptor CR3. The defect lies in the CD11 and CD18 peptides and consequently they cannot respond to C3b opsonins. A defect in the integrins LFA-1 and mac-1 arising from CD11 and CD18 peptides, respectively could also contribute. The patient with defect in these chains cannot effectively respond to chemotactic signals since the integrins (neutrophil adhesion molecules) are pivotal to endothelial adhesion and emigration into tissues. LAD presents with delayed separation of the umbilical cord, recurrent serious bacterial infections, and leukemoid reactions.

Chronic granulomatous disease (CGD): The patients with chronic granulomatous disease that involves defects in intracellular oxidative killing of bacteria have suppurative infections by catalase-positive organisms. Some of these infections include recurrent deep-seated abscesses, oral ulceration, periodontal abscess, and dental caries. Marked lymphadenopathy, hepatosplenomegaly and chronic draining lymph nodes are other features. The defect appears to be in NADPH oxidase (cytochrome b_{558}; $gp91^{phox}$; $gp22^{phox}$ or other cofactor proteins like $gp47^{phox}$ and $gp67^{phox}$. The disease can easily be diagnosed by poor Nitroblue tetrazolium (NBT) reduction test.

Chediak-Higashi syndrome: This syndrome is (as discused above) marked with a reduced intracellular killing and chemotactic movement accompanied by an impaired phagosome-lysosome fusion and lysosomal proteinase deficiency. Respiratory burst is normal. The NK cell and platelet disorders are also seen in these patients.

Complement Dysfunction

Complement disorders, the rarest forms of primary immunodeficiency, represent less than 1% of such diseases. C2-4 deficiency is associated with autoimmune diseases, such as lupus like syndrome and arthritis. C3 deficiency is linked to overwhelming infections with high-grade encapsulated pathogens or unusual strains, or both. Specifically, deficiencies of the late complement (C5-9) predispose to recurrent neisserial infections, such as disseminated gonococcal infection with oligoarticular arthritis or recurrent meningococcal meningitis.

2. ACQUIRED IMMUNODEFICIENCY DISORDERS

Acquired or secondary immunodeficiency often occurs as a complication of other conditions and diseases; and is more common than congenital immunodeficiency. For example, the most common causes of acquired immunodeficiency are malnutrition, malignancy (particularly lymphomas), and infections **(Table 19.2)**. The common infections that can lead to immunodeficiency include chickenpox, cytomegalovirus, German measles, measles, tuberculosis, infectious mononucleosis (Epstein-Barr virus), chronic hepatitis, lupus, and bacterial and fungal infections. The human immunodeficiency virus (HIV) is the virus that causes acquired immunodeficiency syndrome (AIDS). However, this is not the most common cause of acquired immunodeficiency.

The latest addition to the infectious agent responsible for immunodeficiency is the virus causing severe acute respiratory syndrome (SARS) that was first reported in 2003 from China. It eventually affected 8,000 people in Asia and Canada, killing 800 altogether. The virus is characterized by fever, lower respiratory tract symptoms, and abnormal chest X-rays along with immunodeficiency.

Iatrogenic acquired immunodeficiency has also been reported to be caused by particularly immunosuppressive drugs used to control transplant rejection. Similarly, anticancer drugs kill all the rapidly dividing cells including cells of the immune system. During the period of time that these drugs are being taken, the risk of infection increases. It usually returns to normal after the person stops taking the drugs.

The autoimmune disorders like cystic fibrosis, protein malnutrition, malabsorption and protein losing conditions like nephritic syndrome are also associated with immunodeficiency.

Laboratory Evaluation of Immunodeficiency

As with any clinical condition, the clinical presentation is the most important tool for diagnosis and laboratory diagnosis should be planned according to the clinical impression. Recurring infection, particularly by the same agents, is the strong indication for immunodeficiency workup. A complete blood cell count is often helpful. Lymphopenia is characteristic of most forms of SCID, thrombocytopenia is seen in Wiskott-Aldrich syndrome, and an elevated total white blood cell count is a feature of LAD. Giant lysosomal granules in the granulocytes are the feature of Chédiak-Higashi syndrome. Other specialized tests are available for assessing cellular immunity, humoral immunity, phagocytic function, and the complement system.

The **Table 19.3** gives the guidelines for the laboratory workup.

HUMORAL IMMUNITY

Estimation of total protein, albumin and A:G ratio, along with serum protein electrophoresis, is the starting point for evaluating humoral immunodeficiency. The week gammaglobulin band on electrophoresis and increased A:G ratio are indications of reduced immunoglobulins. The values of total proteins and albumin are often reduced in patients with protein-losing states,

Table 19.2: Major causes of secondary immunodeficiency diseases

Causes	***Examples***
Malnutrition	Protein energy malnutrition, malabsorption syndrome
Infection	HIV, congenital rubella, congenital infection with cytomegalovirus, *Toxoplasma gondii,* Epstein-Barr virus
Drugs	Use of corticosteroids, gold salts, penicillamine (Cuprine, Depen), phenytoin sodium (Dilantin), sulfasalazine (Azulfidine), cytotoxic drugs
Chronic medical conditions	Sickle cell disease, cystic fibrosis
Malignancy	Chronic lymphocytic leukemia, non-Hodgkin's lymphoma, B-cell malignancy
Systemic disorders that lead to immunoglobulin loss	Malabsorption (e.g., protein-losing enteropathy), nephrotic syndrome
Chromosomal syndrome	Down syndrome

Table 19.3: Major laboratory investigations for diagnosing immunodeficiency disorders

	Initial	***Advanced***
Humoral immunity	Serum levels of IgG, IgA, IgM and IgE; measurement of isohemagglutinins	• Antibody response to immunization of diphtheria, tetanus, and pneumococcus polysaccharides • IgG subclass determination • B-cell quantitation by flow cytometry • Mitogenic stimulation assay
Cellular immunity	Complete blood cell count; lymphocyte phenotyping; delayed-type hypersensitivity skin testing	• Lymphocyte proliferation in response to mitogens • One-way mixed lymphocyte reaction assay • Cytokine assays • Cytotoxicity assay
Phagocytic function	Complete blood cell count; Nitroblue tetrazolium test	• Phagocytosis assay • Bactericidal assay • Chemotaxis assay
Complement	Total hemolytic complement assay by classical and alternative pathways (CH_{50} and AH_{50})	• Quantitation of individual complement component and regulatory molecules • Serum opsonic and chemotactic assays

such as enteropathies and nephrotic syndrome. The presence of paraproteins on serum protein electrophoresis might indicate malignancy or adult-onset hypogammaglobulinemia. The next step is the measurement of serum IgG, IgA, IgE, and IgM levels. Advanced tests for staging of humoral immune deficiency include B-cell quantitation and antibody responses to antigens. It is essential to demonstrate immune responses to vaccination by measuring antibodies to specific antigens before and 3 to 4 weeks after a patient receives a vaccination (or a booster). Often the postvaccine titers are low as the patients with a primary humoral immune disorder respond poorly to vaccination. Sometimes poor response to pneumococcal vaccination could be observed despite normal levels of total immunoglobulins.

Cellular Immunity

Cellular immunodeficiency may or may not be noticed with simple leukocyte count. Assessment of delayed-type hypersensitivity would be the initial step. Antigens such as purified protein derivative from *Candida,* and diphtheria can be used for this prupose.

The T-cell profiling including T-cells (CD3), helper T-cells ($CD4^+$ T cells), and suppressor and cytotoxic T-cells ($CD8^+$ T cells) by flow cytometry that uses specific antibodies against the T-cell markers giving good information about the condition. Flow cytometry can also detect defective expression of CD40 ligand on the T-cell.

Advanced tests include analyses of T-cell mitogenic responses to plant lectins like phytohemagglutinin or concanavalin A. One-way mixed lymphocyte reaction using radiolabeled thymidine quantifies the proliferative activity of lymphocytes.

Phagocytic Function

The number of phagocytes is evaluated with a complete blood cell count, a white blood cell differential count, and a peripheral smear. The nitroblue tetrazolium (NBT) test is decisive for CGD. In this test, the inability of a patient with CGD to reduce yellow nitroblue tetrazolium to blue formazan pigment is diagnostic. Specialized tests have been developed to assess phagocytosis, chemotaxis, and bactericidal activity. In LAD, a defect in CD18 expression on neutrophils can be demonstrated by flow cytometry.

Complement System

The estimation of total C3 and C4 proteins by immunoassays is the initial step. The complement bioassay forms the basis for evaluating the integrity of the complement system. Measurement of total hemolytic complement (CH50) of classical pathway by using antibody-sensitized sheep erythrocytes is quite informative. Deficiencies of alternative complement activation pathway constituents are evaluated in an assay (AH50) that uses unsensitized rabbit erythrocytes. A very low CH50 or AH50 reading implies deficiency of complement components and may point to a primary, genetic deficiency of complement. Quantitation of individual complement component analysis then would help in classifying the immunodeficiency and staging of the disease.

SUMMARY

Immunodeficiency disorders are characterized by the inadequacy of the immune system to fight tumors or invading organisms. The deficiency thus results in recurrent bacterial or viral infections particularly by organisms that are normally mild, incomplete recovery from illness or poor response to treatment, and an increased incidence of cancer. Immunodeficiency disorders may affect any part of the immune system. Most commonly, this involves decreased functioning of T or B lymphocytes (or both), or deficient antibody production. Inherited immune deficiencies are rare but very severe and are often fatal whereas the acquired deficiencies are relatively mild and many times reversible. The congenital immunodeficiency disorders generally involve either humoral or cellular immunity. Various types of genetic defects lead to the impaired production or incomplete maturation of B-cells or T-cells. Some of the immunodeficiencies are also precipitated by the deficient function of phagocytes or the complement system.

At this time you should know the following:

1. Brief of the immunodeficiency disorders.
2. Their major types and causative factors.
3. Immunodeficiencies affecting humoral immunity.
4. Immunodeficiencies affecting T-cell number and inappropriate activation.
5. Immunodeficiencies due to phagocytic dysfunction.
6. Immunodeficiencies due to inadequate complement activation.
7. Biochemical defects underlying different primary immunodeficiency disorders.
8. Tests available to diagnose and investigate these disorders.

Further Reading

1. Adrian J Thrasher, Hubert B. Gaspar and Christine Kinnon, 1999, Gene Therapy Technologies, Applications and Regulations, Edited by A Meager © 1999 John Wiley and Sons Ltd.
2. Azar AE. Evaluation of the adult with suspected immunodeficiency. Am J Med 2007;120:764-768.
3. Anon, 1993. The clinical presentation of the Primary immunodeficiency diseases, 1993. Available from: http://www.idfnz.org.nz/pub/cms/resources__medical/files/GPPRIM1.pdf
4. Ballow M, 2007. Primary immunodeficiency diseases. In: Cecil Medicine, Goldman L, Ausiello D, eds. 23rd ed. Philadelphia, Pa: Saunders Elsevier; chap 271.
5. Melvin Berger, 2008. Clinical Focus on Primary Immune Deficiencies–Subcutaneous IgG Therapy in Immune Deficiency Diseases. Kathleen Sullivan, Ed., Issue 13, Publisher Immune Deficiency Foundation. Available from: http://www.primaryimmune.org/publications/clinic_focus/cf_feb08.pdf
6. Morimoto Y, 2008. Immunodeficiency overview. Prim Care 35:159-173.

20

CHAPTER

Immunization

(Dr. B K Gupta, Dr. Debapriya Bandyopadhyay and Dr. Mohd. Suhail
anchitbharat@hotmail.com)

OBJECTIVES

1. To learn different types of immunity viz. active and passive immunity and how immunization is inducing immunity.
2. To know the brief history of vaccination and different novel approaches followed to design and develop safe and efficient vaccines.
3. To discuss different types of vaccines and their advantages, disadvantages and other characteristic features.
4. To describe the challenges and concerns in vaccine development and the possible adverse reactions due to vaccination.
5. What are the ongoing research(s) for developing vaccines against different diseases.

"The deviation of man from the state in which he was originally placed by nature seems to have proved to him a prolific source of diseases."

—*Edward Jenner*

INTRODUCTION

Immunization refers to the process of producing immunity in an organism. Our immune system is a remarkably evolved system. It can be taught to fight pathogenic microbes quickly. Immunization starts with the embryonic stage (in the passive form), where mother provides antibodies to the foetus through the placenta. After birth the infant continues to receive readymade antibodies through colostrum, whatever immunity the mother has, is transferred to the baby. To further protect the indiviual against fatal diseases, the vaccines play a very important role. Though vaccines are dependent on many factors like environment, genetic makeup of the host and lifestyle, they still are the most effective agents that save millions of lives. Vaccines have helped to overcome deadly diseases like Diphtheria, Measles, Mumps, Poliomyelitis, Smallpox and many other infectious diseases. Vaccine technology has developed a long way from using conventional 'attenuated' viral/microbial vaccines to nanoparticle mediated DNA vaccines. The advancements in immunotechnology research and molecular biology have led to generation of novel promising vaccines with enhanced activity.

The increasing knowledge about T-cells and B-cells has enabled researchers to design vaccines against both arms of immune system. It is estimated that vaccination has averted about 2 million deaths in 2002. This achievement is a result of hard work of thousands of researchers throughout the world working day and night to provide a tool to fight against those "notorious" little creatures, who have always troubled mankind. A crying need still remains for vaccines against many other diseases. The manufacture of a simple vaccine and its testing may take long time and this effort is fruitful only if vaccines are cost effective, safe, can be delivered to all and are easily accessible. As the molecular understanding of the pathogens improves due to different scientific and research developments, numerous new vaccines are being developed. There is a great hope among the researchers to design vaccines against as many diseases as possible and safeguard the human population from agony, misery and sufferings. However, due to the differences in the genetic makeup, it is difficult to make universal vaccine to provide optimal protection for a polymorphic population in different environment and lifestyle.

Immunity and Immunization

Immunity to micro-organisms can be achieved by active or passive immunization. Immunity is acquired actively when a person is exposed to foreign substances that trigger the immune system to protect against the foreign intruders. On the other hand, immunity is passively acquired when "ready made" antibodies are transferred from one organism to another. In each case immunity can be naturally (usually by antibodies from mother to foetus via placenta or by exposure to antigens) or artificially (by vaccines or by injecting preformed antibodies in the serum) acquired. Passive immunity aims at providing a transient or temporary protection from the existent situation, whereas the aim of active immunity is to provide immunity for subsequent pathogenic attacks (**Table 20.1**).

Active immunity is potentially advantageous for many reasons as this provides a long immunogenic memory, which is lacking in passive immunity. It induces cell-mediated immunity in addition to humoral immunity. In addition, it helps to get rid of the problem of histocompatibility mismatches. In case of passive immunization, there are risks of rejection associated with injection of antibodies produced in species different from the host. The host might elicit a strong response against the foreign antibodies. To overcome this problem, "humanized" antibodies need to be prepared. In today's world the most widespread practice for active immunization is vaccination. The technique has proved to be of real help in saving millions of lives around the globe. It has also helped the mankind to eradicate many lethal diseases like smallpox.

Vaccine means cow?–Historical Background of Immunization

Vaccine is derived from a Latin word "vaccinus" meaning pertaining to cows (but they are in no way related to cows). This name was given by Louis Pasteur in honour of the work done by Edward Jenner with cowpox inoculation. The history of vaccines dates back to 430 B.C. when Thucydides wrote that only those who had recovered of plague could nurse the patients because they would not suffer from the disease a second time. Several reports suggest that Chinese and Turks inhaled or inserted into cuts in skin (a technique called variolation), the dried

Table 20.1: Differences between the events involved in active and passive immunity/immunization effect

Active immunity	*Passive immunity*
Our body develops the antibodies on its own	Antibodies are acquired from some other source
a. Naturally by exposure to infection	a. Naturally by placental transfer
b. Artificially by vaccinations	b. Artificially as in getting antitoxin administration for Rabies, Hepatitis A, Tetanus
Develops slowly but long lasting	Develops fast but temporary
Both humoral and cell mediated responses are generated	Only humoral response is generated

crusts obtained from smallpox pustules to escape the disease.

Edward Jenner, an English physician observed that milkmaids who had contacted cowpox were immune to smallpox. To test this he inoculated an eight years old boy James Phipps with the material derived from a cowpox pustule and later challenged him with the material taken from a smallpox lesion. The boy did not develop the disease. The technique spread quickly throughout Europe. Later Pasteur carried out some experiments with attenuated microbes and showed that weakened germs provide immunity for the second attack. As Jenner and Pasteur are recognized for their contributions in active immunization, similarly Emil von Behry and Hidesaburo Kitasato became pioneers of passive immunization, when they demonstrated that by transfer of serum from immunized animals, unimmunized animals can be protected.

Design Criteria of Safe Vaccine for Effective Immunization

Though vaccines are generating immunity against lethal diseases, not all vaccines are totally safe. Few basic requirements are to be met while designing efficient vaccines. The prime requirement is safety. Some viral vaccines are composed of attenuated or weakened components like polio, hepatitis etc., which have the potential to revert to their fully virulent form that can cause disease in the normal or immunocompromised individuals. The vaccines comprising killed microbes can also be unsafe as in the case of whooping cough where the vaccine though effective is toxic. The second important requirement is the duration of immunity. A vaccine is expected to provide long term immunity. The principle of vaccination is based on the activation of secondary immune response, which is prompt, powerful and prolonged than the primary response. Different organisms have different incubation period as the mode and site of infection varies from organism to organism and it is also based on host. To combat the organisms having shorter incubation period, high antibody titer should be present. This can be achieved by repeated immunizations, which is generally known as booster dose.

Vaccine should be immunogenic. This is the most important consideration for vaccine development as immunogenicity is the property to elicit an immune response. All antigens are not necessarily immunogens. The size of antigens should be greater than 10,000 Daltons in order to mount an immune response. The antigens less than the given molecular weight are labelled 'haptens'. These haptens need to be conjugated with a carrier molecule called adjuvants to be immunogenic.

Haptens are substances which are incapable of inducing antibody formation on their own, but can combine specifically with antibodies. Haptens may be 'simple' or 'complex'. Simple haptens are univalent—they can combine with the specific antibody but they cannot precipitate the same. Complex haptens are polyvalent and they can combine with the specific antibody and also precipitate them. This is as per the assumption that precipitation requires the antigen to have two or more antibody binding sites.

Adjuvants are chemical substances, which enhance the immunogenicity that need to be added as a carrier with low molecular antigens but the problem accounted here is only one adjuvant, i.e., alum (aluminium salt) is approved for human use so far. In order to determine the route of vaccination it is important to have the knowledge about humoral and cell-mediated immune system and their collective response. Moreover, the vaccine should not be immunosuppressive, i.e., to protect the body from one disease it should not make the individual susceptible to others.

As indicated in **Table 20.2**, multiple booster doses at adequate intervals need to be administered to achieve an effective immunity. Depending upon the site of action, route of administration and site of injection needs to be determined.

Table 20.2: Vaccination schedule and their route of administration

Vaccine	*Route of administration*	*Site of injection*	*Birth*	*Age of vaccination*			
				6 weeks	*10 weeks*	*14 weeks*	*9 months*
BCG	Intradermal	Upper left arm	Y				
Oral Polio	Oral	Mouth	Y*	Y	Y	Y	
DTP	Intramuscular	Outer mid-thigh		Y	Y	Y	
Hep B							
Scheme A[a]	Intramuscular	Outer mid-thigh	Y	Y		Y	
Scheme B[a]	Intramuscular	Outer mid-thigh		Y	Y	Y	
Measles	Subcutaneous	Upper left arm					Y[c]
Measles mumps, rubella (MMR)	Subcutaneous	Upper mid-thigh or Upper arm					Y
Yellow fever	Subcutaneous	Upper right arm					Y[b]
Tetanus toxoid # (TT)	Intramuscular	Outer, upper arm		Y		Y	
Haemophilus Influenzae type[b] (Hib)	Intramuscular	Infants–outer mid thigh Older children–upper arm		Y	Y	Y	

Key: * In polio endemic countries; [a] Scheme A is recommended in those countries, where perinatal transmission of hepatitis virus is frequent (e.g. in South-East Asia). Scheme B is recommended for the countries, where perinatal transmission is less frequent (e.g. in Sub-Saharan Africa); [b] in countries, where yellow fever pose the risk; [c] a second opportunity to receive a dose of measles vaccine should be provided for all children; # Primary course - 3 doses of vaccine (usually as combined DTaP/IPV/Hib) at 2, 3 and 4 months of age. Fourth dose - at least 3 years after the primary course, usually pre-school entry (as DTaP/IPV). Fifth dose - aged 13-18 years before leaving school (as Td/IPV)

Vaccines, like other pharmaceutical products, have to undergo sequentially-phased trials to be regarded as safe for use. The trials include preclinical testing, which is conducted in cell cultures and animals and clinical trials, which are conducted on human volunteers once the vaccine appears promising in the preclinical experiments. The clinical trials are divided into four phases. Phase I studies enrol 20 or fewer people and primarily tests for safety. Phase II involves 50 to several hundred people. This is to test the safety as well as to determine the optimal dosage and to gather preliminary data on vaccine's effectiveness. Phase III studies are meant for thorough testing of the vaccine's potency and efficacy to protect against the disease. It includes thousands of people. In addition, most licensed vaccines continue to be evaluated with very large studies that look at tens of thousands of people, who have received the vaccine. These Phase IV studies try to pick up rare or delayed adverse reactions that might not have been apparent in the smaller studies that led to therapeutic approval.

Types of Vaccines

Different strategies have been adopted by researchers for developing effective and safe vaccines. A brief account of how these vaccines work and induce humoral/cell-mediated immunity has been given below. Most of them have been already put to practice but a few like DNA vaccines are still in experimental stages. As the vaccine technology development and discovery is progressing day by day, new prospects like making edible vaccines through plants and therapeutic proteins through milk and egg, which are under research level are quite promising for the affordability of mass vaccination. Due to various technical complexities in designing an ideal vaccine for a particular disease, it is very difficult and cumbersome to formulate a vaccine without any disadvantages (**Table 20.3**).

Table 20.3: Types of vaccines and their advantages and disadvantages. Not all vaccines are having similar characteristics. The performance and efficacy of the vaccines differ based on their type and target

Type	*Disease*	*Advantage*	*Disadvantage*
Live, attenuated	Tuberculosis, Measles, Mumps	Produces a strong immune response. Gives life long immunity. Inexpensive.	Microbe may revert back to its virulent form. Must be kept at low temperature to maintain vaccine potency.
Inactivated and killed	Cholera, Plague, Rabies	Safer and more stable than live vaccines. Can be transported without refrigeration.	High toxicity. Limited duration of immunity. Weaker immune response.
Toxoid vaccine	Diphtheria, Tetanus	Makes body immune to bacterial toxins.	Regular boosters required.
Subunit vaccine	Hepatitis B	Specific in nature. Fewer antigens, so lesser chances of side effects.	Identifying the best antigen may be difficult and time consuming.
Capsular polysaccharide	Meningococcal meningitis	Makes immune system identify some bacteria, which can disguise their antigens using their envelopes.	Poor immunizers. Tremendous structural and serologic variability of antigens.

1. Whole Organism Vaccine

In this strategy whole organisms (either attenuated or killed) are used to induce an immune response and provide vaccination. The organisms used are made avirulent but the important structural components (epitopes), which help immune system to recognize them, are preserved so that the modified organisms can mimic the original virulent type.

a. Live, Attenuated Vaccine:

These vaccines comprise the attenuated, i.e., avirulent bacterial cells or viral particles. Attenuation enables the production of microorganisms that are similar to the original microbe but have no ability to cause the disease. Attenuated viral vaccines are easier to create as compared to attenuated bacterial vaccines because viruses have smaller number of genes and thus, their characteristics can be controlled easily. Attenuation is generally done by growing the pathogen under adverse culture conditions or by the prolonged passage of microorganism through different hosts. Attenuated vaccines generate humoral as well as cell-mediated immune response. This is because of the greater exposure of the host immune system to the epitope of the attenuated microorganisms and the ability of the attenuated vaccine to replicate in the host.

This increased immunogenicity eliminates the need of repeated booster dose of the vaccine which is of great advantage for the developing nations. In spite of its advantages, the major constraint on the use of attenuated vaccine is that there are chances of the live, avirulent microorganism to revert back to its virulent form. In order to prevent this, scientists are employing genetic engineering techniques to bring about irreversible attenuation of the microorganisms to be used as vaccines. This is done by selectively eliminating genes responsible for virulence of the pathogen. For example, it has been done with a herpes virus vaccine for pigs, in which thymidine kinase gene was removed. Another problem with attenuated strains is that they have to be refrigerated to stay potent. Despite its demerits, a large number of diseases are being prevented by the use of attenuated vaccines.

b. Inactivated or Killed Vaccine:

In these vaccines, the ability of the pathogen to cause disease is completely destroyed by inactivation of the pathogen with the help of heat, radiation or chemical treatment. Due to this, the pathogen is no longer able to replicate in the host. It is important to ensure that the surface antigens are not destroyed during the inactivation of pathogen. Thus, heat inactivation is generally avoided. Formaldehyde treatment is the most used technique for inactivation. The inactivated vaccine stimulates a weaker immune response that is mainly humoral as compared to the live, attenuated vaccines. Thus, multiple booster doses are required to maintain immunity against the pathogen. Since inactivated vaccines cannot replicate, they cannot cause any fatal infection. These vaccines are more stable than attenuated vaccines as there is no possibility of these vaccines to revert back to their virulent form.

2. Subunit Vaccines

The whole pathogen sometimes contains antigens that lead to problems by triggering hypersensitivity or by suppressing the immune response to protective antigens. Thus, immunization with the isolated protective antigens (subunits) will prevent these complications. But identification of protective antigens is a challenging task. Mainly three forms of subunit vaccines are in use, the toxoid vaccine, bacterial capsular polysaccharide vaccine, and recombinant antigen vaccine.

a. Toxoid Vaccine:

This vaccine is used, when the bacterial exotoxin is the main cause of illness (for example, in case of diphtheria and tetanus). This toxin is capable of producing the disease symptoms that result from infection. It has been found that these exotoxins can be inactivated by treating them with formalin, a solution of sterilized water and formaldehyde. These detoxified toxins, namely toxoids, are used as vaccines. This detoxification should be done without excessive modifications to the epitope structure as shown in **Figure 20.1**. On encountering the vaccine containing a harmless toxoid, the immune system learns to fight the natural toxin during infection. Nowadays, gene cloning techniques are used to produce large quantities of the pathogenic exotoxin for its use as toxoid vaccine.

b. Capsular Polysaccharide as Vaccine:

These vaccines are used against those pathogenic bacteria, whose virulence mainly depends on the ability of their hydrophilic polysaccharide capsule to disguise the bacterial antigens so that the immune system of the host is not able to recognise or respond to them. This polysaccharide layer prevents the bacterium from being eliminated by opsonophagocytic or lytic killing. Thus, to overcome this bacterial mechanism of resistance, the generation of antibodies against the polysaccharide is required. In capsular polysaccharide vaccines, the antigens or toxoids from a microbe that an infant's immune system can recognize are conjugated to the bacterial polysaccharide. For example, the vaccine for haemophilus influenzae type B (Hib), the major cause of bacterial meningitis in children, consists of type b capsular polysaccharide covalently linked to a protein carrier, tetanus toxoid. This technique has proved to be successful in making these vaccines immunogenic and effective against infections. A major disadvantage with capsular polysaccharide vaccines is the vast structural and serological variability in the antigens along with poor immunogenicity of some of them.

c. Recombinant Antigen Vaccine:

The recombinant antigen vaccines comprise the pathogens protective antigen molecules, which best stimulate the immune system and they are manufactured by Recombinant DNA Technology. The genes encoding surface antigens from virus, bacteria and other microorganisms are cloned into bacterial, yeast, insect or mammalian expression systems. The

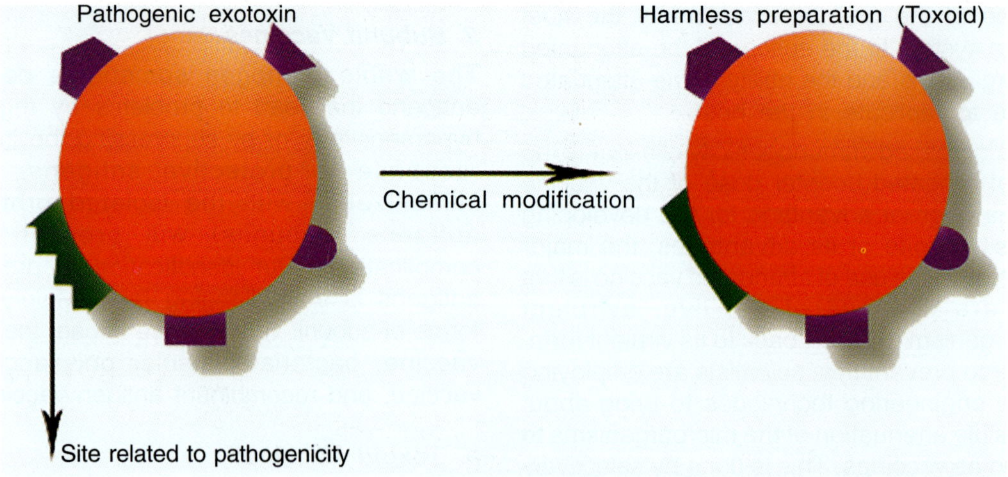

Fig. 20.1: Modification of bacterial toxin to harmless toxoid. Bacterial exotoxin epitopes are shown in green and site responsible for toxicity in red. The pathogenicity related site is altered without changing the epitopes. The modified toxin can be used as a safe vaccine as the modification has rendered it harmless

expressed protein or antigen is then used for vaccine development. Such recombinant vaccine has been made for hepatitis B virus. The vaccine was developed by cloning the gene encoding important surface antigens in yeast cells. The antigens produced were isolated and purified for use in the vaccine development. The potential application of such gene cloning in vaccine production seems very promising to design better vaccines in an economical way.

3. DNA Vaccines

DNA vaccines take immunization to a new technological level. These vaccines contain the genes encoding for the important surface antigens capable of triggering the immune response. In this strategy, plasmid DNA encoding antigenic proteins is introduced into the recipients muscle cells as shown in **Figure 20.2**. The injected gene is expressed in the injected muscle cell and the nearby Antigen Presenting Cells (APCs). These cells then display these antigen molecules on their surface. This leads to the generation of both humoral antibody response and the cell-mediated response as the cells involved in immunity become vaccine manufacturing factories. These DNA vaccines can be administered through conventional methods like syringe or biolistic gun and novel methods like nanoparticle mediated targeted delivery and transport.

The main advantage of DNA vaccine is that the encoded protein is expressed in its natural form in the host. They stimulate good immune response and also generate significant immunological memory. The storage and handling of the plasmid DNA does not require refrigeration. But, as there are two sides of a coin, there are safety issues raised with regard to DNA vaccines. These include the probability of integration of plasmid DNA into the cellular DNA, development of autoimmunity and antibiotic resistance. Naked DNA vaccine being tested in humans includes

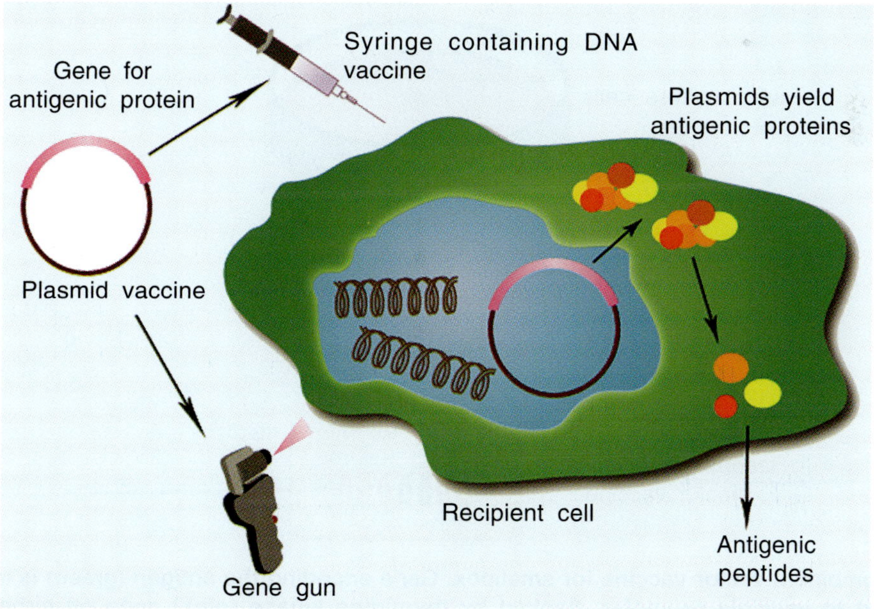

Fig. 20.2: Immunization with DNA vaccine. The gene encoding the antigen (pink) is cloned into a plasmid and inserted in the cell directly or by using a gene gun or through suitable nanocarriers. The plasmid enters nucleus and translates antigens. These antigens produced trigger immunity to the individual

those against malaria, influenza, herpes and HIV. Still in experimenting and testing stages, these vaccines show great promise for future.

4. Recombinant Vector Vaccines

Recombinant vector vaccines are similar to DNA vaccines, but these vaccines do not introduce the pathogenic genes directly into the recipient cells. Instead, they use a bacterial or viral vector system for this purpose. In the preparation of these vaccines, the genes encoding the major antigens of the virulent pathogen are introduced and expressed into an attenuated virus or bacterium. This attenuated organism acts as a vector, replicates in the host and thus, expresses the gene product of the pathogen. Initially, Vaccinia virus were used as a vector because during replication of poxviruses, the DNA recombination occurs extensively and this facilitates the insertion of foreign DNA into the viral genome as described in **Figure 20.3**. Attenuated bacterial vectors are also used. The

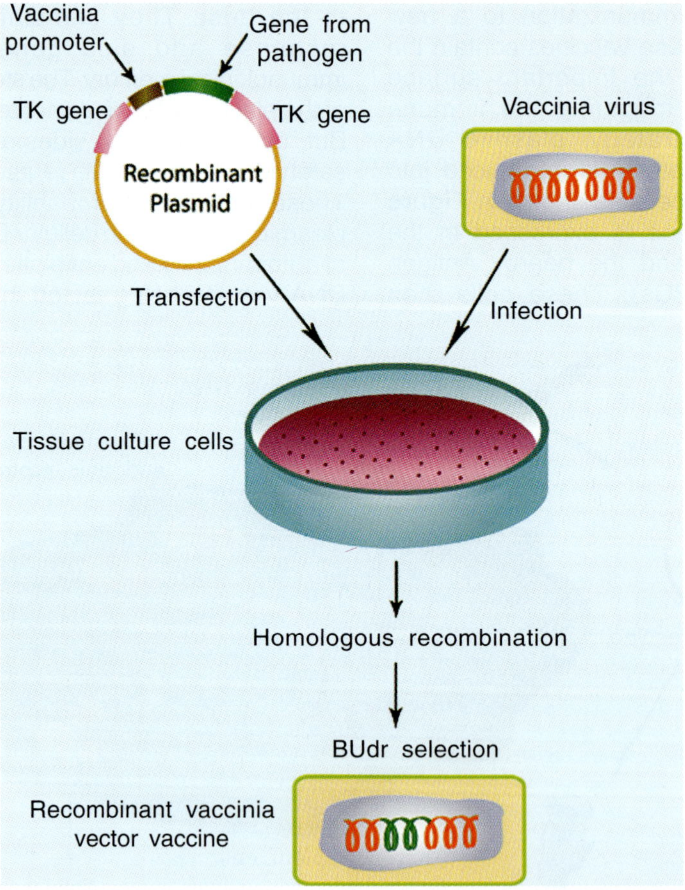

Fig. 20.3: Recombinant vector vaccine for smallpox. Gene encoding the antigen (green) is inserted into a plasmid next to vaccinia promoter, flanked by thymidine kinase (pink) gene on either side. The vaccinia virus and recombinant plasmid are incubated in tissue culture cells simultaneously. The recombinant plasmid is inserted into the virus by homologous recombination at the site of TK gene, resulting in TK^- recombinant virus. These recombinant viruses were then selected by bromodeoxyuridine (BUdr) which kills TK^+ cells

inserted gene of the virulent pathogen causes the bacteria to display the encoded antigens of the pathogen on its surface. Thus, a harmless bacterium mimics a harmful microbe and elicits the immune response.

Other organisms used as vaccine vectors are adenovirus, BCG strain of *Mycobacterium bovis*, attenuated polio virus, and attenuated strains of *Salmonella*. Recombinant vector vaccines can elicit both a strong cellular as well as humoral immune response. But, the major drawback of these vaccines is the generation of a strong immune response against the vector itself.

5. Multivalent Subunit Vaccines

The main limitation of synthetic peptide vaccines is that they do not elicit a strong immune response and the recombinant vaccines sometimes lead to generation of a strong immune response against the vector itself. In order to check these problems, multivalent subunit vaccines are being developed that contain both immunodominant B-cell and T-cell epitopes. Two basic approaches are used to develop these vaccines. The first being the preparation of solid matrix-antibody-antigen (SMAA) complexes having synthetic peptides representing both B-cell and T-cell epitopes (**Figure 20.4**). SMAA complexes induce vigorous humoral and cell-mediated reactions. Various proteins involved in inducing protective immune responses to different viruses can easily be incorporated into SMAA complexes and these complexes act as powerful multivalent immunogens.

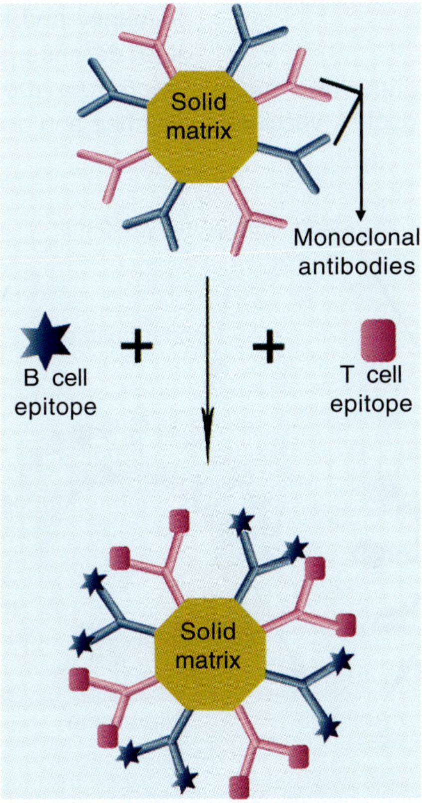

Fig. 20.4: Solid matrix–antibody-antigen (SMAA) comprises a solid matrix on which, the synthetic peptides having B-cell epitopes (blue) and T-cell epitopes (pink) are attached. These complexes act as multivalent immunogens and induce vigorous immune responses

Construction of such SMAA complexes may be one of the most practical and effective ways of producing multivalent subunit vaccines for use in humans and animals. Another means of producing these vaccines is by the use of liposomes, micelles or immunostimulating complexes (ISCOMs), which are particulate antigen delivery vehicles composed of saponin, cholesterol, phospholipids and immunogen. These are lipids carriers prepared by mixing protein with detergent and by a glycoside called Quil A (as shown in **Figure 20.5**). The pathogens, whose membrane proteins have been incorporated into micelles, liposomes or ISCOMs include influenza virus, measles virus, hepatitis B virus and HIV. These vaccines have the ability to deliver the antigen intracellularly, which induces a cell-mediated response and hence increase the immunogenicity.

6. Edible Vaccine

Despite of advances in efficient and safe vaccine development, the noble goal of "vaccines to all" still remains unfulfilled, largely because of constraints like cost of production, transportation and their delivery. So much of research is on the way to solve these limitations by finding ways to produce oral/edible vaccines through transgenic plants (**Table 20.4**). Researchers are now considering plants as bio-factories for the production of immunotherapeutic and bioactive molecules. Like conventional subunit vaccines, edible vaccines can be designed that are comprised antigenic proteins but are devoid of pathogenic genes. Thus, they have no chance in establishing infection, assuring its safety especially in immuno-compromised patients. Edible vaccines are capable of activating both mucosal and systemic immunity and this dual effect provides the first line defense against pathogens like *Mycobacterium tuberculosis*, pathogens causing diarrhea and pneumonia, different STDs and HIV.

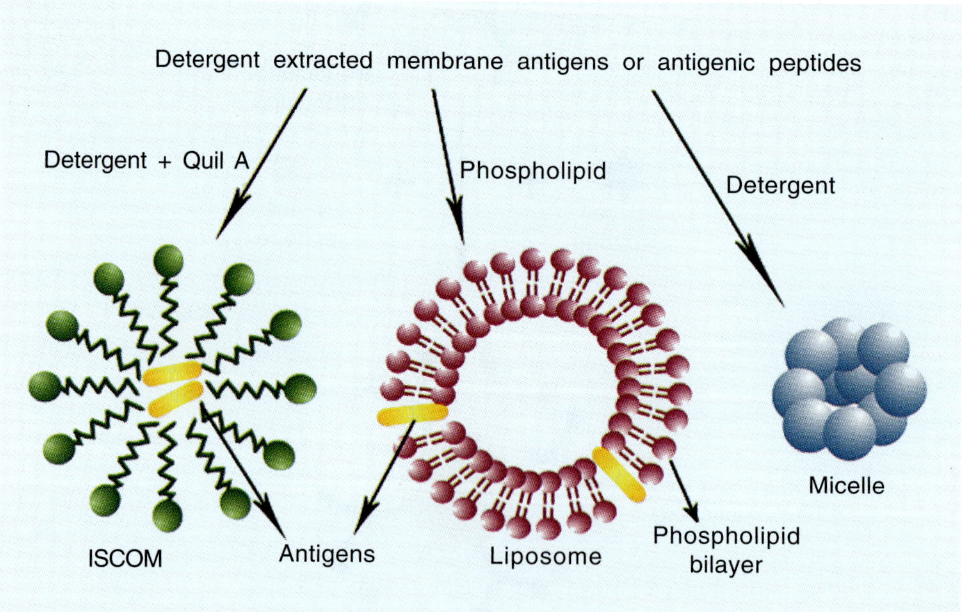

Fig. 20.5: Preparation of multivalent subunit vaccines using immunostimulating complexes (ISCOMs). These delivery vehicles are generally made from lipids and comprise the antigen from the pathogen against which, an immune response is to be elicited

Table 20.4: Plants expressing different antigens that can be used as edible vaccines. As plants are expressing such antigens (epitopes) that can be edible, the cost of vaccine is greatly reduced and the availability and affordability is in the reach. However, the safety aspects of such genetically modified plant/edible vaccine and the effectivity of these expressed antigenic proteins as vaccines has to be validated in all dimensions

Antigenic protein	*Plant*
1. Hepatitis B surface antigen	Tobacco
2. *E.coli* heat labile enterotoxin B subunit	Potato
3. Cholera toxin B subunit	Potato, tobacco
4. Insulin	Potato
5. Rabies virus glycoprotein	Tomato

The concept of edible vaccine may look promising and appealing for generating effective immunization through cost-effective, simple vaccination strategies through fruits and vegetables. However, the host digestive system may digest/degrade the epitopes of the pathogen that is expressed in the edible vaccine. Hence, there is a possibility that the edible vaccine may not generate any immune response as it is not absorbed in the system in its proper structure. In addition, the expressed (antigenic) protein that acts as a vaccine may interact with the native proteins of the plant system that may give rise into an abnormal/unexpected protein folding pattern which may not induce immunization but may be hazardous to the human system. Therefore, safety and efficacy of these vaccines has to be validated and optimized.

Challenges in Vaccine Development

- Vaccine development and production incorporates many medically related as well as technically related tasks, ranging from basic research in immunology, microbiology, human physiology/metabolism and pharmaceutical development to studies of production scaling up, economics of vaccine production and effectiveness.
- The challenges of vaccine development are not just limited to identification of suitable antigens, adjuvants and delivery methods, but

Table 20.5: Important strains of organisms used for vaccination

Mumps vaccine	Jeryl Lynch strain. RIT 4835 is a newer strain derived from the Jeryl Lynch
Measles vaccine	Edmonston Zagreb
Rubella vaccine	RA 27/3
Polio vaccine	*Oral Polio vaccine (Sabin's)* contains Type 1:10 lakh, Type 2:2 lakh and Type 3:3 lakh live attenuated Polio viruses, per test dose. *Injectable polio vaccine (Salk's)* is an inactivated vaccine, not in use in our country.
Typhoid vaccine	Oral Ty 21a live vaccine Injectable Vi polysaccharide vaccine.
Yellow fever vaccine	17D strain, attenuated by growth in chick embryo.
BCG vaccine	Bacille Calmette-Guerin. Danish 1331 strain of Mycobacterium bovis, attenuated by 239 serial subcultures in a glycerine-bile-potato medium over a period of 13 years.
Meningococcal vaccine	Types A,C,Y, W 135 polysaccharide vaccine (indicated in asplenic individuals, terminal complement deficiency and properdin deficiency).
Japanese encephalitis	Nakayama strain (grown in suckling mouse brain) Formaldehyde inactivated and purified.

include many other regulatory, technical and manufacturing hurdles.

- The great serological diversity of the pathogenic microbes and genetic hypervariability of certain pathogens, especially viruses make the universal vaccine development an onerous task.
- Sometimes, the vaccines used in animal trials do not predict the vaccine's effectiveness in humans.
- The effect of the vaccine on the recipient depends upon the genetic variability and the ethnicity, and also on the environment of vaccine application, thus, complicating the development of an effective vaccine.
- Vaccines must be developed with such strategies that they prove to be the most cost-effective interventions available to humanity.

Concerns

- Vaccines are very beneficial but can some times work adversely. There are serious stories aired in some articles, where children have been affected adversely. Some misconceptions and the real facts from such myths are discussed here.
- There is a general view among the common men that the vaccines are not necessary and are useless probably because they have never seen anybody being infected of diseases against which they are getting immunized. The eradication of diseases like smallpox, and the drastic decrease in number of cases of measles, rubella etc. prove that vaccines are working phenomenally well. Vaccines not only protect the individuals but the whole society. Some diseases that occur at a very low rate can take the form of an epidemic if vaccination is stopped.
- Another important concern is pertaining to the age of vaccination. Many vaccines are given to children less than one year of age. This is done to protect them from diseases when their immune system is immature. Young children are surprisingly good at developing immunity and become protected against most diseases they have been immunized against.
- It is often considered that natural infection is better than immunization. Natural infection causes immunity after one infection and is usually life long whereas; vaccines create immunity only after several doses. But the risk associated with natural infections is great. Mental retardation in case of Hib and paralysis in case of polio is a price too high to be paid for immunity. Some times unexpected mortality also occurs, which can not be affordable for any matured civilized society.
- A common misconception existing is that the vaccines may weaken the immune system. Natural infection can sometimes weaken the immune system in the sense that patients infected with one viral disease cannot fight with other viruses but the case of vaccines is different. The viruses are disabled and made into avirulent form to such an extent that they can hardly weaken the immune system.
- Vaccines contain preservatives (thimerosal) having mercury which might harm the infants. Preservatives are needed in multidose vials of vaccines to prevent any bacterial contamination which may cause serious infections. It is true that mercury is harmful for the neural system but only if it is present in high concentration. The amount of mercury present in the vaccines is in acceptable quantities, which is regarded safe.

For efficient vaccination it is necessary to increase the immunization levels because they are the indicators for detecting any problems related to the delivery of vaccines. Few concerns regarding the immunization levels include the childhood immunization rates, which are suboptimal and immunization rates of other age groups, which are even lower. Cost-effectiveness is another important issue. The strategies that can increase immunization levels with least expenditure should be prioritized so that the people in economically backward areas/countries are able to afford the vaccines and get themselves immunized. Sustainable systems for immunization delivery need to be developed so that every individual can be effectively vaccinated.

Vaccine Induced Adverse Reactions and Safety Assessment

Vaccines are intended to produce active immunity to specific antigens in the target system. Adverse reactions resulting from vaccination are the additional effects to the vaccine's primary purpose of providing immunity. The adverse effects resulting from vaccination can be classified by frequency, extent, severity, causality and preventability. These reactions are further divided into the following categories:

- **Vaccine induced:** These effects occur only on vaccination as they are induced by the intrinsic characteristics of the vaccine preparation and the individual response of the vaccine (e.g., vaccine-associated paralytic poliomyelitis).
- **Vaccine potentiated:** This reaction would occur even without vaccines but the effect is intensified on vaccination.
- **Programmatic error:** Adverse effects arising due to technical errors during vaccine preparation, storage, handling or administration.
- **Coincidental:** The effects, which do not result from vaccination but happen by chance or by any other illness.

Recent Developments

1. Human Papilloma Viruses (HPV)

Human papillomaviruses (HPV) are group of DNA-based viruses that infect the skin and the mucous membranes of human and animals. Over 100 different types of HPV have been characterized. They cause benign skin warts or papillomas, which might lead to cancer. Sexually transmitted HPV is the major cause of cervical cancer, which is one of the most important causes of cancer deaths among women in the developing countries. Cervical cancer kills around 240000 women annually. Vaccines consisting of virus like particles (VLPs) can prevent papilloma virus disease in human beings. Gardasil, a prophylactic HPV vaccine which is marketed by Merck was approved by the FDA on June 8, 2006. This vaccine covers the four types of HPV, including the cancer-causing types 16 and 18 and types 6 and 11 of non-cancerous genital warts. As the adolescents are on high risk for HPV infections, the age of vaccination is around 18-25.

2. Meningococcal Meningitis

Meningitis is an inflammation of the meninges, the thin lining surrounding the brain and the spinal cord. Several different bacteria and viruses can cause this infection and *Neisseria meningitidis* is most potent one because of its ability to cause epidemics. Thirteen subtypes or serogroups of *N. meningitidis* have been identified and five of them (*N. meningitidis* A, B, C, Y and W135) are known to cause epidemics. Approximately 5% to 10% of the population carry the meningococcal bacteria in the nose and throat in a harmless state. This carrier state may last for days or months and seems to give those individuals who harbour meningococcus in their upper respiratory tract, some protection from actually developing the disease state. Meningococcal meningitis can be particularly dangerous for two main reasons, it is relatively rare and it can be deceptive.

Polysaccharide vaccines are currently in use, but these are not very effective against infections in young children. These vaccines are unable to develop long lasting immunity and do not confer the 'herd effect', that is they do not prevent the spread of the disease in the non-vaccinated individuals. Meningitis vaccine project (MVP) is an example of an effort to develop "Men A" conjugate vaccine. Toxicology and animal studies have been completed which suggest that the vaccine is highly immunogenic. Other conjugate vaccines, a heptavalent vaccine (DTP Hep B Hib) covering serogroups A and C is under development.

3. Human Immunodeficiency Virus (HIV)

The Acquired Immuno Deficiency Syndrome (AIDS) was first observed in 1981. By the end of 2004 the estimated number of patients reached 39 million worldwide. Some of the commonly used strategies to fight the disease are as described below:

a. Peptide Vaccine–It involves tiny pieces of proteins from HIV virus which act as antigens to provide immunity.
b. Recombinant Subunit Protein Vaccine–In this approach the glycoprotein envelope of HIV is genetically engineered and used as vaccine.

The main problem with HIV is that it is highly mutable. It quickly responds to the selective pressure imposed by the immune system and evolves itself to fight against it. Another problem accounted for is high variability of HIV. Due to this, immune response mounted by one vaccine is not broad enough to fight all the strains and be effective against this high genetic variability.

4. Alzheimer's Disease

It is a progressive, neurodegenerative disorder named after German physician Alois Alzheimer, commonly found in people above 65 years of age. It is characterized by the formation of plaques of misfolded proteins called β-amyloid in the brain, years before the clinical symptoms of the disease appear. These plaques result in the atrophy of the affected regions of brain and reduction in the activity of cholinergic neurons which leads to reduced levels of acetylcholine neurotransmitter. Vaccine for Alzheimer's treats the diagnosed patients rather than preventing the disease spread. The vaccine trains the immune system to target the β-amyloid plaques in the brain which can prevent further deposition of the plaques and thus avoid spread of the disease. Vaccinated patients showed slower progression of the disease due to high levels of antibodies against β-amyloids. AN-1792 is a synthetic form of β-amyloid peptide and it is potent candidate for the Alzheimer's vaccine. It elicits clearance of β-amyloid peptides and plaques in the brain. Onset of microcerebral hemorrhages with passive immunization and meningoencephalitis with active immunization is a threat to this strategy.

Conclusion

The development of vaccines has been one of the most important contributions of Medical research to the community. Vaccines are now widely and routinely used throughout the world. Despite of so many concerns and arguments, vaccines have worked well to protect people from many dangerous diseases in many parts of the world. Due to vaccines, few lethal diseases were eradicated or controlled significantly. While most of the earlier vaccines were developed from live, attenuated or killed micro-organisms, the current technology involves the application of genetic engineering techniques to develop vaccines in the form of DNA vaccine, recombinant vector vaccines and edible vaccines. Hypodermic injections were once the only method of vaccination but now scientists are looking for new, innovative and if possible *non-invasive* methods of delivering vaccines. The immunization campaign carried out by WHO throughout the world against smallpox resulted in its eradication in 1977. According to WHO facts, immunization averted 2 million deaths in 2002.

Since many years, a large number of biomedical and immunological concepts and principles have been explored to facilitate vaccine development including toxoids, purified antigens, killed pathogens, conjugate vaccines, and peptide and DNA vaccines. Still, the diversity and complexity of microbial pathogens, their antigens, and the type of immune response to be elicited by the vaccine presents a challenging task. Vaccine development is often limited by the great serological diversity of protective epitopes expressed by the pathogenic microbes and also by our incomplete understanding of this vast field of science. Sustained research in the field of immunology and vaccinology for the development of new effective vaccines against the emerging infectious diseases is the need of the hour. Though there is a long way to go, the emerging trends in Molecular Biology, Immunotechnology, Nanomedicine and Stem Cell Research may give so many promising prospects towards these objectives of making ideal vaccines for various infectious diseases.

At this time you should know the following:

1. The types of immunity viz. active and passive immunity and how immunization is inducing immunity.
2. Brief history of vaccination and different novel approaches followed to design and develop safe and efficient vaccines.
3. Different types of vaccines and their advantages, disadvantages and other characteristic features.
4. Challenges and concerns in vaccine development and the possible adverse reactions due to vaccination.
5. Ongoing research in vaccinology for developing vaccines against many diseases.

Further Reading

1. Roitt's Essential Immunology: Delves, Martin, Burton and Roitt.
2. Cellular and Molecular Immunology: Abbas, Lichtman, Pillai.
3. Janeway's Immunobiology: Murphy, Travers, Walport.
4. http://www.who.int/topics/immunization/en/
5. http://www.nlm.nih.gov/medlineplus/immunization.html
6. http://www.unicef.org/immunization/index.html

21

CHAPTER

Recent Advances in Immunology

(Dr. Rajinder Chawla chawlarn@cmcludhiana.in)

OBJECTIVES

1. To understand the novel mechanisms involved in elucidating an immune response.
2. To know about the newly discovered immunomodulatory molecules.
3. To apply immuno proteomics in understanding the mechanisms of gene expression and protein-protein interactions at molecular level.
4. To identify the biomarkers for GVHD.
5. To comprehend the molecular mechanisms involved in tumor immunology.
6. To explore the potential of immune therapy to fight cancer.
7. To study the applications of novel techniques in understanding the mechanisms underlying an immune response.

INTRODUCTION

Immunology has come a long way from the time of microscopic observations of the cells involved in immune reaction, when our understanding of immunology was limited to proliferation or depletion of lymphocytes, to a stage where we are able to tailor the specificity of antibodies and use them for specific targeting of the pathological tissue. Today, our knowledge of immunology is not only helping us in diagnosing the diseased state, but is also providing us with tools and protocols to manipulate and kill the target tissues. The demons of cancer and AIDS are being tamed with the help of latest technological advances in the field of immunology. Immunology is not only providing us with newer methods to conquer disease but is also helping us in understanding the mechanisms of gene expression and protein-protein interaction, in normal cellular physiology, at the molecular level. A brief summary of the latest themes of research in the field of immunology is presented in this chapter.

Understanding the Mechanism of Immune Response

Our knowledge of the cells of the immune system has grown multifold over the last few decades. We are able to not only detect and count the number of different types of cells involved in immune activation, but are able to look into their functional hierarchy *in-vivo*. The details of the sequence of immune cell activation, through mutual exchange of regulator cytokines, is being uncovered.

"We see a much more detailed understanding of the action of cells in the immune response in association with a variety of different disease states", says Kristine Kuus-Reichel, director of research for the immunomics business unit at Beckman Coulter. "What is emerging is a more complex understanding of the immunology that involves many fields of science. We are understanding the mechanisms of the immune response and how it plays out in pathogenesis of the disease." We are looking at the post-translational modifications of proteins, with reference to major histocompatibility complex, in a newer light.

Some of the thrust areas of research in understanding the mechanism of immune response are presented in the following text:

Ubiquitin Proteasome System

Ubiquitination of the proteins tags them for degradation by proteasome1. The ubiquitin-proteasome system (UPS) regulates half-life of the endogenous as well as exogenous proteins and is essential for many cellular processes, including cell cycle, regulation of the gene expression, and responses to oxidative stress. The importance of proteolytic degradation inside cells and the role of ubiquitin in proteolytic pathways was acknowledged in the award of the 2004 Nobel Prize in Chemistry to Aaron Ciechanover, Avram Hershko and Irwin Rose.

The proteasome plays a straightforward but critical role in processing and presentation of antigenic peptides bound by the major histocompatibility complex (MHC) class I molecule. The ubiquitinated protein substrate is delivered into the 26S proteasome to be digested and degraded. The proteasome degrading substrate actually involves protein-protein interactions. Research into the prediction of proteasome cleavage site(s) has not been able to give information of the proteasome interacting with its substrate, and so the accuracy and reliability of these proteasome cleavage predictive methods still needs to be improved.

The defective Ub/Ub1 system could change the (MHC) immunological profile of the cells. Inhibitors of ubiquitin system have even been projected to have anti-cancer activity and could make part of the treatment protocol of neurodegenerative diseases. Alzheimer's disease patients exhibit large poly-ubiquitin containing protein aggregates (Lewy bodies).

Due to its role in generating the activated form of NF-κB (an anti-apoptotic and pro-inflammatory regulator of cytokine expression) proteasomal activity has been linked to inflammatory and autoimmune diseases like SLE and rheumatoid arthritis. A number of laboratories are working in this area to develop new tools to identify and study proteins involved in Ub/Ubl modification(s).

Signal Transduction

In biology, *signal transduction* is the process by which an extracellular signaling molecule activates a membrane receptor that in turn alters intracellular molecules creating a response. Certain microbial molecules, e.g., viral nucleotides, bacterial lipopolysaccharides, and protein antigens, are able to elicit an immune system response against invading pathogens, mediated by signal transduction processes. An immune response may occur independent of signal transduction stimulation by other molecules, as is the case for signal transduction by way of the toll-like receptor or with help from stimulatory molecules located at the cell surface of other cells, as is the case for T-cell receptor signaling.

Research is being carried out to understand the intracellular changes occurring in response to various stimuli such as cytokines or pathogen-derived molecules. The intracellular signaling alters the differentiation state of cells in the immune system. Failure to respond to the specific signals (cytokines) may manifest as a disease state. The quantitative assessment of components involved in immune cell signaling networks, is being carried out under different conditions.

Post-translational modifications play a very important role in the regulation of cell signaling and quantification of these modifications during the signal transduction is another thrust area of research in immunology. Scientists are developing tools to delineate the signaling pathways of toll-like receptor (TLR) in macrophages or the downstream pathways of T-cell antigen receptors.

Phosphorylation / dephosphorylation of proteins is one of the key mechanism of functional regulation of a number of proteins and has significant implications in cell proliferation, differentiation, and migration. The abnormal phosphorylation of proteins can disrupt the signaling cascade and can precipitate in the form of a disease. At a given time only a fraction of the protein is phosphorylated and estimating the degree and dynamics of phosphorylation is quiet a tedious job. Tools of proteomics coupled with mass spectroscopy have made it possible not only to generate a large amount of phospho-proteomics data but to correlate and interpret it with a greater degree of sensitivity and accuracy. Phosphoproteomics has, therefore, developed as an essential component of system biology and is unraveling a number of mysteries of the cell signaling in immune system.

Immunological Synapse

Different cells in the immune system need to communicate with each other to mount an effective immune response. One way in which this is done is by the formation of immuno-logical synapses between cells. The immuno-logical synapse has created a frenzy of research since the term was first coined by Bill Paul to describe the directed secretion of cytokines into a "small space between the two interacting cells", synapses are formed between both T cells and B cells with their cognate antigen-presenting cells (APCs), and both are characterized by a dramatic reorganization of the receptors involved in recognition and adhesion. The immunological synapse has been an area of very active scientific interest over the last decade. Surprisingly, much about the synapse remains unknown or is controversial. Recent progress in understanding the formation of the immunological synapse has been facilitated by the use of artificial planar lipid bilayers as well as a method of imaging known as total interference reflection microscopy (TIRFM). Elucidating the signaling function of the synapse, and the cSMAC in particular, has proven to be difficult because there are many competing effects and components at play, which makes it difficult to intuit mechanisms from experimental observations of a few variables. Computational and theoretical models have been applied to complement experimental studies to help unravel the interplay of complex-competing effects in various aspects of T-cell signaling.

Immunomodulatory Molecules

SLAM Family

The 'signaling lymphocyte activation molecule' (SLAM) family is a newly appreciated group of immune cell-specific receptors that has the ability to regulate the function of several immune cell types. Members of the SLAM family of receptors are expressed in multiple cells of the immune system, including natural killer cells, T cells and B cells. SLAM receptors interact with SH2 domain-containing, cytosolic adaptor proteins such as SAP, EAT-2, and SH2D1A, and mediate tyrosine phosphorylation events that contribute to immune cell activation. The SLAM family proteins belong to the CD2 subset of Ig superfamily cell surface receptors. They have extracellular domains containing an Ig V- and a C2-like domain. The SLAM-associated protein, SAP, was first identified as the protein affected in most cases of X-linked lymphoproliferative (XLP) syndrome, a rare genetic disorder characterized by abnormal responses to Epstein-Barr virus infection, lymphoproliferative syndromes, and dysgammaglobulinemia.

SLAM family members are now recognized as important immunomodulatory receptors with roles in cytotoxicity, humoral immunity, autoimmunity, cell survival, lymphocyte development, and cell adhesion. The cytoplasmic domains of the receptors contain multiple copies of ITSM (immunoreceptor tyrosine based switch motifs). The SAP interacts with SLAM at its cytoplasmic domains. The binding of the ligand to the extracellular domain of SLAM induces the phosphorylation of ITSMs. The SAP-related adaptors, SAP and EAT-2, dock onto the ITSM and then recruit Fyn through its SH3 domain **(Figure 21.1)**. The activated Fyn phosphorylates the tyrosine residues on the cytoplasmic domain of SLAM that triggers the downstream cell signaling. SLAM family proteins participate in the development, differentiation, activation, and regulation of effector functions of B cells, T cells, NK cells and NKT cells. The finding that mutations in SAP are associated with an X-linked lymphoproliferative disorder suggests that signaling through SLAM receptors can influence the development and effector functions of immune cells.

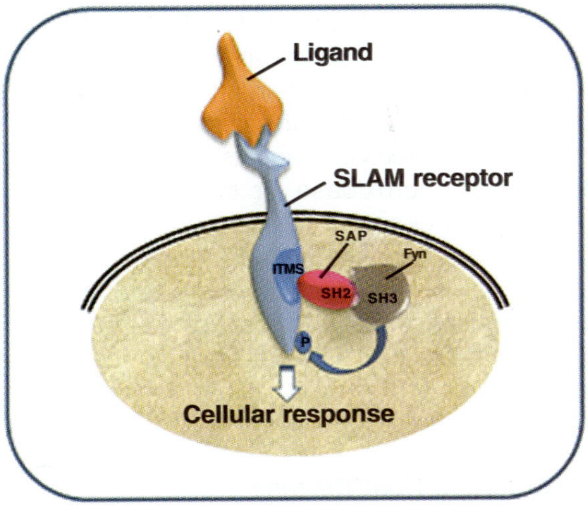

Fig. 21.1: Fyn-mediated phosphorylation of SLAM receptor via SAP coupling

Semaphorins–Immune and Tumor Regulators

Semaphorins are soluble or membrane bound proteins that are products of a large family of genes comprising 30 members. These were initially implicated in the guidance of neuronal cell migration during development. A number of the semaphorins, particularly Sema3, Sema4, Sema6 and Sema7 series are now proved to be involved in the regulation of immune system. Sema3A and Sema3C inhibit activation and migration of T cells or monocytes. The transmembrane proteins, Sema4A, Sema4D and Sema6A, influence the differentiation or activation of T cells, B cells, dendritic cells, and Langerhans cells. Sema7A, a GPI-linked member, stimulates monocytes yet inhibits T cell functions. All the semaphorins act through multimeric transmembrane receptors known as Plexin receptors, except the class-3 semaphorins that act through neurophilins/plexins. TIM-2, a member of the T cell immunoglobulin and mucin (TIM) gene family, is the only well characterized immune receptor for Sema4A, although a Plexin family member has also been implicated.

Recently, semaphorins have been found to play a role in cell motility, cell adhesion, tumor progression and angiogenesis. They modulate the migratory properties of the malignant cells and hence could be responsible for metastasis. Interestingly, semaphorins have been shown to function on both sides of oncogenesis – they could play a role as tumor suppressors and anti-angiogenic factors; or could be involved in angiogenesis, invasion and metastasis of cancer cells. Semaphorins, thus, display divergent activities in different cell types. The class-3 semaphorins semaphorin-3B (s3b) and semaphorin-3F (s3f) function as potent inhibitors of tumor development in small cell lung carcinoma. Recent evidence indicates that S3f as well as semaphorin-3A (s3a) function as inhibitors of angiogenesis, and it was shown that the anti-angiogenic properties of s3f contribute significantly to its anti-tumorigenic properties. In contrast with these inhibitory semaphorins, there is some evidence indicating that semaphorins such as semaphorin-3C (s3c), semaphorin-3E (s3e), semaphorin-4D (s4d), semaphorin-5C (s5c) semaphorin-6A (s6a) and semaphorin-6b (s6b) may contribute to tumorigenesis or to tumor progression.

These multifaceted functions may be explained by the involvement of different kinds of semaphorin receptor complexes, and by the consequent activation of multiple signaling pathways, in different cells or different functional stages.

Immuno-Proteomics

The accumulation of research data over the last century, particularly over last two decades, has been mind boggling. The changes in hundreds of proteins in response to a challenge, e.g., a disease state, is difficult to comprehend; and to determine the cause and effect relationship out of this data is an astronomical task. Proteomics is a tool that helps us to study the changes in the expression and levels of multiple proteins in a cell under specific conditions.

The antigen presentation by the mammalian immune system involves processing of multiple proteins or peptides by proteolytic cleavage followed by presentation on the cell surface in conjunction with the MHC molecules. The presented MHC-peptide complexes are then scrutinized by effector T cells that express clonally distributed T cell receptors. Since the antigen presentation is a continuous phenomenon, every cell displays an array of antigen-derived peptides on its surface. Any change in the *peptide landscape of cells* is perceived by the immune effector cells that set into motion a sequence of events that result in the elimination of the causative agent. The changes in the peptide landscape of the cell surface could be associated with infection, malignant transformation, or abnormal metabolism. Therefore, study of this peptide-landscape of the immune cell surface would be a great help to identify the disease or cancer status. By combining the increasing range of selective specific antibody reagents available, in part due to advances in antibody engineering technology, and the resolving power available, using mass spectrometry, immunoproteomics is the latest magnificent tool in the hands of immunologists that is ideally suited for the study of the immune responses at a molecular level.

Proteome Profiler Cytokine Array

The microarray based proteomics tools are being developed and a number of commercial companies are coming up with tailor-made microarrays for the simultaneous detection of a number of proteins. An example of a cytokine array (for mouse) is shown below. The array detects the relative levels of 40 different cytokines, chemokines and other proteins in a single sample. Simplicity of the technique is just astonishing–no specialized equipment is necessary and there is no need for multiple immunoprecipitation/Western blot experiments.

The microarray incorporates specific capture antibodies impregnated on specific locations (in duplicate) on the plate (a nitrocellulose membrane). The sample (cell culture fluid, plasma or cell lysate) is mixed with detection antibodies labelled with biotin. The mixture is incubated with the microarray that results in the binding of the target proteins (if present) to the captured antibodies on the membrane **(Figure 21.2A)**. The detection reagents like Streptavidin-horseradish peroxidase or chemiluminescent ligands then generate a signal in proportion to the amount of analyte bound to the microarray. The signal is processed through the software that identifies the cytokines being expressed by the immune cell. The software can generate the histograms **(Figure 21.2B)** to represent the cytokine profile of the cell.

Graft Versus Host Disease

Graft versus Host Disease (GVHD) is a complex disease resulting from donor T cell recognition of a genetically disparate recipient that is unable to reject donor cells after allogeneic hematopoietic stem cell transplantation (HSCT). The factors responsible for the GVHD are not very well characterized. The gene expression profile of the donor has been proved to have a deep impact on the occurrence of GVHD in the recipient. A pre-transplant microarray assay of gene expression profiles of CD_4^+ and CD_8^+ T cells can segregate donors

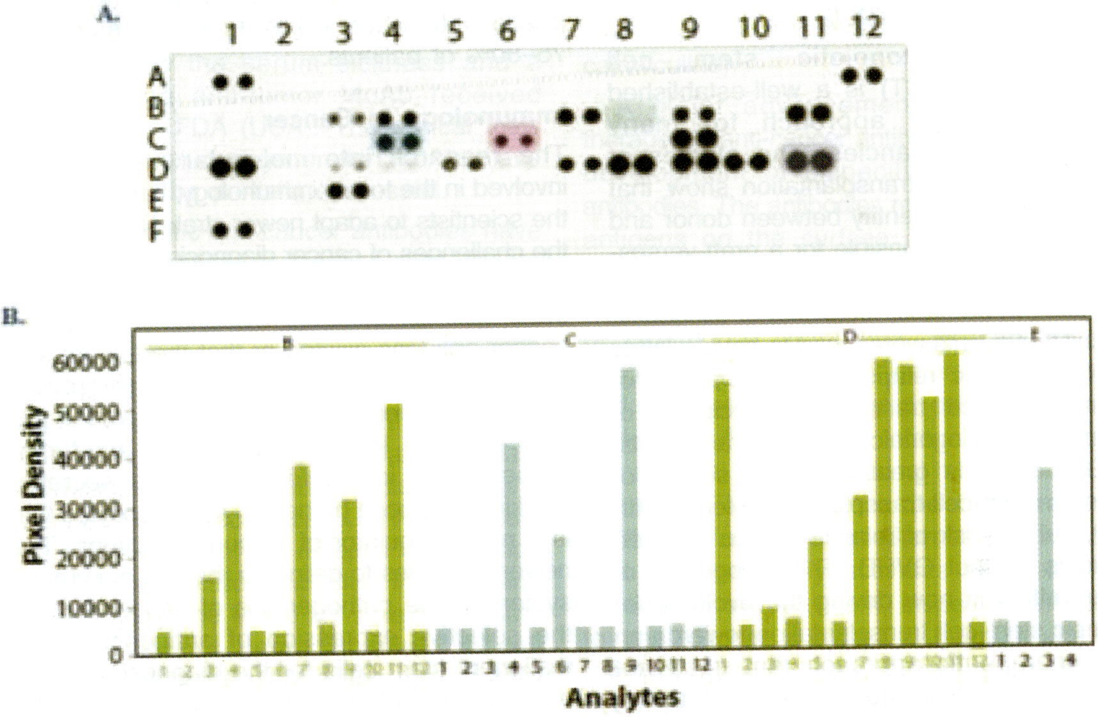

Fig. 21.2: (A) The qualitative microarray data showing the presence/absence of the cytokines in the sample; (B) The data quantified by the software to generate a protein profile

based on whether their transplant recipient suffered from chronic GVHD. Some latest studies have revealed that the "dangerous donor" trait (occurrence of GVHD in the recipient) is under polygenic control. The proteomic and gene profiling are now being utilized to define the disease in real perspective and to construct predictive models for acute GVHD.

Proteomic tools are being used to explore the synthesis and secretion of different proteins that reflect the GVHD. Answers are being found to the questions like - What are the pathophysiologic mechanisms responsible for late-onset acute GVHD seen after reduced intensity conditioning?; or What are the mechanisms underlying steroid-resistant disease?

Socie´ and Bruce R. Blazar have recently (2009) applied proteomics to screen for plasma proteins specific for GVHD in a mouse model and identified a peak that discriminated the GVHD subjects from the normal controls. The peak was later analyzed by mass spectrometry and was identified to correspond to CCL8, a member of a large chemokine family. The serum concentration of the cytokine, CCL8, also showed good correlation with the severity of GVHD in humans. Various attempts have been made to identify the proteins that could serve as biomarkers for GVHD. Different antibody microarrays have been used to screen for more than hundred proteins or polypeptides on a large number of patient samples, and to determine their significance with respect to patient outcome. Initially, eight potential biomarkers of GVHD were identified, which were further tested by ELISA in 400 transplant patients to close down on 4 proteins, viz. IL-2 receptor-α, TNF receptor-1, IL-8 and hepatocyte growth factor.

team at Cambridge created a transgenic mouse model with established Lewis lung carcinomas. A total of only 2% of the tumor cells expressed FAP. They found that when they destroyed all FAP-expressing cells (stromal and cancerous), the tumor began to die rapidly. By unmasking an immune response to cancer, immunizing against fibroblasts in tumors can provide us with another potential target for anti-cancer therapy.

Autologous Immune Enhancement Therapy (AIET)

In the multipronged approach to cancer, one very useful latest weapon is **AIET** (Autologous Immune Enhancement Therapy), which is in clinical practice in Japan since 90s with good efficacy. Several clinical trials and researches using AIET have been reported from institutions all over the world including the US, though there have not been any publications in this field from Indian institutes or hospitals.

The AIET involves an *ex-vivo* immune-potentiation (activation) of the immune cells and then re-injecting them into the patient **(Figure 21.3)**. During the *ex-vivo* enhancement, the immune cells are cultured and processed to be activated or to acquire additional anti-cancer functions. Researchers have found that post injection, the activated immune system so formed is now better able to differentiate between cancerous and non-cancerous cells and provide better opportunity to eliminate the cancer cells from the body.

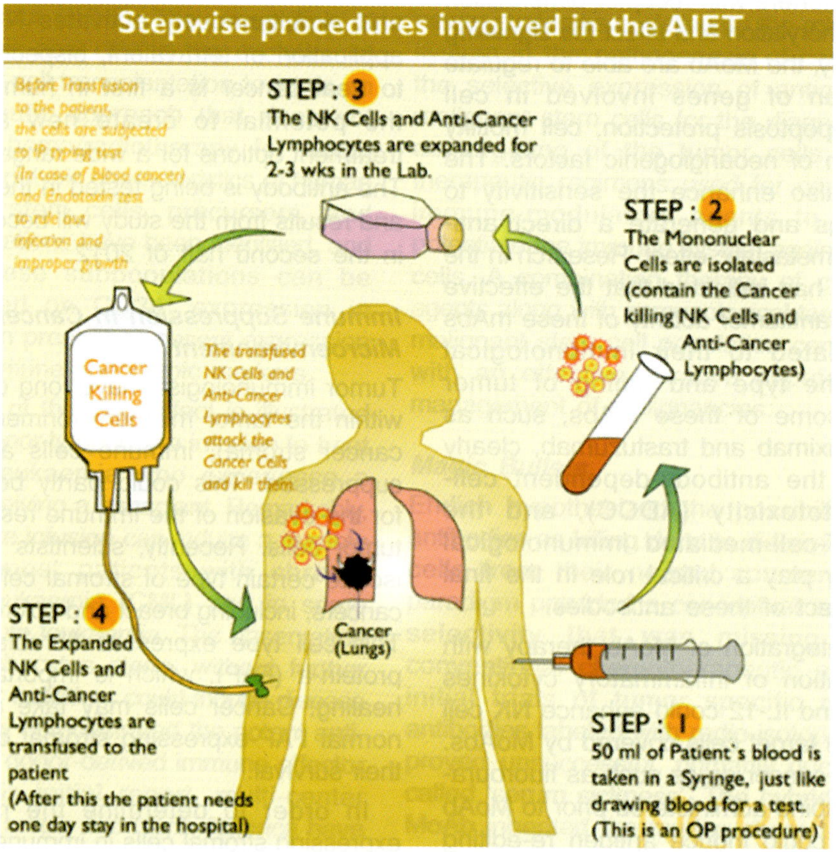

Fig. 21.3: Schematic presentation of Autologous Immune Enhancement Therapy (AIET) (Adapted from www.ncrm.org/aiet/wellness.htm)

Peripheral blood of the cancer patients (who received chemotherapy and are in remission) is drawn and by proven methods, the peripheral blood mononuclear cells are separated and processed *in vitro*. The processing technology specifically expands lymphocytes and NK cells to 25-30 folds in about 2-3 weeks. After expansion, the activated lymphocytes and NK cells are injected back into the patient's body wherein these cells act against the cancer cells effectively and also repopulate the patient's peripheral blood cells thereby recharging the immune system.

Technological Advances in Immunology

The conceptual advancement in any field is fuelled by the parallel advances in the technology applied to it. Researchers rely on new and improved technologies of several types to advance their understanding of immunological processes and to apply that understanding to practical ends. As discussed above, the advent of genomics, proteomics and microarray techniques have revolutionized the research in the field of immunology. Another technique that has shown tremendous flights is flowcytometry and immunology has been the backbone to this technique in the form of development of highly specific antibodies to label the cells.

The development of newer tools have made it possible to measure the cytotoxic T cells against infected targets in human with utmost precision. The activation of T cells by recognition of various epitopes on the antigens can now be monitored with the help of *ELISPOT assays*. The evaluation of T cell epitope recognition has further achieved a major boost by the development of *Tetramer assays* that helps in identification of T cells with a given specificity. Tetramers consist of four HLA molecules of a specific type bound to a particular peptide. They bind to and thus identify T cells that recognize a particular HLA molecule and particular peptide.

These days we don't have to use antigen stimulation to study the antigen-specific T cell activation. The cells are directly detected from the circulation by ELISPOT assays or by flowcytometry. Both these assays enable us to measure any number of cytokines that activated T cells produce. Because they allow for both quantitative and qualitative assessment, these can allow us to compare various vaccines under investigation.

Tetramer Assay and Flowcytometry

Identification and separation of an antigen specific T cell population in response to a disease or immunogen exposure is very difficult by the traditional methods. The major glitch is that the T cell has to recognise not only the antigen but also the MHC complexed with the peptide after processing in the APC. The problem has been solved with the development of tetramer assays.

A tetramer is a complex formed of four MHC α/β dimers bound to a central (fluorescence labelled) streptavidin molecule through the biotin-streptavidin binding. All the MHC units carry the same target peptide (**Figure 21.4**), which increases the avidity of binding with the T cells. These tetramers allow the direct visualization of CD4+ (by using class II MHC tetramers) or CD8+ (by using class I MHC tetramers) cells with the desired antigen specificity. After incubating the cells with the specific tetramers, flowcytometry is utilized for the final visualization of the T cells **(Figure 21.4)**. Class I tetramers bind more tightly than the Class II tetramers because the CD8 cells show a stronger cooperative binding than CD4 cells.

The tetramer assays can be utilized for detecting the presence of T cell population specific for either a self or a foreign antigen. They have been used for understanding the role of CD4+ T cells in immune response.

ELISPOT Assay Principle

ELISPOT assays are the latest development in real-time testing of cytokine secretion by stimulated T cells. The technique is basically a

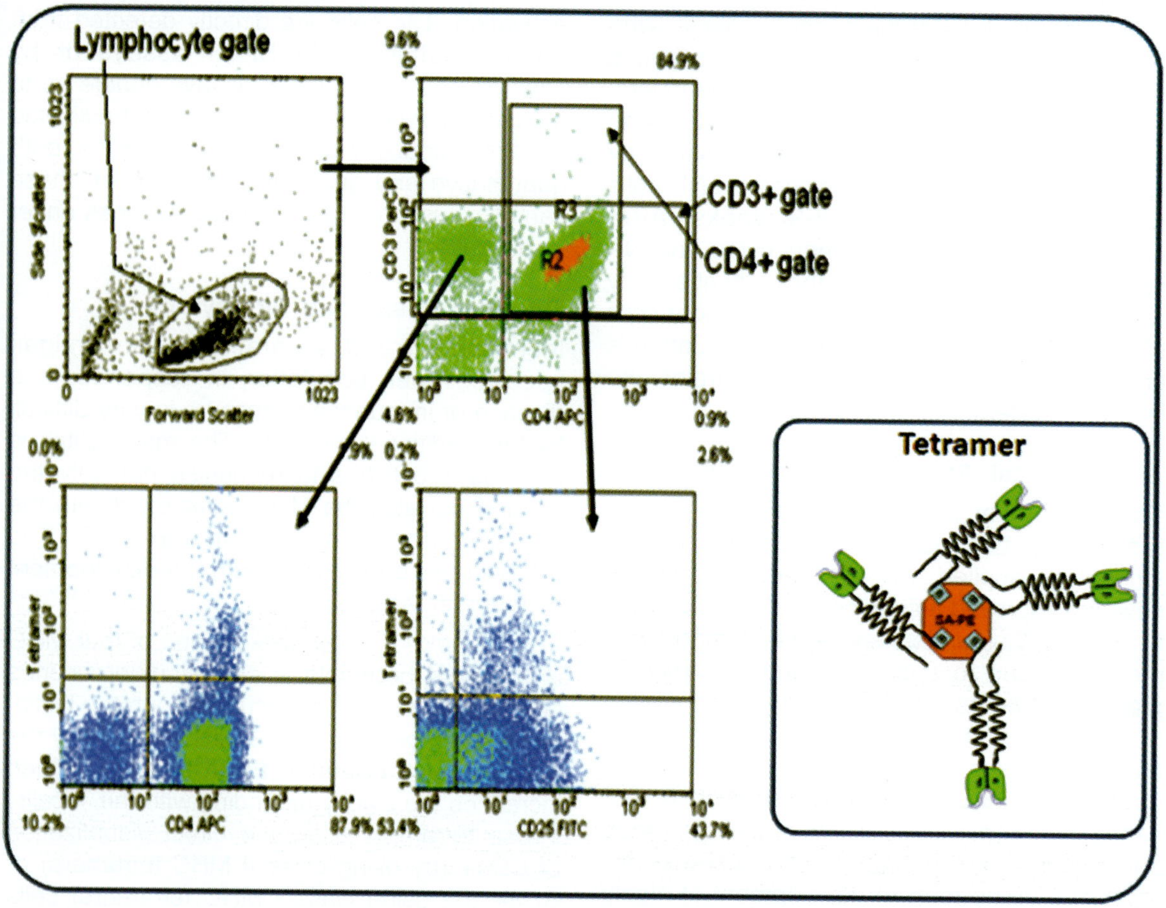

Fig. 21.4: Flowcytometric visualization of T cells with selected specificity labelled by MHC class II tetramer. Inset: A Tetramer–The red core represents the streptavidin-PE molecule. The green and black extensions represent the MHC class II α/β dimers. The complex is joined by the high affinity interaction between biotin and streptavidin
(Source: Adapted from James *et al.*, 2009 : URL: http://www.jove.com/index/Details.stp?ID=1167. DOI: 10.3791/1167)

modification of the sandwich enzyme-linked immunosorbent assay (ELISA). The elispot plates are coated with capture antibodies specific for the cytokine to be tested. The cells are stimulated with the required antigen and are then incubated in a humidified 37°C CO_2 incubator for a specified period of time. The cytokines secreted from the stimulated T cells are captured by the immobilized antibody, in the immediate vicinity of the secreting cells. The cells and the unbound reagents are washed away and a biotinylated polyclonal antibody specific for the chosen cytokine is added to the wells. Following a wash to remove any unbound biotinylated antibody, alkaline-phosphatase conjugated to streptavidin is added. Unbound enzyme is subsequently removed by washing and a substrate solution is added. A blue-black colored precipitate forms and appears as spots at the sites of cytokine localization, with each individual spot representing a foot-print of the individual analyte-secreting cell. The spots can be counted with an automated ELISPOT reader system or manually, using a stereomicroscope **(Figure 21.5)**.

Applications of the ELISPOT assays include analysis of the frequency of T cell precursors producing the cytokines (TH1, TH2, TH3 ....) in response to a specific antigen stimulation; and identification of the T lymphocytes with characterization of their polarization. Sensitivity of the ELISPOT assays has been claimed to be upto 1 in 10^5 cells. The newer ELISPOT assays can even characterize cells simultaneously producing multiple cytokines.

At this time you should know the following:

1. The role of ubiquitin proteasome complex in antigen processing and presentation.
2. The processes like signal transduction and post translational modifications that take place subsequent to the invasion of pathogens.
3. Formation and signalling at the immunological synapse.
4. Newly discovered immunomodulatory molecules: SLAM and Semaphorins.
5. The application of immuno-proteomics in studying the changes in protein expression associated with immune response.
6. Understand the proteomic and genetic factors responsible for GVHD.
7. The role of immune system in pathogenesis of cancer and the use of immune modulatory

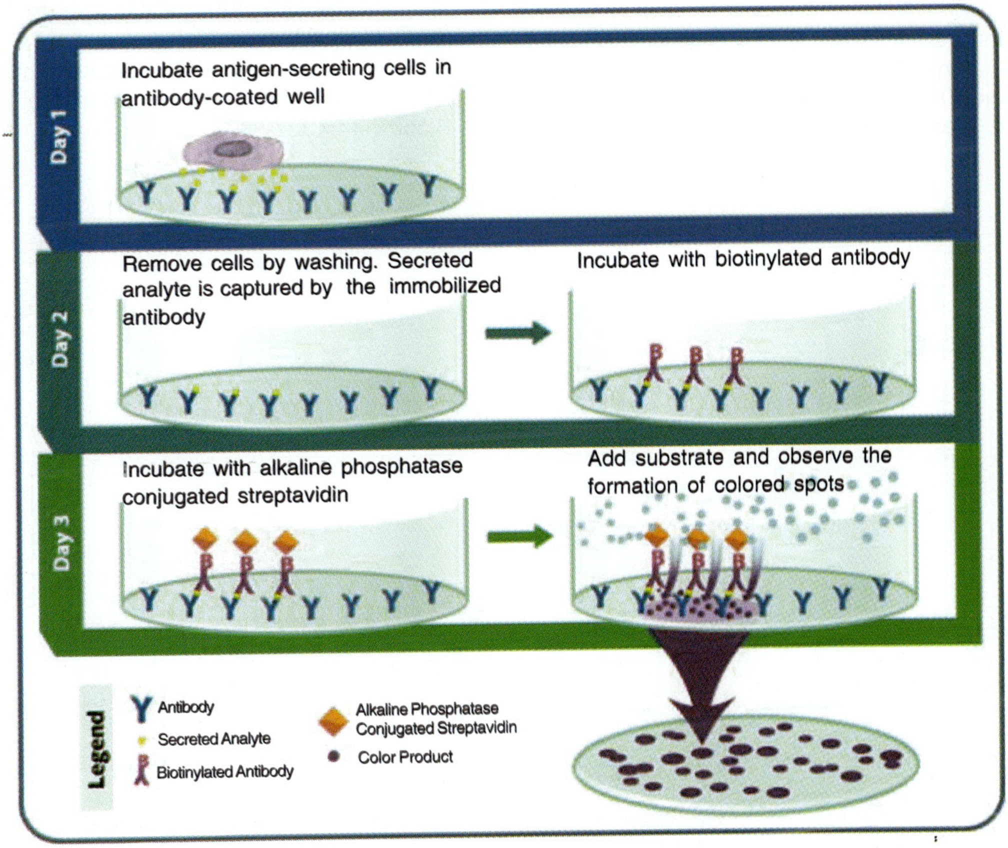

Fig. 21.5: Schematic diagram depicting principle of the ELISPOT assay (Adapted from RnD System.com)

agents (Abs, immune suppression, AIET) as therapeutic agents against tumor cells.

8. The application of new technologies (Flow-cytometry, ELISPOT and tetramer aasay) in understanding the immune response and as tools in diagnosing diseases, and identifying molecules of biological or medical interest.

Further Reading

- Catherine J. Wu Immunologic targeting of the cancer stem cell. StemBook 2008, ed. *The Stem Cell Research Community*, StemBook, doi/ 10.3824/stembook.1.21.1, http://www.stembook.org.
- Correale P., Cusi M.G. and Tagliaferri P. Immunomodulatory properties of anticancer monoclonal antibodies: Is the 'magic bullet' still a reliable paradigm? *Immunotherapy* 2011, 3(1): 1–4.
- Demaria S., Pikarsky E., Michael K., Coussens L.M., Yen-Ching Chen, J. Emad M. El-Omar, Giorgio Trinchieri, Steven M. Dubinett, Jenny T. *et al.* Cancer and Inflammation: Promise for Biologic Therapy. *J Immunotherapy* 2010, 33(4): 335-351.
- Hans-Jochem Kolb Graft-versus-leukemia effects of transplantation and donor lymphocytes. *Blood* 2008, 112 (12): 4371-4383.
- Hillen N.S. Contribution of mass spectrometry-based proteomics to immunology. *Expert Rev Proteomics* 2006, 3(6):653-64.
- R&D systems. ELispot Assays. Available at http://www.rndsystems.com/product_detail_objectname_ELISpotAssayPrinciple.aspx Accessed on 15th Feb. 2011.
- Veillette Andre´. SLAM-Family Receptors: Immune Regulators with or without SAP-Family Adaptors. *Cold Spring Harb Perspect Biol* 2010;2:a002469. Downloaded from cshperspectives.cshlp.org on January 28, 2011.
- Yazdani U. and Terman J.R. The semaphorins. *Genome Biology* 2006, 7:211 (doi:10.1186/gb-2006-7-3-211).
- Socie G, Blazar BR (2009). Acute graft-versus-host disease: From the bench to the bedside. Blood 114:4327-36.

22 CHAPTER

Immunohistochemistry—An Introduction

(Dr. Poonam Elhence docpoonam@yahoo.co.in)

OBJECTIVES

1. Definition, introduction and historical background.
2. To learn the principles of immunohistochemistry.
3. To know the various factors which can influence results.
4. Pitfalls in immunohistochemistry.
5. Application and interpretation of different markers.

Definition

Immunohistochemistry (Immunocytochemistry) is a group of procedures used for identifying and demonstrating various cellular proteins by specific antigen-antibody interactions and to understand the localization, amount and distribution of these target proteins in the cells and tissues. It has immense advantage over special enzyme staining (histochemical) techniques which identify only a limited number of proteins, enzymes and tissue structures. Immunocytochemistry is widely used in pathology, microbiology, medical research laboratories and clinical diagnostics.

Much of medical treatment for cancer depends on the pathologist's interpretation of histopathology, hematology and cytology specimens. Immunocytochemistry is a group of techniques used to identify and classify difficult tumors and other entities. It guides the clinicians to offer recent treatment modalities aimed at molecular level of tumor histogenesis. For instance, many tumors show increased expression of Her-2-neu (also referred to as erb-B2). Hence, monoclonal antibodies (MAb) against Her-2/neu have been developed which are targeted specifically for the treatment of cancers with Her-2-neu upregulation (Example: For treating patients with breast cancer who show increased Het-2-neu receptors).

Historical Background

Albert H. Coons and his colleagues[1] were the first to label antibodies with a fluorescent dye, and used it to identify antigens in tissue sections. This was the **immunofluorescence** technique. Subsequently, it was found that immunologic complexes formed by enzymes and homologous antibodies allow the cellular antigens to be demonstrated. This formed the basis of **immunohistochemical** procedures. With the expansion and development of immunohistochemistry techniques, various enzyme labels have been introduced such as horse radish peroxidase[2,3] and alkaline phosphatase.[4] Colloidal gold has also been used as a label to identify immunohistochemical reactions at both light and electron microscopic level.[5] Guedson et al. and Hsu *et al.* developed Avidin-Biotin labeling.[6,7] The use of Avidin-Biotin especially with peroxidase is currently the most popular method used. Radioactive elements can be used as labels and the subsequent reaction can

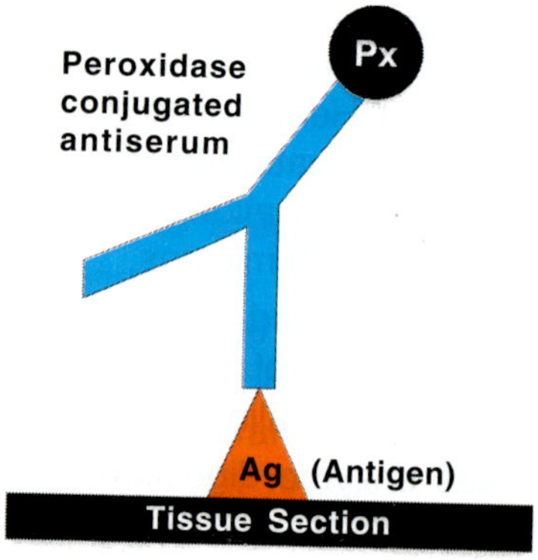

Fig. 22.1: Direct immunostaining method

- This procedure is short, relatively simple to perform and quick.
- However, it is insensitive due to little signal amplification and rarely used since the introduction of indirect method.
- Also, it would be necessary to make custom labelled antibodies against every antigen of interest.

Indirect Immunostaining Method

- It utilizes an unlabelled primary antibody (first layer) which reacts with tissue antigen, and a labeled secondary antibody (second layer) which reacts with the primary antibody.
- The secondary antibody must be against the IgG of the animal species in which the primary antibody has been raised.
- This method is more sensitive due to signal amplification through several secondary antibody reactions with different antigenic sites on the primary antibody.
- The second layer antibody may be labeled with an enzyme such as horse radish peroxidase or alkaline phosphatase and the subsequent reaction is visualized with bright field microscopy after staining with a chromogen (DAB, AEC etc.). This is referred to as the *indirect immunoenzyme method*.
- DAB (3, 3' Diaminobenzidine tetrahydrochloride) produces a brown precipitate at the reaction site. This reaction can be enhanced using nickel, cobalt chloride, imidazole etc.
- AEC (3-Amino-9-ethyl carbazole) produces a crisp red colour at the site of antigen antibody binding. AEC is a lower risk carcinogen as compared to DAB.
- The mounting medium used for DAB chromogen slides is DPX (Distrene 80, Dibutyl phthalate, Xylene) and for AEC, glycerol is used to mount slides.
- When a fluorescent dye such as FITC, rhodamine etc is used for labeling, the fluorescence emitted by the bound antibody is detected by fluorescent microscopy and this is known as the *indirect immuno-fluorescence method* **(Figure 22.2)**.

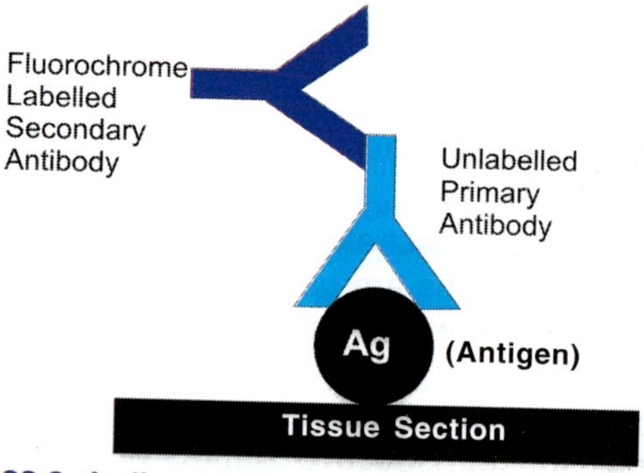

Fig. 22.2: Indirect immunofluorescence method

- Advantages of indirect fluorescent method are that no deparaffinisation is required as frozen sections are used. No chromogen or peroxidase block is required.
- Disadvantage of indirect fluorescent method is that specialized equipment is required for visualization.

Detection Systems

These have evolved from the direct immuno-histochemical assay introduced by Coons in 1941 to the most recent ones in which multiple bridging antibodies are used.

1. PAP Method (Peroxidase-Antiperoxidase Method): (Figure 22.3)

- PAP method is a further development of the indirect technique.

histogenesis and SMA for smooth muscle differentiation. Further, in some cases in which site of primary tumor is not known, a definite tissue of origin may be suggested by the use of antibody to tissue-specific antigens.e.g. Positive staining for thyroglobulin or calcitonin provides good evidence of thyroid origin in a metastatic deposit,CK7 is commonly present in all adenocarcinomas (~100% positive in lung adenocarcinoma and tumors of salivary gland) except for those of gastrointestinal origin. The gastrointestinal adenocarcinomas are usually positive with CK20.Prostate Specific Antigen (PSA) positivity is a very helpful indicator of prostatic primary. To subclassify lymphomas, antibodies to CD3, CD 20, MUM-I, CD 10, bcl-2 etc are used. For malignant small round cell tumors—commoner in childhood, the panel of antibodies uses may comprise CD99, EMA (Epithelial Membrane Antigen), Synaptophysin, Desmin, LCA, Chromogranin, Neuron Specific Enolase (NSE), Myoglobin etc. Mic-2/CD 99 is used as a specific marker for Ewing's sarcoma, Myoglobin and Desmin are specific for Rhabdomyosarcoma, NSE, Chromogranin and Synaptophysin etc are markers of neuroendocrine differentiation such as neuroblastoma and PNET (Peripheral Neuro Ectodermal Tumor).

For germ cell tumors, for example as in seminoma and yolk sac tumor, markers such as α-Fetoprotein (AFP), β-Human Chorionic Gonadotrophin (β-HCG) and Placental alkaline phosphatase (PLAP) are often used. AFP is useful for the identification of yolk sac or endodermal sinus component, hepatoblastoma and hepatocellular carcinoma. β-HCG is used to identify the trophoblastic component and PLAP for the identification of the seminomatous component. CD31, FVIII-related Antigen, CD34 and Blood Group Antigens UEA1 (Ulex europaeus I agglutinin) serve as endothelial/vascular markers. Estrogen Receptor (ER), Progesterone Receptor (PR) and her-2-neu are used for breast carcinomas. Breast cancer which are immunopositive for ER/PR respond better to treatment with antiestrogenic drugs like Tamoxifen. Meningiomas are graded according to their MIB-1 proliferation fraction as having atypical or atypical morphology in the WHO classification system. Pituitary adenomas are further classified according to the hormone which they secrete as demonstrated by immunostaining for various hormones such as Growth Hormone (GH), Prolactin (PRL), Follicle Stimulating Hormone (FSH) etc. The judicious choice of a panel of antibodies allows the identification of many anaplastic and poorly differentiated tumors thereby providing definitive clues to diagnosis and chances of more precisely targeted treatment modalities. Various antibodies are commercially available for immunohistochemical diagnosis of infectious diseases such as antibody against CMV (Cytomegalovirus), HBsAg (Hepatitis B surface Antigen), Pneumocystis carinii, EBV (Epstein Barr Virus), BK virus etc.

Specific antibodies are also available against pathogenic organisms like Cryptococcus, Aspergillus, Toxoplasma, Giardia etc. which helps to diagnose and initiate early treatment.

Congenital myopathic disorders are categorised as dystrophinopathy, sarcoglycanopathy etc. depending on the lack of expression of specific sarcolemmal membrane proteins.

Skin diseases such as epidermal bullous lesions are further subdivided according to the antigens expressed in the basement membrane, when stained by Direct Immuno Fluorescence (DIF). Characteristic staining patterns for immunoglobulins and complement are seen in certain glomerulonephritides.

Hence, properly and judiciously planned immunohistochemical markers and panels aid in the resolution of diagnostic dilemmas and thereby help in treatment and patient care.

References

1. Coons AH and Kaplan MH Localization of Antigen in Tissue Cells: II. Improvements in a Method for the Detection of Antigen by means of Fluorescent Antibody. The Journal of Experimental Medicine 1950, Vol 91, 1-13.
2. Nakane PK, Pierce GBJ. Enzyme-labelled antibodies for the light and electron microscopic localization of tissue antigens. J Cell Biol 1967; 33:307.

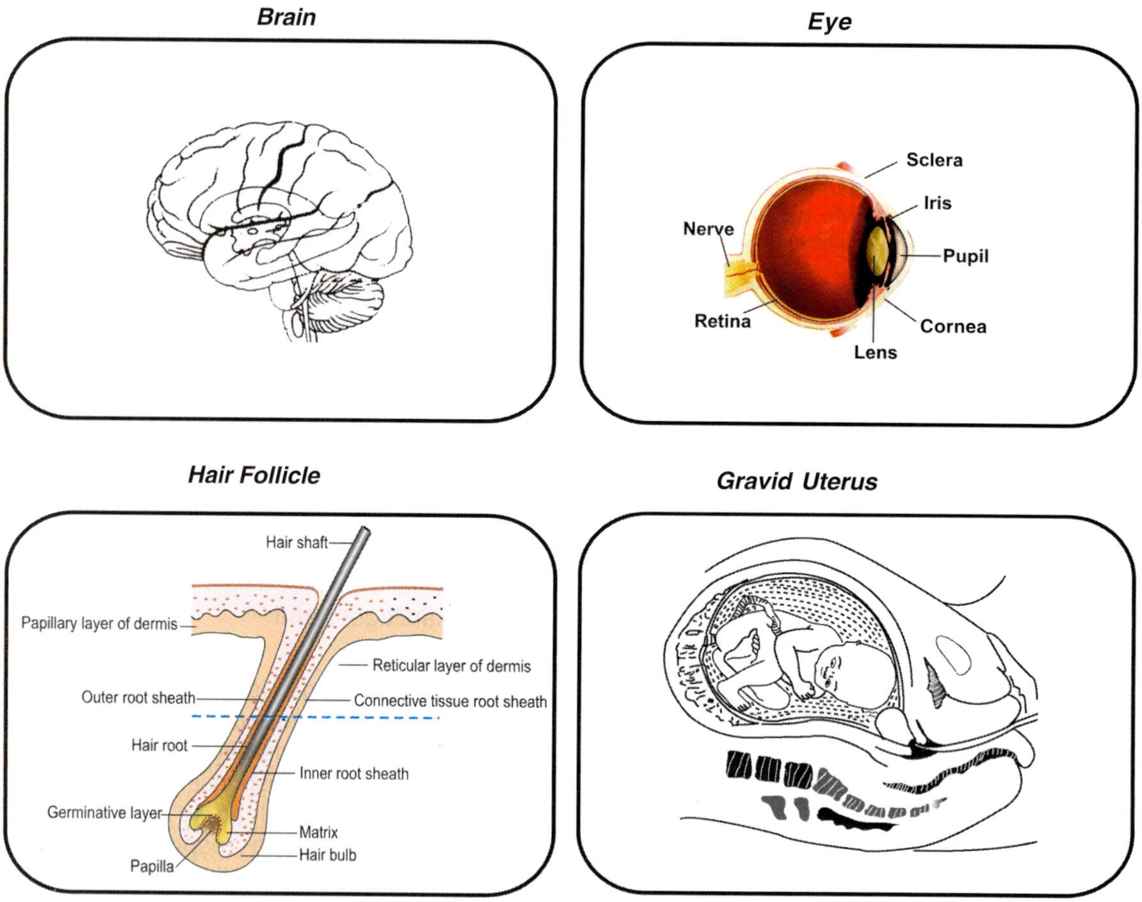

Fig. 23.1: Showing immunologically privileged site

- Low expression of MHC molecules.
- Increased expression of surface molecules that inhibits complement activation.
- Local production of immunosuppressive cytokines such as TGF-β.
- Presence of neuropeptides.
- Constitutive expression of Fas ligand (FasL) that controls the entry of Fas-expressing lymphoid cells.[1]

Antigens from immune privileged regions have been found to interact with T cells in an unusual way inducing tolerance as opposed to a destructive response.[2] Immune privilege has emerged as an active rather than a passive process.

The nature of isolation of immunologically privileged sites from the rest of the body's immune system can cause them to become targets of autoimmune diseases or conditions, including sympathetic ophthalmitis in the eye.

Immune Privileged Tissue

Certain tissues tend to provoke little or no immune response. These are called immune privilege tissue. Testis grafts containing Sertoli cells and corneal tissue deprived of epithelium inherently possess this unique property. For example, when allogeneic testis grafts are placed under the kidney capsule they survive well, whereas allogeneic grafts of skin and islets of Langerhans are quickly rejected from the same site. Similarly, corneal allografts (within species) survive indefinitely under the kidney capsule. Both these tissues express CD95L, which protect them from immune rejection. FasLigand (also called FasL, CD95L or Apo-1L) induces apoptosis in cells that bears its receptor FasR. FasL expressing cells include cells of the immune system. Thus tissues that naturally express FasL, kill infiltrating lymphocytes and inflammatory cells and therefore become an immune privilege tissue. Several ocular cells express CD95L, including the Retinal Pigment Epithelium (RPE), the presence of CD95L on these cells suggest that they may possess inherent immune privilege. RPE transplantation is being tried as a possible treatment of certain types of retinal degeneration.

The strategy of expressing FasL or other molecules with similar function in donor tissue to make them immune privileged is being tried. Such a tissue will be able to wade off invading immune cells.

Mechanism for Maintenance of Site Specific Immune Privilege (Figure 23.2)

FasL expression plays an important role in maintenance of immune privilege.

Important characteristics of immune privileged tissues:

- Absence of lymphatic vessels.
- In some cases absence of blood vessels (lens of eye).
- Consequently, the alloantigens of the graft are not able to sensitize the recipient's

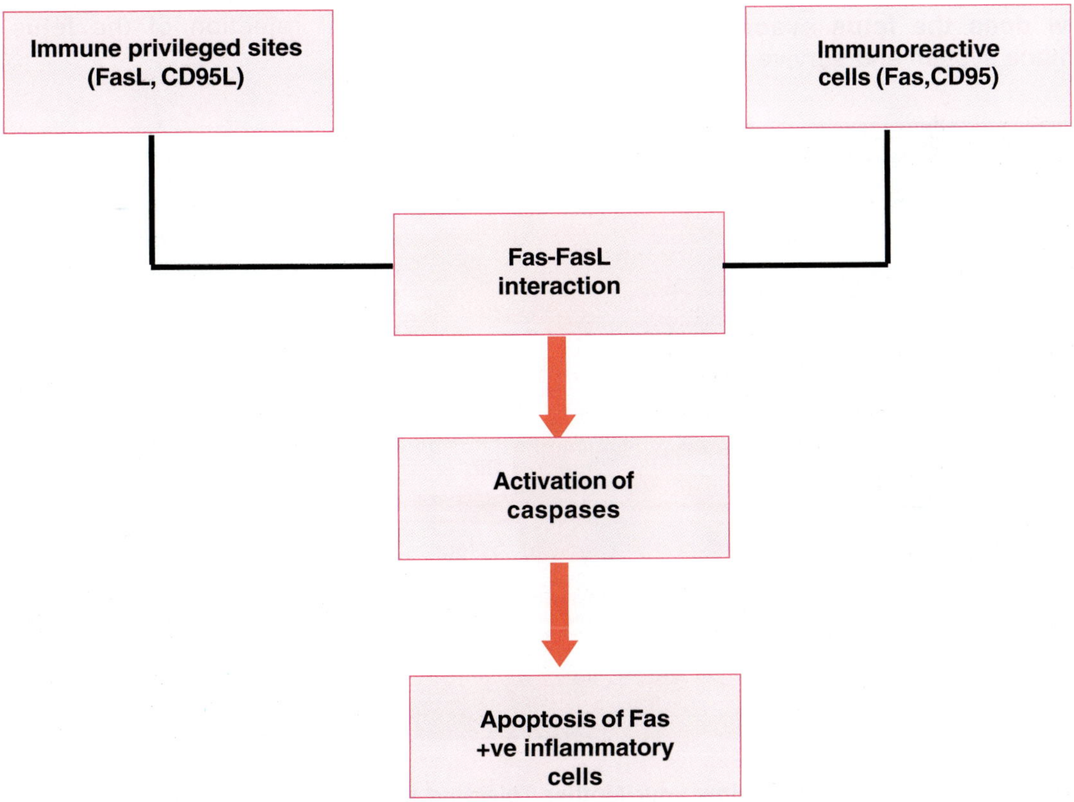

Fig. 23.2: Showing mechanism for maintenance of immune privilege

lymphocytes and the graft has an increased likelihood of acceptance even when HLA antigens are not matched.

- Presence of barriers (blood-brain barrier, blood testis barrier, trophoblast of placenta etc.).

Pregnant Uterus

The genome of the fetus that mammalian mothers carry within their wombs is half maternal and half paternal. Thus, fetal tissues expressing paternally inherited alloantigens would be considered foreign by the mother's immune system. The fetus should trigger an immune response and therefore should be eliminated. However, the presence of billions of humans on the earth and the continued growth of the human population disproves this hypothesis.

How does the fetus evade the maternal immune system and survive for nine months in an environment that considers it foreign (Figure 23.3)?

A successful pregnancy may be mediated in two ways: the maternal immune system may be prevented from recognizing the fetal tissue as foreign and/or the cells of the maternal immune system may be prevented from mounting an immune response.

To avoid being detected as a foreign body, the fetal cell hides its antigens by not presenting them on its surface. T cells cannot detect the presence of a pathogen or a foreign body if antigens are not presented to them via MHC molecules and therefore, no T cell mediated response can be mounted. Moreover, a subset of T cells called Regulatory T cells (Tregs) appears to be important in the maintenance of tolerance to fetal antigen. Tregs counts are found to increase during normal pregnancy and their decreased numbers is associated with immunological rejection of the fetus and miscarriage.[3]

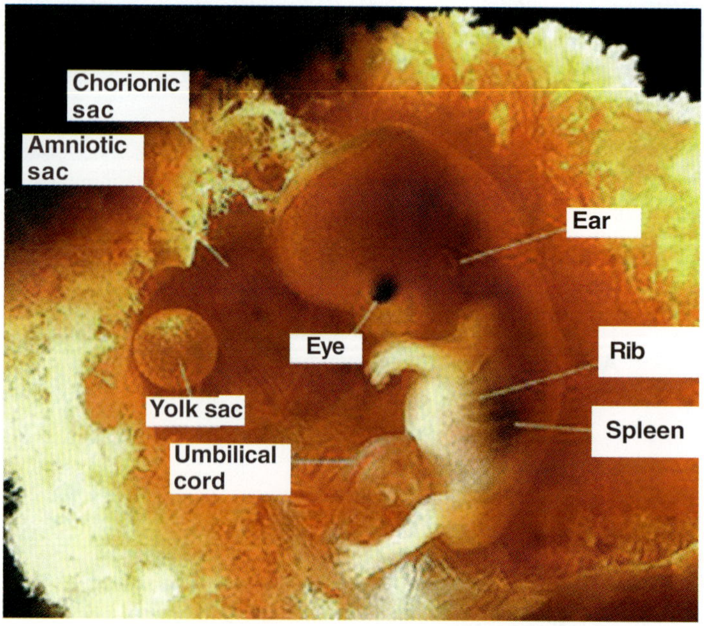

Fig. 23.3: A child developing in the womb carries foreign antigens from its father as well as from its mother, and might be expected to trigger a graft rejection. But one source of protection appears to be a substance produced by the child, perhaps in response to antibodies from the mother, which promotes the development of special white blood cells in the uterus, and these cells release a factor that blocks the actions of IL-2. Another source of protection appears to be a substance produced by the pregnant uterus which helps in changing the antigens on the fetal surface of the placenta, shielding them from the mother's immune defenses and so the uterus is an "immunologically privileged" site where immune responses are subdued

(Source: Madona A de Lemos. How your Mother Tolerated you for Nine Months BioTeach Journal. Fall 2003, Vol-1, 27-30)

There are specialized lymphoid cells called Natural Killer cells (NK cells) which destroy cells which do not have any MHC molecules on their surface. The fetal cells devoid of antigens presented by MHC molecules would be eliminated by NK cells. To prevent such cytotoxic destruction by NK cells, fetal tissue displays a unique type of MHC class I molecule encoded by the gene HLA-G. This molecule is considered to be a non-classical MHC molecule because of its low allelic variation (only two polymorphs are known) and restricted tissue distribution (found only in the placenta). The expression of HLA-G is restricted to the trophoblast cells, the embryonic contribution to the placenta.[4] Its function in the placenta may be to prevent the activation of decidual cytotoxic T cells and NK cells. Trophoblasts also express Fas ligand: a proposed mechanism for immune privilege in placenta and preventing maternal immune invasion.

Studies have shown that cells expressing HLA-G are unable to activate T cells and inhibit cytotoxic lysis mediated by NK cells in the decidua: the maternal contribution to the placenta. It has also been shown that NK cells have receptors called killer inhibitory receptors (KIRs), that upon binding to MHC molecules, inhibit the cytotoxic activities of the maternal NK cells.

Eye

The eye contains active immune cells that act upon the detection of foreign antigens. These cells interact with the immune system to induce unusual suppression of the systemic immune system response to an antigen introduced into the eye. This is known as Anterior Chamber Associated Immune Deviation (ACAID).[6, 7] The main features of this deviation include suppressed delayed hypersensitivity, preserved humoral immunity, and primed cytotoxic T cell responses. ACAID is made possible by unique characteristics of the anterior segment of the eye and those of the spleen.

Sympathetic ophthalmitis is a rare disease, which results from the isolation of the eye from the systemic immune system. Usually, trauma to one eye induces the release of eye antigens, which are recognized and picked up by local antigen presenting cells (APC) such as neutrophils and dendritic cells. These APC carry the antigen to local lymph nodes to be sampled by T cells and B cells. Entering the systemic immune system, these antigens are recognized as foreign and an immune response is mounted against them. The result is the sensitization of immune cells against a self-protein, causing an autoimmune attack on both, the damaged eye and the non-damaged eye.[2]

In this manner, the immune-privileged property has served to work against the eye instead. T cells normally encounter self-antigens during their development, when they move to the tissue draining lymph nodes. Anergy is induced in T cells, which bind to self-antigens, deactivating them and preventing an auto-immune response in the future. However, the physical isolation of eye antigens results in the body's T cells never having encountered them at any time during development. Studies in mice have shown that the lack of presentation of eye self-antigens to specific T cells will fail to induce a sufficient amount of anergy to the self-antigens. While the lack of antigen presentation (due to the physical barriers) is sufficient to prevent the activation of auto reactive immune cells to the eye, the failure to induce sufficient anergy to T cells has detrimental results as well. In the case of damage or chance presentation to the immune system, the antigen presentation and immune response will occur at elevated rates.[8]

Mechanisms of immune privilege of the eye is a result of:

1. Special anatomical features of the anterior chamber.
2. Presence of blood-ocular barrier.
3. No blood supply to lens.
4. Other immune privileges within eye like; the presence of unique immunomodulatory molecules in the ocular fluids as well its expression by the ocular cells.

These factors modify how antigenic material placed in the anterior chamber is recognized by the systemic immune system. These factors alter the responses of immune effector molecules and cells to foreign and antigenic material in the eye eventually limiting the development of intra ocular inflammation.

Blood-Ocular Barriers in the Expression of Ocular Immunity

The anatomical barriers of the eye play a major role in the lack of expression of adaptive immunity in the eye. Blood aqueous barrier represent this barrier. This barrier is a selectively permeable barrier that is formed by the tight junctions between cells of nonpigmented layer of the ciliary epithelium and the endothelium of the iris blood vessels. The blood-aqueous barrier bars relatively large molecules such as plasma proteins from entering the eye. Similar barrier exists in the posterior segment of the eye, which prevents large molecules from entering the retina. It is called the blood retinal barrier. It is formed by tight junctions between the cells of the retinal pigment epithelium and the retinal vascular endothelium. Owing to these barriers the plasma proteins within aqueous is extremely low (about 1% of plasma concentrations). T and B lymphocytes are present only in the tissues around the anterior chamber. When the blood-aqueous ocular barrier is broken down, the T cells from the blood are able to gain access to the eye and allow the expression.

Immune Tolerance of Eye-derived Antigens

The deviant immune response of the anterior chamber is called anterior chamber-associated immune deviation (ACAID). It is a selective, antigen-specific response characterized by T cell deficiency. These cells are responsible for delayed hypersensitivity and secretion of complement-fixing antibodies. Both of these functions trigger immune inflammation. In ACAID antigen-specific regulatory T cells (CD4+ and CD8+) are generated. These cells inhibit pro-inflammatory effector mechanisms but have no effect on other effector mechanisms thus leaving cytotoxic T cells and non-complement-fixing antibodies intact.

The ocular environment plays a pivotal role in the generation of ACAID. Cells in the stroma of iris and ciliary body are the indigenous antigen presenting cells of the eye. They express CD1. These cells respond to soluble molecules in the ocular environment, including transforming growth factor beta2 (TGF-beta2). Upon capturing antigen, these cells process and present peptides on class I and II MHC molecules. Although they express certain costimulatory molecules such as B7-1, they do not secrete IL-12, thus, fail to upregulate important costimulatory molecules such as CD 40 that are essential for the induction of T cells. On the other hand, ocular antigen presenting cells (APCs) secrete TGF-beta2. Certain ocular APC leave the anterior chamber via trabecular meshwork and reach venous circulation by passing the lymphatic and reach the marginal zone of the spleen. In spleen they secrete macrophage inflammatory protein (MIP-2), which attracts NK cells. NK cells now conjugate with the CD1 expressing ocular APC. NK cells in the conjugate secrete additional chemokines attracting antigen-specific T cells. The regulatory T cells of ACAID emerge from this multicellular aggregate.

In brief, the ACAID confers immune privilege to the eye by pre-emptying the systemic immune response against eye-derived antigens.

This implies molding all subsequent responses to such an antigen in a way that it does not cause inflammation. This is made possible by TGF-beta2, which confers special costimulatory properties to the APCs arising from the eye and possibility of ocular APCs to by pass lymphatics and directly reach the spleen by joining the blood circulation (via trabecular meshwork). Spleen plays a key role in inducing ACAID, which fails to develop in the absence of spleen.

Modification of Ocular Adaptive Immunity

In addition to anatomical factors, a number of soluble factors in the anterior chamber modify adaptive immune effectors that are able to reach the ocular environment. *In vitro* experiments have shown that aqueous humor inhibits the activation of T lymphocytes. A large number of soluble factors that mediate this have been identified. These factors include TGF-beta2, vasoactive intestinal peptide (VIP), and alpha-Melanocyte-stimulating hormone (alpha-MSH). The concentration of TGF-beta2 and VIP in the aqueous is sufficient to prevent T-cell from proliferating in response to antigen. Alpha-MSH selectively inhibits any T cells that get activated from producing either IFN-gamma or IL-4. Interestingly, these soluble factors present in the aqueous do not prevent cytotoxic T mediated lysis of specific targets. This suggests that the negative effects of aqueous on adaptive immune selectively target T cells that are likely to cause inflammation. Aqueous also does not interfere with the effectiveness of antibodies in neutralizing viruses. Immune effectors such as complement-fixing antibodies, which cause inflammation, are the target of soluble factors in aqueous. These immunomodulatory factors are possibly secreted by the pigmented epithelium cells of the ciliary body and by the corneal endothelial cells. The autonomic nerves in iris and ciliary body are another possible source.

Constitutive expression of FasLigand (FasL) on parenchymal cells in immune privileged sites play an important role in imparting the immune privilege. The FasL is a type II transmembrane protein belonging to the tumor necrosis factor (TNF) family. Cleaving of membrane-bound FasL by the external serine matrix metalloproteinase produces soluble FasL. FasL binds to its receptor (FasR), which comprises of three cysteine-rich pseudorepeats, a transmembrane domain, and an intracellular death domain. Another Fas receptor, called decoy receptor 3 (DcR3) has recently been discovered. DcR3 is a soluble receptor. It also belongs to the tumor necrosis factor superfamily. It binds to FasL but has no signal transduction capabilities. Thus, it mitigates Fas R-FasL interactions.

Fas-Fas ligand triggered apoptosis plays a central role in the immune system regulation. In addition to immune privilege, its functions include homeostasis of T-cell to prevent excessive immune response and to remove autoreactive T-cells. Fas-induced apoptosis (in addition to perforin pathway), are used by cytotoxic T cells to induce cell death in cells expressing foreign antigens such as viral infected or tumor cells. Tumors express Fas ligand and kill infiltrating lymphocytes. This permits the tumor to escape immune response. Some tumors upregulate Fas ligand during chemotherapy causing tumor immune escape.

FasL plays a very important role in immune privilege, also in ocular tissue and induces apoptosis of Fas-positive inflammatory cells. Similarly, Sertoli cells of the testis express FasL that prevents graft rejection. However, recent studies have indicated a paradoxical role of FasL in immune privilege. For example, transgenic expression of FasL on islet cells in pancreas causes a rapid rejection of this tissue associated with granulocyte or neutrophilic infiltration. Other molecules are also important for the immune privilege/deviation. These molecules include cytokines such as TGF-beta.

Also, the infiltrating precursor CTLs are not directly cytotoxic in the privileged sites. In the eye, immune responses on re-encountering the antigen are tilted toward a T_H2-like response.

Brain

The brain is a sensitive organ with a limited capacity for regeneration. This makes immune privilege in the brain essential for the limitation of inflammation and maintenance of function. The blood-brain barrier is important in maintaining the brains separation from the systemic immune system but it is not on its own responsible for the maintenance of immune privilege.[9] Immune privilege of the brain varies throughout different compartments and is most pronounced in the parenchymal tissue or "white matter".[9]

The brain is limited in its capacity to deliver antigen to local lymph nodes and causes T-cell activation.[10] In normal tissues antigen is taken up by antigen presenting cells (dendritic cells), which migrate to the lymph nodes, or soluble antigen can drain by itself into the lymph node. Dendritic cells have not been found in normal parenchyma tissue or perivascular space although they are present in the meninges and choroid plexus.[9]

Although there is no conventional lymphatic system in the brain, the drainage of antigen from the brain to cervical lymph nodes has been demonstrated. The response elicited in the lymph nodes to brain antigen is skewed towards B cells. Dendritic cells from cerebrospinal fluid have been found to migrate to B cell follicles of cervical lymph nodes.[11] The skewing of the response to antigen from the brain is a means that a more dangerous inflammatory T cell response can be avoided.

The induction of systemic tolerance to an antigen introduced into the brain has been proven.[12] This was seen in the absence of the T cell mediated inflammatory "delayed type hypersensitivity reaction" (DTH) when the antigen was reintroduced in another part of the body. This response is analogous to ACAID in the eye.

Fas ligand expression by astrocytoma *in vivo*: maintaining immune privilege in the brain

Astrocytomas are among the most common brain tumors that are usually fatal in their malignant form. They appear to progress without significant impedance from the immune system, despite the presence of intratumoral T cell infiltration. To date, this has been thought to be the result of T cell immunosuppression induced by astrocytoma-derived cytokines. Cell contact-mediated events also play a role, since *in vivo* expression of Fas ligand (FasL/CD95L) by human astrocytoma and the efficient killing of Fas-bearing cells has been demonstrated. Functional FasL is expressed by human, mouse, and rat astrocytoma and hence, may be a general feature of this nonlymphoid tumor. In the brain, astrocytoma cells can potentially deliver a death signal to Fas+ cells, which include infiltrating leukocytes, and, paradoxically, astrocytoma cells themselves. The expression of FasL by astrocytoma cells may extend the processes that are postulated to occur in normal brain to maintain immune privilege. FasL-induced apoptosis by astrocytoma cells may play a significant role in both immunosuppression and the regulation of tumor growth within the central nervous system.

Tumor

The anterior chamber (AC) of the murine eye has been studied extensively for its property as an immune privileged site. The experiments of Niederkorn *et al.*[13] first documented that minor histoincompatible tumor cells injected into the AC formed progressively growing tumors that never experienced immune rejection. Moreover, these allogenic tumors induced a deviant systemic immune response, termed anterior chamber associated immune deviation (ACAID), which has proved to be a characteristic feature of systemic immunity induced by a wide variety of antigens injected intracamerally.

Since unrelenting tumor growth coincided temporally with sustained ACAID in recipients of AC tumor cell injections, the concept emerged that deviant immunity and immune privilege are mechanistically linked.

This concept was further strengthened by the observations that major histocompatibility complex (MHC) incompatible tumor cell grafts injected into the AC experienced immune privilege only transiently and correspondingly, the ACAID induced by MHC incompatible tumors also proved to be evanescent.

Immune privilege is also a feature of the vitreous cavity. The initial pattern of growth of tumor cells injected in this compartment of eyes of mice has been found to be essentially similar to that observed for tumors placed within the AC, and tumors growing within the vitreous cavity readily induced ACAID.

The subretinal (SR) space is a third intraocular compartment with the potential to be an immune privileged site. There has been a long-standing interest in promoting the survival of retina-derived grafts in the SR space; to aid in this goal researchers have begun to examine the extent to which this intraocular compartment displays immune privilege. Several years ago Jiang *et al.*,[14] reported that allografts of retinal pigment epithelium (RPE) as well as of neonatal neuronal retina experienced immune privilege within the SR space.

It is evident that several molecular pathways are likely to be involved in the establishment of tumor immune privilege. Several hypotheses have been suggested that involve the inability of mutant p53 to up-regulate Fas expression within the tumor. Increased p53 activity has been correlated with Fas expression. FasL-mediated depletion of tumor-infiltrating immune cells contributes to tumor immune privilege.[15]

Lymphocyte apoptosis induced by CD95 (APO-1/Fas) ligand-expressing tumor cells—A mechanism of immune evasion

The CD95 (APO-1/Fas) system is an important mediator of T-cell cytotoxicity. Scientists have investigated this system in hepatocellular carcinomas (HCCs) from patients. All HCCs had partially or completely lost the expression of the CD95 receptor constitutively expressed by normal liver cells and might thus evade CD95-mediated killing.

It has been suggested that tumor cells can evade immune attack by down-regulation of the CD95 receptor and killing of lymphocytes through expression of CD95L.

TRANSPLANTS TO IMMUNOLOGICALLY PRIVILEGED SITES

Corneal graft is among the most successful transplantation and it needs no immuno-suppressive therapy.[16]

Allogenic grafts may provoke a lesser immunological response in these immunologically privileged sites. Foreign grafts are well tolerated in these sites. The absence of lymphatic drainage in these areas is believed to block the afferent limb of the immune response and thus prevent sensitization of the graft. But the mechanism of reduced immune responses in these areas is now known to be more complex than it was thought earlier.[16,17]

The cells in the immunologically privileged sites express high level of FasL on their surface. It is suggested that the high level of FasL expression may protect these cells from immunological attack. The FasL on the cells of immunologically privileged sites bind to Fas molecules on the T cells that infiltrate the sites and destroy the T cells.

The FasL mediated protection of the cells in immunologically privileged sites is now being researched as a possible way of preventing organ rejection after transplantation. Before transplantation, the organ cells to be transplanted will be made to express high levels of FasL on their surface. The FasL molecules on transplanted cells are expected to induce apoptotic death of Fas receptor bearing cytotoxic T cells, which attack the transplanted cells. Eventually the transplanted organ cells live for longer periods,[17] by escaping immune rejection.

At this time you should know the following:

1. Why at all some organs of human body has privileged immunity status?
2. How these organs react when need be?
3. How these mechanisms are useful in defense?
4. How these applications of immune privilege are useful in understanding the complexities of life and treating diseased states?

References

1. Hong Seokmann, Van Kaer Luc (1999). Immune Privilege: Keeping an Eye on Natural Killer T Cells. The Journal of Experimental Medicine 190 (9): 1197-1200.
2. Janeway CA Jr., Travers P, Walport M, Shlomchik MJ (2005). Immunobiology, the immune system in health and disease 6th Edition, Garland Science.
3. Zenclussen AC (2006). Regulatory T cells in pregnancy. Springer Seminars in Immunopathology 28(1): 31-39.
4. Kovats S, Main EK, Librach C, Subblebine M, Fisher SJ, DeMars R. "A class I antigen, HLA-G, expressed in human trophoblasts "Science 1990, 248: 220-223.
5. Madona A de Lemos. "How your Mother Tolerated you for Nine Months" BioTeach Journal, Fall 2003, Vol-1, 27-30.
6. Keino H, Takeuchi M, Kezuka T, Hattori T, Usui M, Taguchi O, Streilein JW, Stein-Streilein J (2006). Induction of Eye-Derived Tolerance Does Not Depend on Naturally Occurring CD4+CD25+ T Regulatory Cells. Investigative Ophthalmology and Visual Science 47:1047-1055.
7. Streilein JW, Stein-Streilein J (2002). Anterior chamber associated immune deviation (ACAID): Regulation, biological relevance and implications for therapy. International Reviews of Immunology 21(2-3):123-52.
8. Lambe T, JCH, Leung H, Ferry T, Bouriez-Jones K, Makinen T L, Crockford HR Jiang JM Nickerson L Peltonen J V Forrester, and RJ Cornall (2007), Limited Peripheral T Cell Anergy Predisposes to Retinal Autoimmunity. The Journal of Immunology 178:4276-4283.
9. Galea I, Beckmann I, Perry VH (2007). What is Immune Privilege (not)? Trends in Immunology 28(1): 12-18.
10. Mendez-Fernandez YV *et al.* (2005) Anatomical and cellular requirements for the activation and migration of virus-specific CD8+ T cells to the brain during Theiler's virus infection. Journal of Virology 79: 3063-3070.
11. Hatterer E *et al.* (2006) How to drain without lymphatics? Dendritic cells migrate from the cerebrospinal fluid to the B-cell follicles of cervical lymph nodes. Blood 107: 806-812.
12. Wenkel H *et al.* (2000), Systemic immune deviation in the brain that does not depend on the integrity of the blood-brain barrier. Journal of Immunology 164: 5125–5131.
13. Niederkorn J Y, Brieland J K and Mayhew E (1983). Enhanced natural killer cell activity in experimental murine encephalitozoonosis. Infect Immun, July 41(1): 302-307.
14. Jiang Lin, Eric A Althoff, Fernando R Clemente Lindsey Doyle, Daniela Röthlisberger, Alexandre Zanghellini, Jasmine L, Gallaher, Jamie L Betker, Fujie Tanaka, Carlos F Barbas, III, Donald Hilvert, Kendall N Houk, Barry L. Stoddard, David Baker (2008). De Novo Computational Design of Retro-Aldol Enzymes. Science 7 March 2008: Vol. 319. no. 5868, 1387-1391.
15. F Michael Yakes, Barbara D. Wamil, Fenglei Sun *et al.* "CM101 Treatment Overrides Tumor-induced Immunoprivilege Leading to Apoptosis" Cancer Research 2000, 60, 5740–5746.

16. Roit's Essential Immunology (2004),10th Ed 362-363.
17. Richard A G, Thomas J, Kuby Immunology (2003), 5th Ed.,Transplants to immunologically previliged sites, Transplantation immunology 517-537.

Future Research Areas

1. Role of immunologically privileged sites in transplantation of organs.
2. Role of immunologically privileged sites in rejection of transplantation.

Further Reading

1. Janeway CA Jr., Travers P, Walport M, Shlomchik. MJ (2005). Immunobiology, the immune system in health and disease 6th Ed., Garland Science.
2. Madona A de Lemos. How your Mother Tolerated you for Nine Months. BioTeach Journal. Fall 2003, Vol-1, 27-30.
3. Keino H, Takeuchi M, Kezuka T, Hattori T, Usui M, Taguchi O, Streilein JW, Stein-Streilein J (2006). Induction of Eye-Derived Tolerance Does Not Depend on Naturally Occurring CD4+CD25+ T Regulatory Cells. Investigative Ophthalmology and Visual Science 47:1047-1055.
4. Wenkel H. *et al.* (2000). Systemic immune deviation in the brain that does not depend on the integrity of the blood.brain barrier. Journal of Immunology 164: 5125.5131.
5. Galea I, Beckmann I, Perry VH (2007). What is Immune Privilege (not)?. Trends in Immunology 28(1): 12-18.
6. Roit S Essential Immunology (2004),10th Ed.,362-363.
7. Richard AG, Thomas J, Kuby Immunology (2003), 5th Ed.,Transplants to immunologically previliged sites, Transplantation immunology 517-537.

GLOSSARY

Antigen: A foreign substance (usually a protein or carbohydrate) capable of triggering an immune response in an organism.

Antibody: A protein on the surface of B cells that is also secreted in large amounts into the blood or lymph in response to an antigen, a component within an invader such as a bacterium, virus, parasite, or transplanted organ. Antibodies neutralize the antigen, and thereby the invader, by binding to it, often directing it toward a macrophage for destruction. Also called an immunoglobulin.

B cell: A type of lymphocyte that produces antibodies, which bind to free-floating microbes circulating in the blood so that they cannot infect other cells.

CD (Cluster of differentiation): This is a designation used to catalogue surface molecules (antennae) on lymphocytes (white blood cells). It tells what the cell is and how activated it is. For example, Natural Killer cells have CD 56+.

Cytotrophoblast : This is a specialized cell of the placenta (also a trophoblast) whose function is to attach the baby to the mother's uterus. It provides the anchor. It grows deeply into the lining of the uterus (decidua) and firmly attaches the placenta for the duration of pregnancy.

Immunoglobulin class: There are five different classes or families of antibodies (immunoglobulins). IgM is the first antibody produced when an immune response is initiated. It lives in the blood system. IgG lives in the lymphatic system and is made by IgM. IgA lives in the organs and protects them. IgD which is present as a memory antibody in the blood once a person is immune or immunized. IgE is the antibody that causes allergies and asthma. It is present throughout the body.

Lymphocyte: A type of white blood cell involved in the human body's immune system, of which there are two broad categories, T cells and B cells. Lymphocytes are an integral part of the body's defenses because they are highly specific for antigens associated with microbes, tumor cells, transplants, allergies and tissues attacked in autoimmune diseases. The immune system comprises clones of lymphocytes, each with a single specificity, and exposure to antigens leads to clonal expansion, the acquisition of helper and killer functions, and formation of immune memory.

Major histocompatibility complex (MHC) molecules: A group of molecules that help the immune system distinguish between harmful and safe foreign substances in the body.

Regulatory T cells (Treg cells): Special T cells that regulate or suppress immune responses, preventing autoimmunity for example.

T cell: A type of lymphocyte that possesses highly specific cell-surface antigen receptors; types include CD4+ helper T cells, regulatory T cells and CD8+ killer T cells.

Tolerance: The capacity of the body to become less responsive to a substance or a physiological insult. Tolerance to components of the self prevents or suppresses autoimmunity.

APPENDIX

The Nobel Laureates and Immunology

(Dr. Parul Goel, Dr. Mohd. Suhail and Dr. Madhvi Gupta parul006@gmail.com)

Sl. No.	Year of award	Name of the Nobel Laureate	Country	Work
1.	1901	Emil A Von Behring	Germany	For his work on serum therapy especially against diphtheria
2.	1905	Robert Koch	Germany	For his work in tuberculosis
3.	1908	Ilya Metchnikoff and Paul Ehrlich	Russia, Germany	In recognition of their work on immunity; phagocytosis, cellular theory and humoral theory
4.	1912	Alexis Carrel	France	In recognition of his work on vascular suture and the transplantation of blood vessels and organs
5.	1913	Charles Robert Richet	France	In recognition of his work on anaphylaxis
6.	1919	Jules Bordet	Belgium	For his discoveries relating to immunity; work on complement
7.	1930	Karl Landsteiner	Austria / USA	For his discovery of human blood groups
8.	1951	Max Theiler	South Africa/ USA	For the work concerning yellow fever
9.	1957	Daniel Bovet	Italy/ Switzerland	For the work related to histamine, anti-histamine compounds and other substances

Contd.

Contd.

10.	1960	Sir Frank Macfarlane Burnet and Peter Brian Medawar	Australia / Great Britain	For discovery of acquired immunological tolerance
11.	1972	Gerald M. Edelman and Rodney R. Porter	USA, Great Britain	For their discoveries concerning the chemical structure of antibodies
12.	1977	Rosalvn Yalow	USA	For the work on radioimmunoassays of peptide hormones
13.	1980	Baruj Benacerraf, Jean Dausset and George D. Snell	USA / France / USA	For their discoveries concerning genetically determined structures on the cell surface that regulate immunological reactions
14.	1982	Sune K. Bergstrom, Bengt I. Samuelsson and John R. Vane	Sweden / Sweden / UK	For their work concerning prostaglandins and related biologically active substances
15.	1984	Niels K. Jerne	Denmark/ Switzerland	For the work concerning the specificity in development and control of the immune system
16.	1984	Georges J.F. Köhler and César Milstein	Denmark / Germany Argentina and United Kingdom	For the discovery of the principle for production of monoclonal antibodies
17.	1987	Susumu Tonegawa	Japan/USA	For his discovery of the genetic principle for generation of antibody diversity
18.	1990	Joseph E. Murray and E. Donnall Thomas	USA / USA	For their discoveries concerning organ and cell transplantation in the treatment of human disease
19.	1996	Peter C. Doherty and Rolf M. Zinkernagel	Australia / Switzerland	For their discoveries concerning the specificity of the cell mediated immune defence
20.	1997	Stanley B. Prusiner	USA	For the work on prions as a new biological principle of infection
21.	1999	Gunter Blobel	USA	For work concerning signal transduction

Contd.

Contd.

22.	2001	Leland H Hartwell, Tim Hunt and Sir Paul Nurse	USA / UK / UK	For their discoveries of key regulators of the cell cycle
23.	2002	Sydney Brenner, H. Robert Horvitz and John E. Sulston	UK / USA / UK	For their discoveries concerning genetic regulation of organ development and programmed cell death
24.	2006	Andrew Z. Fire and Craig C. Mello	USA / USA	For their discoveries of RNA interference – gene silencing by double-stranded RNA
25.	2007	Mario R Capecchi, Oliver Smithies and Sir Martin J Evans	USA / USA / UK	For their discoveries of principles for introducing specific gene modifi-cations in mice by the use of embryonic stem cell called gene targeting technology, helps in understanding gene-disease relationship
26.	2008	Herald Zur Hausen, Fraincose Barre Sinoussi and Luc Montagnier	Germany / France / France	For their discovery of human papilloma viruses causing cervical cancer for their discovery of the human immunodeficiency virus
27.	2008	Osamu Shimomura, Martin Chalfie and Roger Y. Tsien	USA / USA / USA	For their work on green fluorescent protein (GFP)
28.	2009	Venkat Raman Rama Krishnan, Thomas A. Steitz and Ada E. Yonath	UK / USA / Israel	For their work on elucidation of structure and function of ribosomes
29.	2011	Bruce A. Beutler Jules A. Hoffmann	USA / France	For their discoveries concerning the activation of innate immunity
30.	2011	Ralph M. Steinman	Canada	For his discovery of dendritic cell and its role in adaptive immunity

Further Reading

www.nobelprize.org/**nobel**_prizes/**medicine/laureates/**

www.medindia.net › Nobel Prize in Medicine

www. nobelprizes.com/**nobel/medicine**

INDEX

A

B

C

I

T

U

V

W

X

Z